Dental Charting: A Standard Approach

Jill Jaroski-Graf, RDH, BSDH, MS

Chair, Department of Biology
Associate Professor of Biology and Forensic Science
Mount Senario College
Ladysmith, Wisconsin

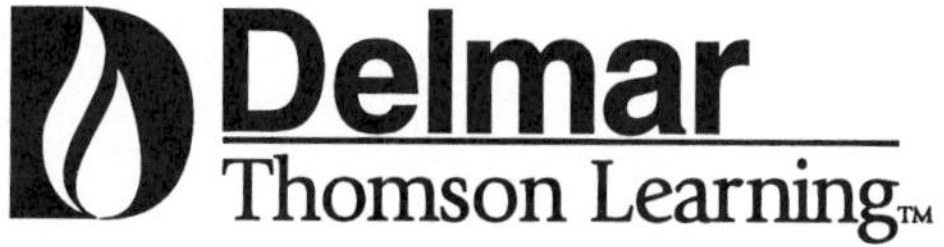

Africa • Australia • Canada • Denmark • Japan • Mexico • New Zealand • Phillipines
Puerto Rico • Singapore • Spain • United Kingdom • United States

NOTICE TO THE READER

Publisher does not warrant or guarantee any of the products described herein or perform any independent analysis in connection with any of the product information contained herein. Publisher does not assume, and expressly disclaims, any obligation to obtain and include information other than that provided to it by the manufacturer.

The reader is expressly warned to consider and adopt all safety precautions that might be indicated by the activities herein and to avoid all potential hazards. By following the instructions contained herein, the reader willingly assumes all risks in connection with such instructions.

The Publisher makes no representation or warranties of any kind, including but not limited to, the warranties of fitness for particular purpose or merchantability, nor are any such representations implied with respect to the material set forth herein, and the publisher takes no responsibility with respect to such material. The publisher shall not be liable for any special, consequential, or exemplary damages resulting, in whole or part, from the readers' use of, or reliance upon, this material.

Cover Design: William Finnerty

Delmar Staff
Publisher: William Brottmiller
Executive Editor: Cathy L. Esperti
Developmental Editor: Helen Yackel
Executive Marketing Manager: Dawn Gerrain
Marketing Coordinator: Nina Lontrato
Editorial Assistant: Maria Perretta
Production Manager: Linda Helfrich
Project Editor: Judith Boyd Nelson
Art/Design Coordinator: Richard Killar

Printed in Canada
1 2 3 4 5 6 7 8 9 10 XXX 05 04 03 02 01 00

For more information, contact Delmar, 3 Columbia Circle, PO Box 15015, Albany, NY 12212-0515; or find us on the World Wide Web at http://www.delmar.com

Library of Congress Cataloging-in-Publication Data
Jaroski-Graf, Jill.
Dental charting : a standard approach / Jill Jaroski-Graf
p. cm.
Includes bibliographical references and index.
ISBN 0-7668-0625-1 (alk. paper)
1. Dental records—Standards. 2. Dentistry—Practice. I. Title.
[DNLM: 1. Dental Records—standards. 2. Documentation—methods.
WU 95 J82d 2000J
RK59.5.J67 2000
651.5'04261-dc21
DNLM/DLC 99-30235
for Library of Congress CIP

Dedication

TO THE MEMORY OF MY MOST DEVOTED TEACHERS

mother and grandfather

ANNA M. and GILBERT VENNE

and

professor

MICHAEL CHARNEY, Ph.D., D-ABFA

TO MY BELOVED FAMILY

husband and daughter

STEPHEN E. and SAVANNAH BROOK GRAF

Contents

Preface

Throughout my many years as a dental professional, associate professor of biology and forensic science, chief deputy coroner, and board certified examiner, I have utilized dental charting as a key component of my work. It has become evident that, although dental charting methods are taught in every dental, dental hygiene, and dental assisting program in the United States, there is a lack of publications written specifically for the purpose of introducing students to dental charting techniques. The existing books provide some information on dental charting but there is a wide variation in the information and methods presented. Furthermore, in compiling the styles of dental charting used in every dental school in the United States and Canada, I discovered there is no one standardized and accepted method for dental charting. Instead, I found numerous ways to chart different types of dental restorations and conditions.

This book is intended to introduce dental, dental hygiene, and dental assisting students to dental charting using standardized techniques. Other professionals who desire to become familiar with dental charting, and routinely use these procedures in their work, will also find this text useful. Understanding and using this knowledge will enable students and professionals to provide the most consistent service to their patient or client and their community.

Developmental Approach

Before beginning the process of writing this book, I compared all the charting methods used in schools in both the United States and Canada. I noted how different schools had charted each specific restoration and selected the most commonly used method across my sample.

This book is an attempt to remedy the incongruity that currently exists in dental charting. The reasons for the need for standardization of dental charting come to mind immediately:

1. To facilitate the maintenance of complete and current dental records for patients.
2. To support and enhance education and training.
3. To improve the efficiency and effectiveness of the process of human identification through standardized techniques.

The content of this book supports the needs of clinical evaluation courses and will aid the student as well as dental and medico-legal professionals in recognizing the importance of thorough and consistent dental charting.

Organization

The organization of material begins with coverage of dental anatomy, tooth numbering, and charting fundamentals (Chapters 1 through 4). It follows with charting for restorations, crowns, sealants, and prostheses (Chapters 5 through 12). The remaining material continues with normal and abnormal charting of dental conditions (Chapters 13 through 22).

The basic information covered on the oral cavity and the teeth include such topics as: anatomy and anatomic positions; tooth numbering systems; dental examination records and the principles of dental charting; radiographic interpretation; silver amalgam, gold, non-precious metal, and resin restorations; and fixed and removable prosthesis and dental implants. Other topics discussed are charting manifestations associated with hard and soft dental tissues, occlusion and malocclusion, dental anomalies, and developmental malformations.

This standard approach uses the primary and secondary codes from the Computer-Assisted Postmortem Identification, Version 4 (CAPMI4) system developed by the United States Army Institute of Dental Research (USAIDR) and the Armed Forces Institute of Pathology (AFIP), and the WinID© program developed by Dr. James B. McGivney. The CAPMI4 and WinID© computerized systems use abbreviations that represent individual tooth surfaces, dental restorations, and abnormal conditions referred to as primary and secondary codes.

The charting of each restoration and/or dental condition has been presented and illustrated using three types of dental charting forms: anatomic, geometric, and numeric coding systems, along with an accompanying photograph and/or radiograph for each. Additionally, all of the teeth shown on each dental radiograph and photograph are represented using Universal/National (American Dental Association), Palmer Notation, and International Standards Organization/Fédération Dentaire Internationale (ISO/FDI) tooth designation systems that are adjacent to each image.

Features of this Text

Dental Charting: A Standard Approach includes many pedagogical features that promote learning and accessibility of information:

- **Capitalization of primary and secondary codes.** All primary and secondary codes are capitalized throughout the text to facilitate the comprehension of the procedures through reinforcement.
- **Dental charts.** Three types of dental charting are covered. Included are step-by-step instructions on how to correctly chart anatomic, geometric, and numeric dental charts. Each is explained in enough depth and detail to help students understand the methods.
- **Photographs and radiographs.** Where possible, we have included a radiograph along with each photograph of the same region to help develop the skills necessary for dental charting from radiographs.
- **Tooth notation information adjacent to photographs and radiographs.** This information provides feedback to the reader on tooth notation information using the three different formats to aid the learning process.
- **Review questions and answers.** Review questions have been included at the end of each chapter to help readers test their comprehension of chapter material. Answers are provided for immediate feedback.
- **Online forensic material.** With this book, you also get online access to several appendices of forensic material. We have also included a direct link

to the website for the WinID© Dental Computer System, which is used for matching unidentified persons to dental characteristics. Online appendices include:

A Bite Mark Analysis

B Missing and Unidentified Persons: A Disaster of Immense Magnitude

C Guidelines for Mass Fatality Dental Identification Plan

D Forensic Anthropology: The Purpose and Value of Facial Restoration in Human Skeletal Identification

- **Online dental charting exercises.** Five groups of dental charting review exercises are included online. Each group of exercises consists of the three types of dental charting formats: anatomic, geometric, and numeric coding systems. Answer sheets are included for each exercise.

  To access the online materials, just point your browser to: http://www.delmaralliedhealth.com/dental and click on the Online Companion for *Dental Charting: A Standard Approach*.

I hope that this book encompasses all aspects relevant to dental charting and meets the needs of the profession through its comprehensive scope and systematic approach to dental charting.

Jill Jaroski-Graf

Acknowledgments

I would like to acknowledge several professionals from the dental and forensic profession who made content contributions to this project.

Marilyn M. Beck, RDH, BSDH, MEd
Associate Professor of Dental Hygiene
College of Health Sciences
Marquette University
Milwaukee, Wisconsin

Gary L. Bell, DDS
Forensic Odontologist Board Certified
American Board of Forensic Odontology
Seattle, Washington

David E. Cadle, ASP
Forensic Scientist Advanced
Forensic Photography
Wisconsin State Crime Laboratory—Milwaukee
Milwaukee, Wisconsin

Michael Charney, PhD, D-ABFA
Diplomat American Board of Forensic Anthropology
Emeritus Professor of Anthropology
Director Forensic Science Laboratory
Colorado State University
Forensic Science Officer University Police Department
Deputy Coroner Larimer County
Fort Collins, Colorado

Donald J. Ferguson, DMD, MSD
Executive Director and Professor of Orthodontics
Head, Division of Orthodontics
Center for Advanced Dental Education
St. Louis University
St. Louis, Missouri

Ronald L. Groffy, ASP
Forensic Scientist Advanced
Forensic Photography and Crime Scene Investigation
Wisconsin State Crime Laboratory—Madison
Madison, Wisconsin

Kathleen D. Heiden, RDH, MSPH
Health Education Specialist
Centers for Disease Control and Prevention (CDC)
National Center for Chronic Disease Prevention and Health Promotion
Division of Oral Health
Atlanta, Georgia

L. Thomas Johnson, DDS
Forensic Odontologist Board Certified
American Board of Forensic Odontology
Milwaukee, Wisconsin

John A. Lewis Jr., DDS,
Forensic Odontologist Board Certified
American Board of Forensic Odontology
Jacksonville, Florida

James McGivney, DMD
Forensic Odontologist Board Certified
American Board of Forensic Odontology
St. Louis, Missouri

Donald O. Simley, II, DDS
Forensic Odontologist Board Certified
American Board of Forensic Odontology
Madison, Wisconsin

Reviewers

Robin Caplan, CDA, EFDA, DRT
Medix College
Towson, Maryland

Ellen Dietz, CDA, AAS, BS
Formerly at:
University of North Carolina
School of Dentistry
Chapel Hill, North Carolina

Patricia Frese, RDH, MEd
University of Cincinnati
Raymond Walters College
Cincinnati, Ohio

Darlene Hunziker, CDA, RDA
Eton Technical Institute
Everett, Washington

Sheila Semler, RDH, BA
Blinn College
Bryan, Texas

Marianne Watts, CDA
Tarrant County Jr. College
Hurst, Texas

I wish to acknowledge all the people who helped make this project possible. For help in preparing the manuscript I would like to extend my thanks and appreciation to Victoria Stanke Tainter, Cynthia L. Reinert, W. Alexander Wheeler, Ph.D., Barbara Gremban-Renc, R.D.H., Dr. Paul Johnson, Gina Catlin, Wendy Bresina, Cynthia Hart, and Annette Havlik-Berns, R.D.H.

Special thanks is given to Dr. Blaine Christman, and Jenny J. Knight, R.D.H. for taking many of the dental radiographs used in this book. For their assistance in locating references my appreciation goes to Kathy Stempf and Ann M. Stolarzyk. Further acknowledgments go to Eastman Kodak Company and Rinn Corporation for use of their radiographs and illustrations.

Thanks to David Zimmer, Artan Nikaj, and Radenko Ritan for computer assistance.

Thanks to the staff at Delmar Publishers: Marlene Pratt, Helen Yackel, Maria Peretta, Richard Killar, and Judith Boyd Nelson. Thanks also to the staff at Argosy.

CHAPTER 1

Dental Anatomy

Key Terms

- Anatomic Crown
- Anatomic Root
- Apical Foramen
- Cementoenamel Junction (CEJ)
- Cementum
- Cervical Line
- Dental Pulp
- Dentin
- Dentinocemental Junction
- Enamel
- Mandibular
- Maxillary
- Pulp Canal
- Pulp Cavity
- Pulp Chamber
- Pulp Horns
- Reparative Dentin

The arrangements of the natural teeth in the dental arch are referred to as dentition. There are two classifications: primary (deciduous) and secondary dentitions. The primary dentition refers to the first set of teeth; deciduous implies the teeth will be shed. There are twenty teeth present in the primary dentition. Each of the four quadrants includes the following teeth: a central incisor, lateral incisor, canine, first molar, and second molar (Figure 1–1).

The secondary or permanent dentition refers to the thirty-two natural teeth that are present throughout life and include the following: central and lateral incisors, canines, premolars, and molars (Figure 1–2). These teeth are also referred to as succedaneous, the teeth succeed and replace the primary central and lateral incisors, canines, and molars.

When the first permanent teeth erupt into the primary dentition, the combination of teeth present from both dentitions is referred to as the mixed dentition (described in Chapter 2).

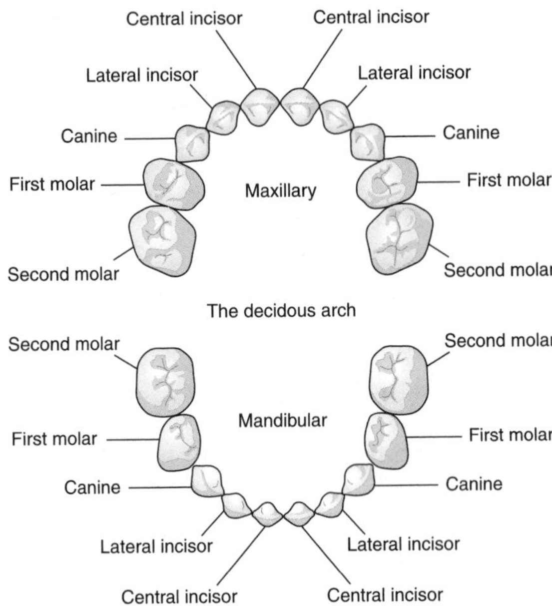

Figure 1–1 The deciduous arch

Anatomical Surfaces of the Teeth

The anatomical crown is that part of the tooth covered by **enamel**. The five tooth surfaces that form the crown of the tooth are named according to the direction in which they face. The anterior teeth include the central and lateral incisors and canines and have Mesial, Distal, Labial (Facial), and Lingual tooth surfaces, and Incisal edges. The posterior teeth consist of the premolars and molars and their crowns are comprised of Mesial, Distal, Facial (Buccal), Lingual, and Occlusal tooth surfaces (Figure 1–3).

The **maxillary** and **mandibular** arches are divided in half by an imaginary line called the midline. The tooth surfaces of the anterior and posterior teeth that face the midline are referred to as the Mesial surface. The Distal surface is the tooth surface that faces away from the midline and these two tooth surfaces located next to each other in a dental arch are referred to as a proximal surface.

The anterior and posterior teeth tooth surfaces facing the lips and cheeks are collectively called the Facial surfaces. If the tooth surface being referred to involves only an anterior tooth, the Facial surface is then referred to as the

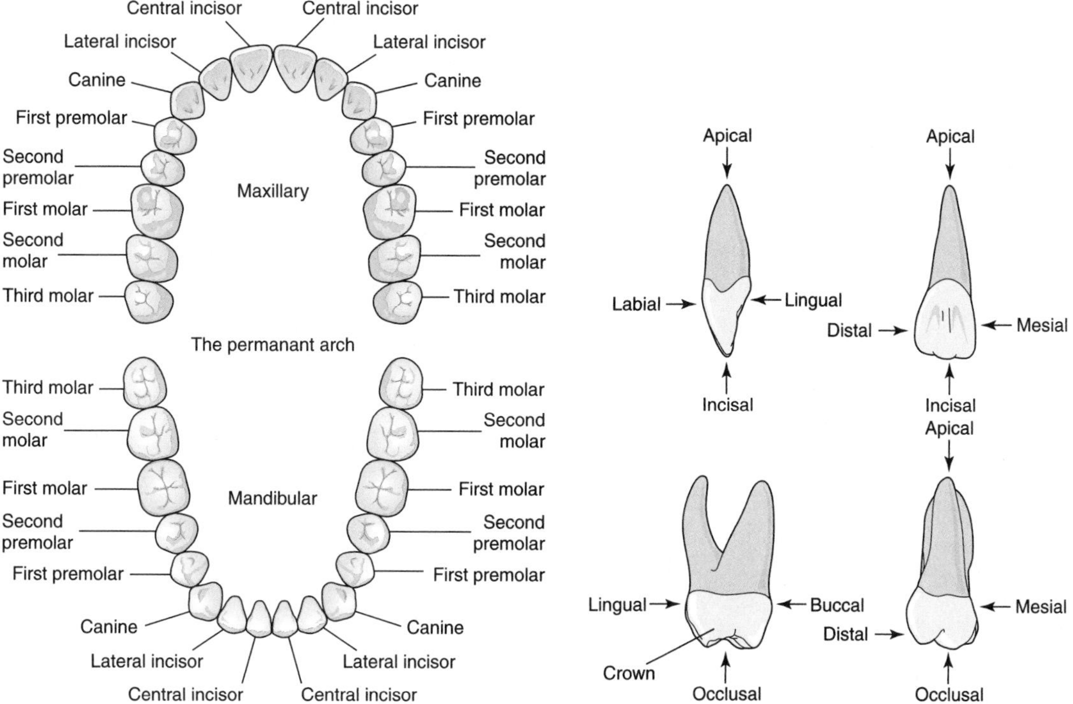

Figure 1–2 The permanent arch

Figure 1–3 The surfaces of the teeth

Labial surface. If the designated tooth is a posterior tooth, the tooth surface is called the Buccal surface. Tooth surfaces of the anterior and posterior teeth that face the tongue are referred to as the Lingual surfaces. The biting edge of the anterior tooth is known as the Incisal edge. The biting and chewing surface of a posterior tooth is referred to as the Occlusal surface. Figure 1–4 illustrates the anatomical surfaces of the teeth.

Tooth Division

For the purpose of describing a specific area on a tooth's surface, the Mesial, Distal, Facial (Labial and Buccal), and Lingual tooth surfaces are divided into thirds.

Figure 1–4 Anatomical surfaces of the teeth (Reproduced with modification from M. Massler and I. Schour, 1958, *Atlas of the Mouth,* by permission of the American Dental Association, Chicago.)

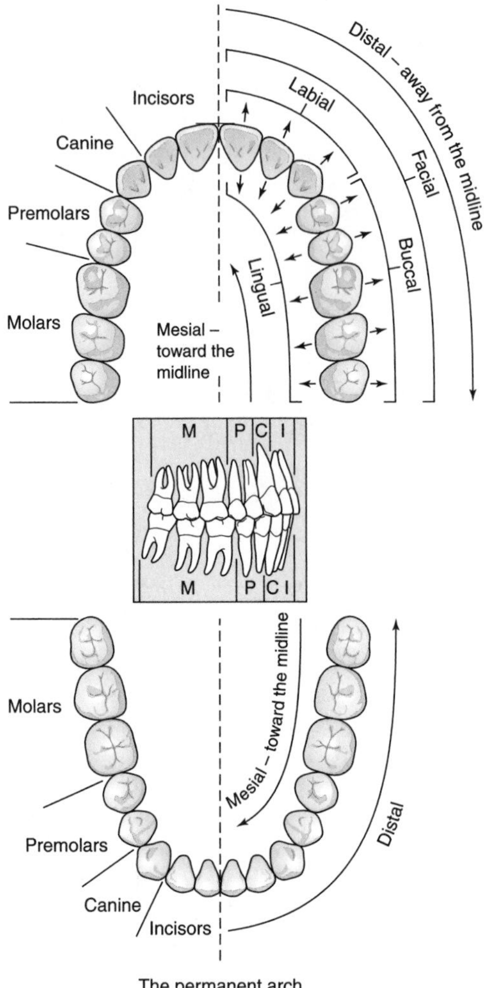

The Labial and Lingual surfaces of central and lateral incisors and canines have three vertical divisions designating the Mesial, middle, and Distal thirds of the tooth's surface. The horizontal divisions delineated on the Labial and Lingual surfaces comprise the Incisal, middle, and cervical thirds (Figure 1–5).

The root surface is also divided into thirds on the Labial and Lingual tooth surfaces and includes horizontal lines depicting the cervical, middle, and apical thirds. Apical is a term that refers to the tip or apex of the root.

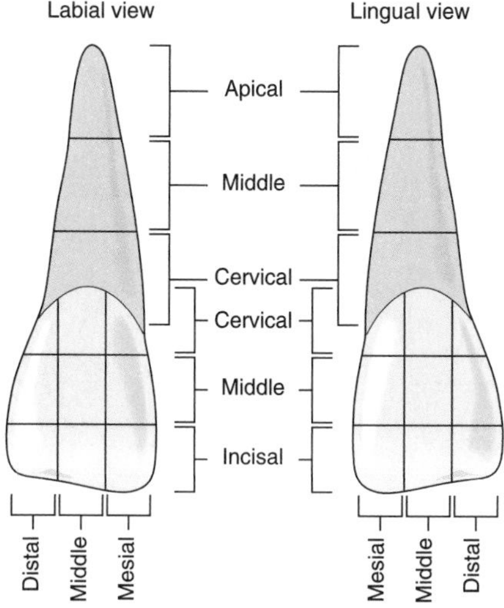

Figure 1–5 Labial and Lingual views of a maxillary right central incisor, which shows the division of the tooth surfaces into thirds

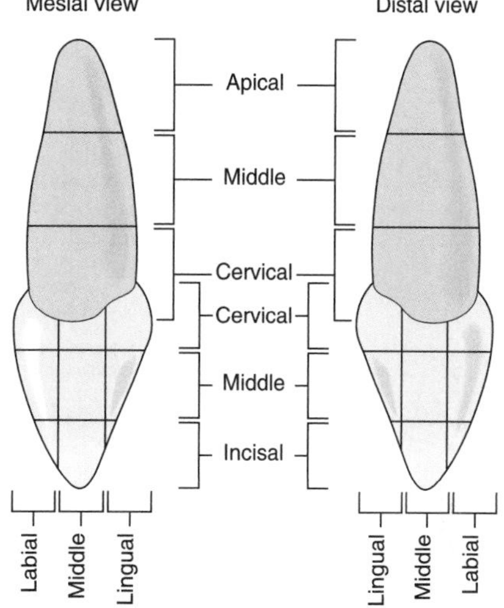

Figure 1–6 Mesial and Distal views of a maxillary right central incisor, which shows the division of the tooth surfaces into thirds

The Mesial and Distal surfaces of the anterior teeth are divided with vertical lines indicating Labial, middle, and Lingual thirds. The Incisal, middle, and cervical thirds of the central and lateral incisors and canines are depicted with horizontal lines (Figure 1–6).

The Buccal and Lingual surfaces of posterior teeth, premolars and molars, have three vertical divisions designating the Mesial, middle, and Distal thirds of the tooth's surface. The horizontal divisions delineated on the Buccal and Lingual surfaces comprise the Occlusal, middle, and cervical thirds (Figure 1–7).

The root surface is divided into thirds on the Buccal and Lingual tooth surfaces and includes horizontal lines depicting the cervical, middle, and apical thirds. The Mesial and Distal tooth surfaces of premolars and molars are divided with vertical lines indicating Buccal, middle, and Lingual thirds. The Buccal, middle, and cervical thirds of the posterior teeth are depicted with horizontal lines.

The divisions for the root surfaces for anterior and posterior teeth on the Mesial and Distal views are identical and are portrayed with horizontal lines indicating cervical, middle, and apical thirds as illustrated in Figures 1–6 and 1–8.

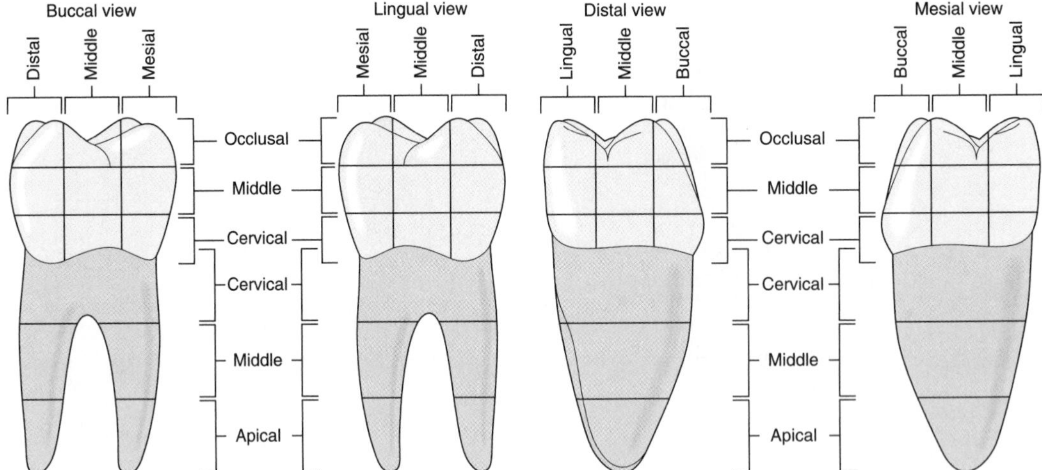

Figure 1–7 Buccal and Lingual views of a mandibular right molar, which shows the division of the tooth surfaces into thirds

Figure 1–8 Mesial and Distal views of a mandibular right molar, which shows the division of the tooth surfaces into thirds

The Tooth: Structure, Function, and Terminology

The teeth are unique structures that develop within the maxillary and mandibular alveolar processes. The alveolar process is that part of the bone located in the maxilla and mandible that forms the tooth sockets.

Each tooth consists of two main parts: the **anatomic crown**, which is that portion of the tooth covered by enamel, and the **anatomic root**, which is the part of the tooth covered by **cementum**. The enamel of the crown and the cementum of the root are joined together to form an area called the **cementoenamel junction** or **CEJ** and the line formed by this junction is called the **cervical line**.

Each tooth undergoes a series of developmental phases during its formation. Beginning with the formation of a tooth bud, the cells of the enamel organ proliferate and differentiate into specialized cells called ameloblasts and odontoblasts. Following histodifferentiation, morphogenesis occurs providing the shape to the crown of the tooth. Then after the deposition of a matrix consisting of enamel and **dentin** (apposition), the structure becomes hardened by calcium salts forming the future tooth as illustrated in Figure 1–9.

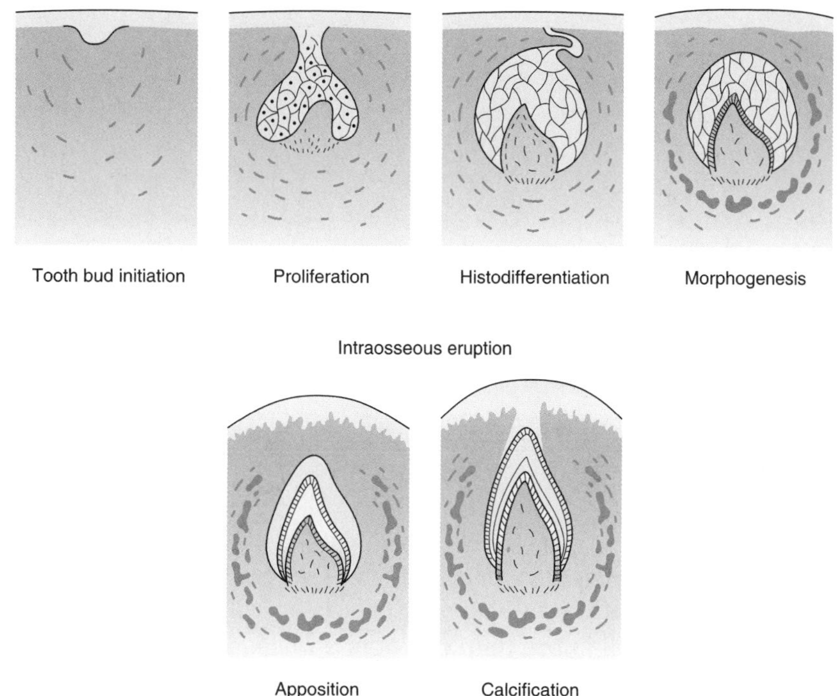

Figure 1–9 Developmental phases of tooth formation and intraosseous eruption

Prior to the complete calcification of the crown, root formation is initiated after the contour of the crown has been established. Eruption begins as the developing root lengthens and the tooth moves through the alveolar bone to the surface into the oral cavity (Figure 1–10).

The structure of a tooth is comprised of four tissues: enamel, dentin, cementum, and pulp. The crown of a tooth is covered by enamel, a mineralized structure composed of calcium salts (hydroxyapatite) and is the hardest substance in the body. This tissue has some limited ability to repair itself if it becomes damaged due to abrasion, trauma, or dental caries, and tends to wear away with age. The process of normal wear on the crown of a tooth is called attrition (see Figure 1–10).

The bulk of the tooth is composed of a densely calcified tissue called dentin. It is located beneath the enamel and forms the body of the tooth. Unlike

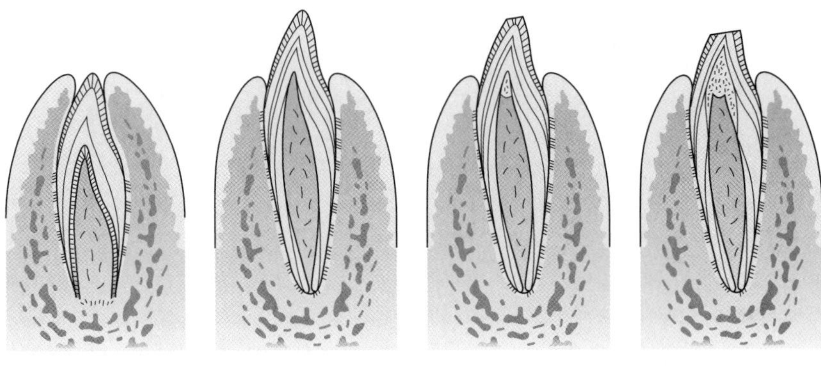

Figure 1–10 Tooth eruption and attrition

enamel, dentin is capable of repairing itself by laying down additional dentin in response to trauma or dental caries; this is called **reparative dentin**. Another type of dentin, secondary dentin, will, from the time of eruption, continuously fill in the pulp chamber and canal.

The root of the tooth is covered by a bonelike connective tissue called cementum. There are two types of cementum: acellular and cellular. The anatomical root surface is composed of acellular cementum, which is formed by cementoblasts (cementum-building cells) but these cells are not deposited into the root structure so the tissue cannot be reproduced. The apical third of the root consists of cellular cementum, which consists of cementoblasts embedded into the cementum and it has the ability to reproduce itself. Functional changes, such as attrition, will influence the reproductive activity of cellular cementum.

The function of cementum is to provide attachment sites for the periodontal ligament fibers, which connect the root of the tooth to the alveolar process. Beneath the cementum is the dentin and the area where the two tissues are joined together is called the **dentinocemental junction** (Figure 1–11).

The **dental pulp** is located beneath the dentin and occupies the **pulp cavity**. The pulp cavity is the area located within the center of the tooth and includes the **pulp chamber** and **pulp canals**. The walls of the cavity contain odontoblasts, which are responsible for producing and laying down primary and

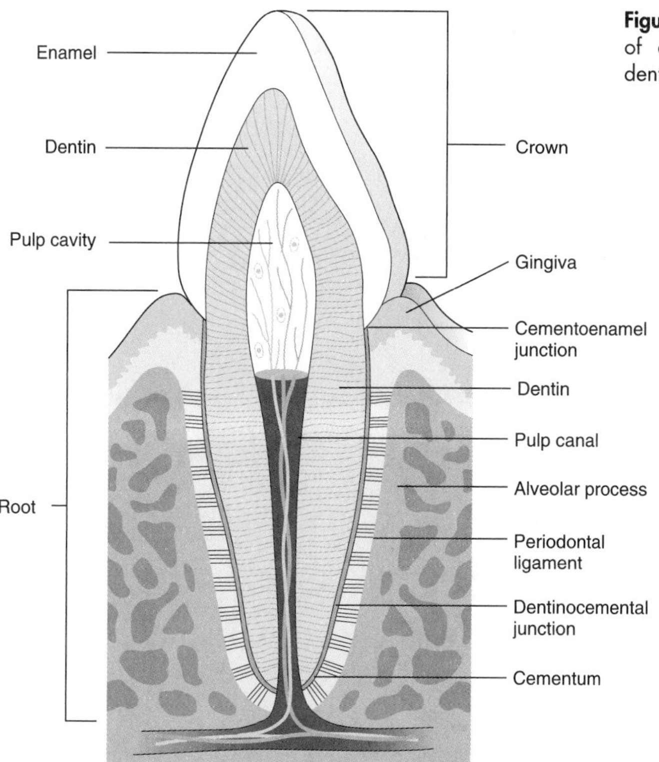

Figure 1–11 Longitudinal section of a tooth shows the enamel, dentin, and cementum

secondary dentin. All of the soft tissues are located inside this cavity. The tissues provide sensory innervation, nutrients, immunity, and repair processes and include the following: nerves, blood vessels, lymph vessels, and mesenchymal or connective tissues.

The pulp chamber is located in the crown of the tooth and contains most of the dental pulp. There are pointed extensions of pulp tissue projecting up from the top of the pulp chamber and they are called **pulp horns** (Figure 1–12).

The other portion of the pulp extending down from the pulp chamber located within the root of the tooth is called the pulp canal. Located at the base or apex of the root is an opening in which the nerve and blood vessels of the pulp pass through and this area is referred to as the **apical foramen** as illustrated in Figure 1–12.

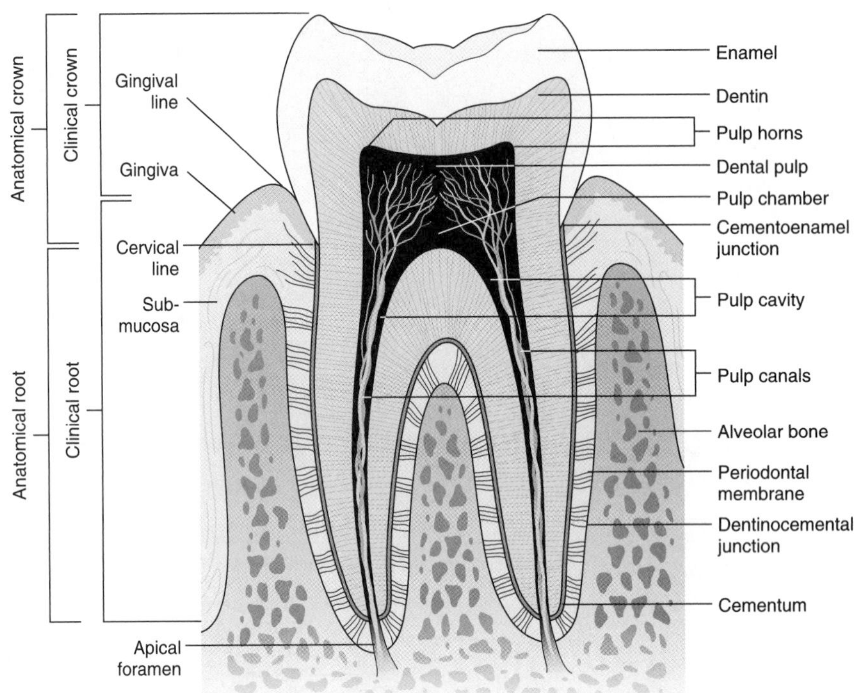

Figure 1–12 Longitudinal section of a tooth shows the dental pulp and other soft tissues

Review Questions

Multiple Choice

Directions: Select the letter of the choice that *best* answers the question.

1. Deciduous implies:
   a. the second set of teeth.
   b. it has more teeth than the permanent dentition.
   c. the teeth will be shed.
   d. there are only ten teeth.
2. Succedaneous refers to:
   a. the primary dentition.
   b. a mixed dentition.

c. the permanent dentition.
d. all of the above.

3. How many tooth surfaces are there to a tooth?
   a. 2
   b. 3
   c. 4
   d. 5
4. The midline refers to:
   a. an imaginary line down the center of each tooth from the Mesial to the Distal.
   b. an imaginary line that divides the maxillary and mandibular arches in half.
   c. an imaginary line down the center of each tooth from the Facial to the Lingual.
   d. an imaginary line that divides the maxillary and mandibular arches in half from between the first and second premolars on both sides.
5. The alveolar process:
   a. is a part of the bone located in the maxilla.
   b. is a part of the bone located in the mandible.
   c. forms the tooth sockets and supports the teeth.
   d. is all of the above.
6. The developmental phases of a tooth, in order, are:
   a. tooth bud, ameloblasts or odontoblasts, morphogenesis, matrix, calcium salts.
   b. matrix, ameloblasts or odontoblasts, tooth bud, morphogenesis, calcium salts.
   c. tooth bud, ameloblasts or odontoblasts, morphogenesis, calcium salts, matrix.
   d. calcium salts, matrix, morphogenesis, ameloblasts or odontoblasts, tooth bud.
7. The hardest substance in the body is:
   a. enamel.
   b. dentin.
   c. cementum.
   d. pulp.

8. The tissue that does not have the ability to reproduce if damaged is:
   a. enamel.
   b. cellular cementum.
   c. all of the above.
   d. none of the above.
9. The pulp cavity contains the:
   a. dental pulp.
   b. pulp chamber.
   c. pulp canal.
   d. all of the above.
10. The pulp chamber:
    a. is located in the crown of the tooth.
    b. contains most of the dental pulp.
    c. has pulp horns projecting out of the top.
    d. all of the above.

Answers

1. **c,** 2. **c,** 3. **d,** 4. **b,** 5. **d,** 6. **a,** 7. **a,** 8. **a,** 9. **d,** 10. **d**

References

Ash, M. M. (1993). *Wheeler's dental anatomy, physiology, and occlusion* (7th ed.). Philadelphia: W. B. Saunders Company.

Avery, J. K., & Steele, P. D. (1992). *Essentials of oral histology and embryology: A clinical approach*. St. Louis: Mosby.

Bhaskar, S. N. (1991). *Orban's oral histology and embryology* (11th ed.). St. Louis: Mosby.

Dorland's illustrated medical dictionary (28th ed.). (1994). Philadelphia: W. B. Saunders Company.

Fehrenbach, M. J., & Herring, S. W. (1996). *Illustrated anatomy of the head and neck*. Philadelphia: W. B. Saunders Company.

Melfi, R. C. (1988). *Permar's oral embryology and microscopic anatomy* (8th ed.). Philadelphia: Lea and Febiger.

CHAPTER 2

Tooth Notation Systems

Key Terms

American Dental Association Universal/National System
Eruption
Exfoliation
International Standards Organization/Fédération Dentaire Internationale System (ISO/FDI System)
Mixed Dentition
Quadrant
Sextant
Tooth Notation Systems
Zsigmondy-Palmer Notation System

The three **tooth notation systems** in general use are the **Zsigmondy-Palmer Notation system**, the **American Dental Association Universal/National system**, and the **International Standards Organization/Fédération Dentaire Internationale system (ISO/FDI system)**. Each of these notation systems has a method of identifying primary and permanent teeth.

The first system for designating the position of the teeth originated in 1861 by Viennese dentist, Adolf Zsigmondy. His method consisted of dividing the maxilla and mandible at the midline into **quadrants** (four regions) with each permanent tooth, starting at the central incisor, specified by the numbers 1 through 8. Several years later, in 1870, an American dentist, Corydon Palmer, reintroduced the Zsigmondy eight-tooth quadrant system as the Palmer system. The American Dental Association Committee on Nomenclature adopted the quadrant tooth numbers 1 through 8 symbolic system in 1947 and referred to it as the Zsigmondy-Palmer Notation system. This system was widely used internationally.

The Universal/National system is used primarily in the United States and was officially adopted by the American Dental Association House of Delegates in 1984. The method consists of continuous numbers, #1 through #32, for the permanent dentition and uppercase letters A through T for the primary dentition.

The Fédération Dentaire Internationale (FDI) system developed by Dr. Jochen Viohl uses a two-digit code to identify each tooth. The first digit indicates the quadrant, 1 through 4 for permanent teeth and 5 through 8 for primary teeth. The second digit designates the type of tooth, 1 through 8 for permanent teeth and 1 through 5 for primary teeth. It is important to be familiar with each of the three tooth notation systems.

In 1994, the American Dental Association (ADA) adopted the International Standards Organization (ISO) Designation System for Teeth and Areas of the Oral Cavity. The maxilla and mandible are divided either into quadrants or **sextants** (six regions). A two-digit number designates the areas of the oral cavity and one of the two digits is always a zero, as follows:

- 00 Designates the entire oral cavity as a whole.
- 01 Designates the maxillary arch.
- 02 Designates the mandibular arch.
- 10 Designates the upper right quadrant.
- 20 Designates the upper left quadrant.
- 30 Designates the lower left quadrant.
- 40 Designates the lower right quadrant.
- 03 Designates the upper right sextant.
- 04 Designates the upper anterior sextant.
- 05 Designates the upper left sextant.
- 06 Designates the lower left sextant.
- 07 Designates the lower anterior sextant.
- 08 Designates the lower right sextant.

The ISO uses a two-digit code to designate the teeth. The ISO and the FDI systems use the same two-digit designation codes and currently they are referred to as the ISO/FDI Tooth Designation System.

In January 1995, the Commission on Dental Accreditation adopted the ADA-approved tooth designation systems. They recommend all commission-accredited educational programs inform and indoctrinate students about both systems.

Zsigmondy-Palmer Notation System for the Permanent Dentition

The Zsigmondy-Palmer Notation system divides the maxillary and mandibular teeth at the midline forming four corresponding sections; each component is referred to as a quadrant. Every quadrant is designated by a symbol (Table 2–1). A number located within the symbol (Table 2–2) represents each tooth.

Table 2–1

Quadrant	Symbol
Maxillary right	┘
Maxillary left	└
Mandibular left	┌
Mandibular right	┐

The permanent teeth, beginning with the central incisor to the third molar, are numbered 1 through 8 for the maxillary and mandibular arches right and left (Figure 2–1). The corresponding symbol indicating the quadrant must be placed adjacent to the designated tooth number. For example, the maxillary right first molar is 6┘, the mandibular right lateral incisor is 2┐, and the

Table 2–2: Zsigmondy-Palmer Notation System

Permanent Dentition

MAXILLARY TEETH	QUADRANT SYMBOL DESIGNATION	MANDIBULAR TEETH	QUADRANT SYMBOL DESIGNATION
Right Third Molar	8┘	Left Third Molar	┌8
Right Second Molar	7┘	Left Second Molar	┌7
Right First Molar	6┘	Left First Molar	┌6
Right Second Premolar	5┘	Left Second Premolar	┌5
Right First Premolar	4┘	Left First Premolar	┌4
Right Canine	3┘	Left Canine	┌3
Right Lateral Incisor	2┘	Left Lateral Incisor	┌2
Right Central Incisor	1┘	Left Central Incisor	┌1
Left Central Incisor	└1	Right Central Incisor	1┐
Left Lateral Incisor	└2	Right Lateral Incisor	2┐
Left Canine	└3	Right Canine	3┐
Left First Premolar	└4	Right First Premolar	4┐
Left Second Premolar	└5	Right Second Premolar	5┐
Left First Molar	└6	Right First Molar	6┐
Left Second Molar	└7	Right Second Molar	7┐
Left Third Molar	└8	Right Third Molar	8┐

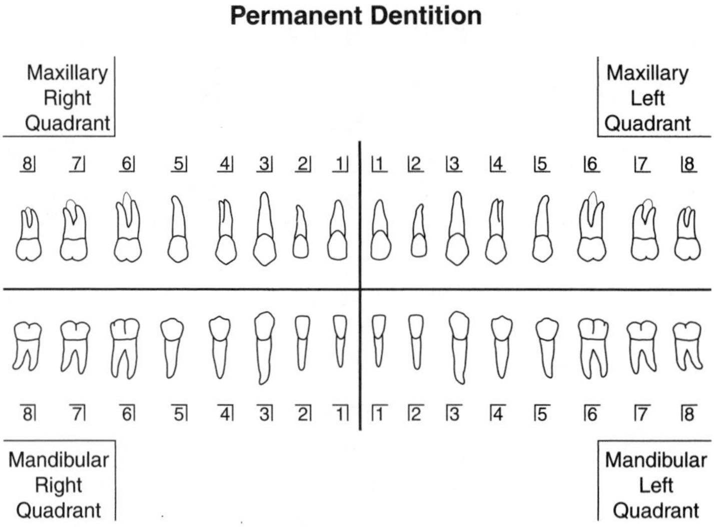

Figure 2–1 Zsigmondy-Palmer Notation system for permanent teeth

Permanent Dentition

Maxillary Right Quadrant | Maxillary Left Quadrant

8⌋ 7⌋ 6⌋ 5⌋ 4⌋ 3⌋ 2⌋ 1⌋ ⌊1 ⌊2 ⌊3 ⌊4 ⌊5 ⌊6 ⌊7 ⌊8

8⌉ 7⌉ 6⌉ 5⌉ 4⌉ 3⌉ 2⌉ 1⌉ ⌈1 ⌈2 ⌈3 ⌈4 ⌈5 ⌈6 ⌈7 ⌈8

Mandibular Right Quadrant | Mandibular Left Quadrant

maxillary left lateral incisor is ⌊2. When referring to several teeth located in the same quadrant, consecutively write the tooth identification numbers next to each other adjacent to one quadrant symbol. The maxillary left lateral incisor, canine, and premolar would be identified as ⌊234. To represent an entire quadrant, place an uppercase letter Q adjacent to the corresponding symbol. For example, the mandibular left quadrant would be identified as ⌈Q.

Zsigmondy-Palmer Notation System for the Deciduous Dentition

To distinguish between deciduous and permanent teeth using the Zsigmondy-Palmer Notation system, uppercase letters A through E are used instead of numbers (Table 2–3).

Beginning with the central incisor to the second molar, the teeth are identified by the letters A through E (Figure 2–2). Examples are the maxillary right first molar D⌋ and the mandibular left lateral incisor ⌈B, which are represented with uppercase letters adjacent to the quadrant symbols.

Table 2–3: Zsigmondy-Palmer Notation System

Deciduous Dentition

MAXILLARY TEETH	QUADRANT SYMBOL DESIGNATION	MANDIBULAR TEETH	QUADRANT SYMBOL DESIGNATION
Right Second Molar	E⌋	Left Second Molar	⌈E
Right First Molar	D⌋	Left First Molar	⌈D
Right Canine	C⌋	Left Canine	⌈C
Right Lateral Incisor	B⌋	Left Lateral Incisor	⌈B
Right Central Incisor	A⌋	Left Central Incisor	⌈A
Left Central Incisor	⌊A	Right Central Incisor	A⌉
Left Lateral Incisor	⌊B	Right Lateral Incisor	B⌉
Left Canine	⌊C	Right Canine	C⌉
Left First Molar	⌊D	Right First Molar	D⌉
Left Second Molar	⌊E	Right Second Molar	E⌉

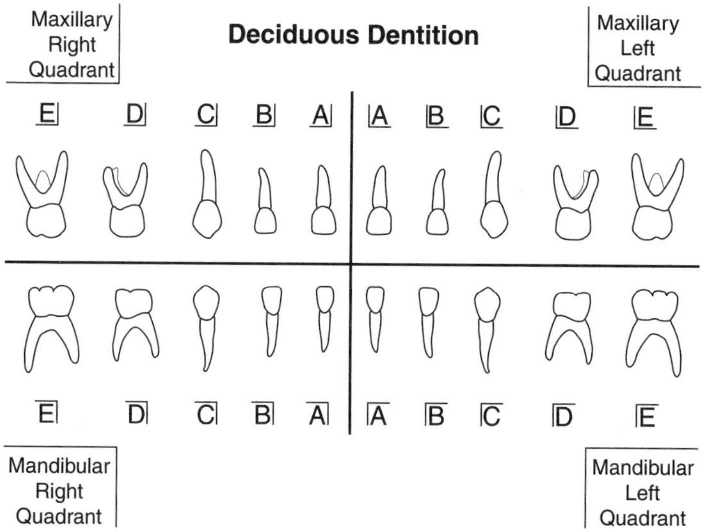

Maxillary Right Quadrant

Deciduous Dentition

Maxillary Left Quadrant

E⌋ D⌋ C⌋ B⌋ A⌋ ⌊A ⌊B ⌊C ⌊D ⌊E

E⌉ D⌉ C⌉ B⌉ A⌉ ⌈A ⌈B ⌈C ⌈D ⌈E

Mandibular Right Quadrant

Mandibular Left Quadrant

Figure 2–2 Zsigmondy-Palmer Notation system for deciduous teeth

American Dental Association Universal/National System for the Permanent Dentition

The American Dental Association Universal/National system is a sequential tooth numbering system designated by the numbers 1 through 32 for the permanent dentition (Table 2–4).

Begin with the maxillary right third molar, which represents tooth #1, and continue numbering to the maxillary left third molar, which is designated as tooth #16. Descend down to the mandibular left third molar, represented as tooth #17, and follow around the mandibular arch to the right third molar, identified as tooth #32 (Figure 2–3).

Table 2–4: American Dental Association (ADA) Universal/National System

Permanent Dentition

MAXILLARY TEETH	ADA TOOTH NUMBER	MANDIBULAR TEETH	ADA TOOTH NUMBER
Right Third Molar	1	Left Third Molar	17
Right Second Molar	2	Left Second Molar	18
Right First Molar	3	Left First Molar	19
Right Second Premolar	4	Left Second Premolar	20
Right First Premolar	5	Left First Premolar	21
Right Canine	6	Left Canine	22
Right Lateral Incisor	7	Left Lateral Incisor	23
Right Central Incisor	8	Left Central Incisor	24
Left Central Incisor	9	Right Central Incisor	25
Left Lateral Incisor	10	Right Lateral Incisor	26
Left Canine	11	Right Canine	27
Left First Premolar	12	Right First Premolar	28
Left Second Premolar	13	Right Second Premolar	29
Left First Molar	14	Right First Molar	30
Left Second Molar	15	Right Second Molar	31
Left Third Molar	16	Right Third Molar	32

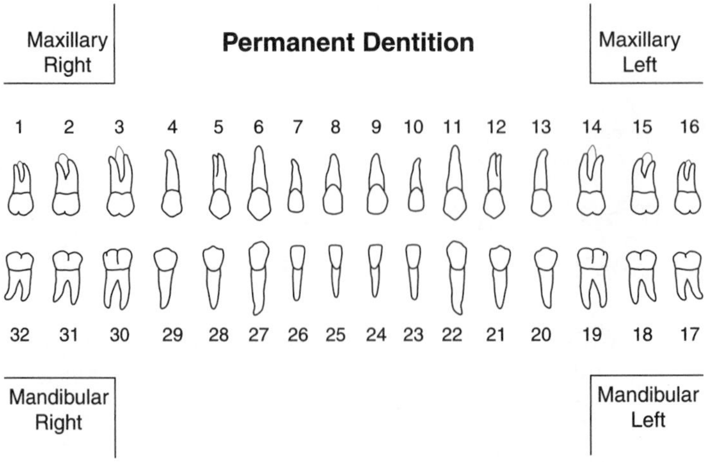

Figure 2–3 American Dental Association (ADA) Universal/National system for permanent teeth

Maxillary Right

Permanent Dentition

Maxillary Left

1 2 3 4 5 6 7 8 9 10 11 12 13 14 15 16

32 31 30 29 28 27 26 25 24 23 22 21 20 19 18 17

Mandibular Right

Mandibular Left

American Dental Association Universal/National System for the Deciduous Dentition

To distinguish between deciduous and permanent teeth using the ADA Universal/National system, uppercase letters A through T are used instead of numbers (Table 2–5). The deciduous right second molar is represented with the letter A and the sequence of letters continues around the maxillary arch to the right second molar (J). Descend to the mandibular left second molar, represented with the letter K, and progress to the right second molar that represents tooth letter T (Figure 2–4).

Table 2–5: American Dental Association (ADA) Universal/National System

Deciduous Dentition

MAXILLARY TEETH	ADA TOOTH LETTER	MANDIBULAR TEETH	ADA TOOTH LETTER
Right Second Molar	A	Left Second Molar	K
Right First Molar	B	Left First Molar	L
Right Canine	C	Left Canine	M
Right Lateral Incisor	D	Left Lateral Incisor	N
Right Central Incisor	E	Left Central Incisor	O
Left Central Incisor	F	Right Central Incisor	P
Left Lateral Incisor	G	Right Lateral Incisor	Q
Left Canine	H	Right Canine	R
Left First Molar	I	Right First Molar	S
Left Second Molar	J	Right Second Molar	T

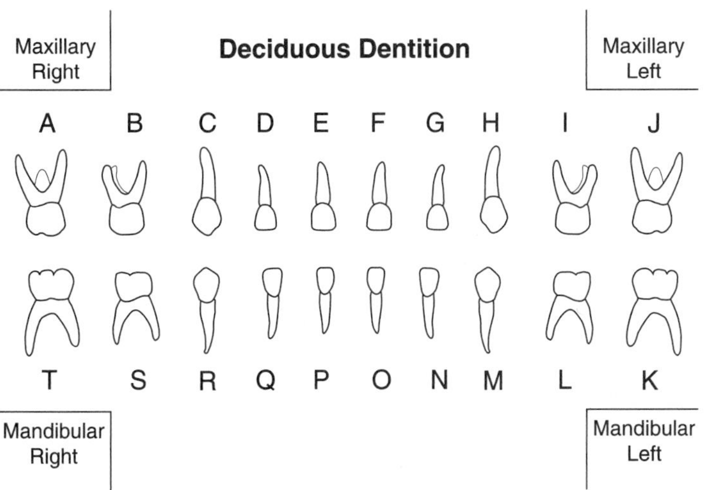

Figure 2–4 American Dental Association (ADA) Universal/National System for deciduous teeth

International Standards Organization/Fédération Dentaire Internationale System for the Permanent Dentition

The International Standards Organization/Fédération Dentaire Internationale (ISO/FDI) system uses a two-digit system of designating teeth for the permanent and deciduous dentitions (Table 2–6).

The maxillary and mandibular teeth are divided at the midline forming four corresponding sections; each component is referred to as a quadrant. The first digit identifies the quadrant. Each quadrant is numbered 1 through 4, with quadrant number 1 the maxillary right, and continuing clockwise, quadrant number 2 the maxillary left, quadrant number 3 the mandibular left, and quadrant number 4 the mandibular right. The second digit designates the tooth within the quadrant. The permanent teeth, beginning with the central incisor to the third molar, are numbered 1 through 8 for the maxillary and mandibular arches right and left (Figure 2–5).

Table 2–6: International Standards Organization/Fédération Dentaire Internationale (ISO/FDI) System

Permanent Dentition

MAXILLARY TEETH	ISO/FDI TWO-DIGIT DESIGNATION	MANDIBULAR TEETH	ISO/FDI TWO-DIGIT DESIGNATION
Right Third Molar	18	Left Third Molar	38
Right Second Molar	17	Left Second Molar	37
Right First Molar	16	Left First Molar	36
Right Second Premolar	15	Left Second Premolar	35
Right First Premolar	14	Left First Premolar	34
Right Canine	13	Left Canine	33
Right Lateral Incisor	12	Left Lateral Incisor	32
Right Central Incisor	11	Left Central Incisor	31
Left Central Incisor	21	Right Central Incisor	41
Left Lateral Incisor	22	Right Lateral Incisor	42
Left Canine	23	Right Canine	43
Left First Premolar	24	Right First Premolar	44
Left Second Premolar	25	Right Second Premolar	45
Left First Molar	26	Right First Molar	46
Left Second Molar	27	Right Second Molar	47
Left Third Molar	28	Right Third Molar	48

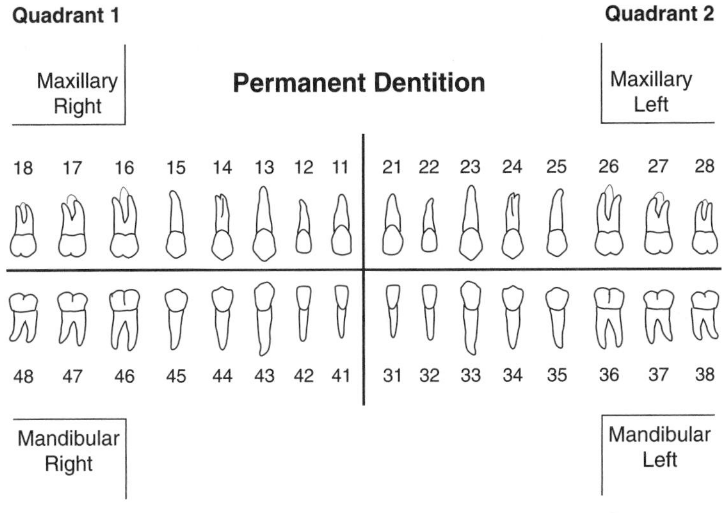

Figure 2–5 International Standards Organization/Fédération Dentaire Internationale (ISO/FDI) system for permanent teeth

The maxillary right first molar is written as 16. In speech, the digits are pronounced separately, "one-six." The maxillary left lateral incisor is written as 22 and correctly pronounced as "two-two," not "twenty-two."

To prevent confusion between the ISO/FDI and ADA-Universal Tooth Designation systems, the use of the symbol "#" always precedes the designated tooth number when using the Universal system; for example, Universal tooth #24 (twenty-four) as opposed to ISO/FDI tooth 24 (two-four).

International Standards Organization/Fédération Dentaire Internationale System for the Deciduous Dentition

To distinguish between deciduous and permanent teeth using the International Standards Organization/Fédération Dentaire Internationale (ISO/FDI) system, the quadrants are consecutively numbered 5 through 8, the same order as the permanent teeth. The designations for the individual teeth are 1 through 5 (Table 2–7).

As shown in Figure 2–6, the first digit represents the quadrant and the second digit the type of tooth within the quadrant. The mandibular right first molar is written as 84 and the digits are pronounced "eight-four."

Table 2–7: International Standards Organization/Fédération Dentaire Internationale (ISO/FDI) System

Deciduous Dentition

MAXILLARY TEETH	ISO/FDI TWO-DIGIT DESIGNATION	MANDIBULAR TEETH	ISO/FDI TWO-DIGIT DESIGNATION
Right Second Molar	55	Left Second Molar	75
Right First Molar	54	Left First Molar	74
Right Canine	53	Left Canine	73
Right Lateral Incisor	52	Left Lateral Incisor	72
Right Central Incisor	51	Left Central Incisor	71
Left Central Incisor	61	Right Central Incisor	81
Left Lateral Incisor	62	Right Lateral Incisor	82
Left Canine	63	Right Canine	83
Left First Molar	64	Right First Molar	84
Left Second Molar	65	Right Second Molar	85

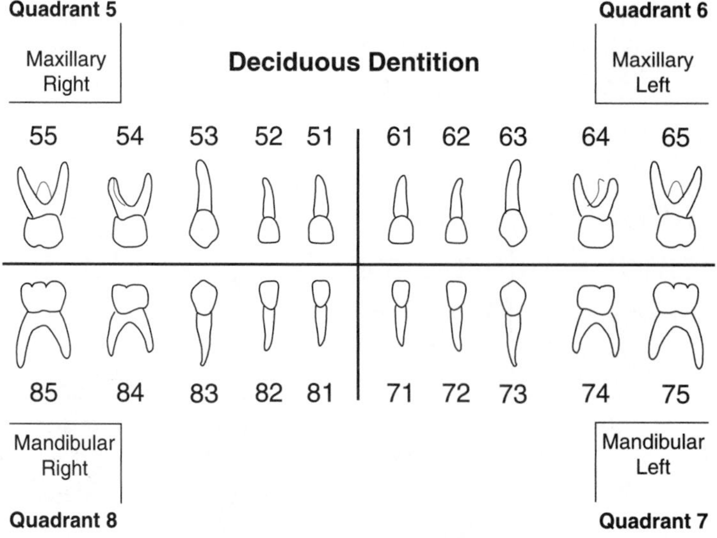

Figure 2–6 International Standards Organization/Fédération Dentaire Internationale (ISO/FDI) system for deciduous teeth

Tooth Eruption

The development of the deciduous teeth begins with the hard tissue formation and calcification of the crowns between 4 to 6 months *in utero* (Table 2–8).

Table 2-8: Tooth Development and Eruption

Tooth	Hard tissue formation begins	Enamel completed	Eruption	Root Completed
DECIDUOUS DENTITION				
Maxillary				
Central incisor	4 mos. in utero	1 1/2 mos.	7 1/2 mos.	1 1/2 yrs.
Lateral incisor	4 1/2 mos. in utero	2 1/2 mos.	9 mos.	2 yrs.
Cuspid	5 mos. in utero	9 mos.	18 mos.	3 1/4 yrs.
First molar	5 mos. in utero	6 mos.	14 mos.	2 1/2 yrs.
Second molar	6 mos. in utero	11 mos.	24 mos.	3 yrs.
Mandibular				
Central incisor	4 1/2 mos. in utero	2 1/2 mos.	6 mos.	1 1/2 yrs.
Lateral incisor	4 1/2 mos. in utero	3 mos.	7 mos.	1 1/2 yrs.
Cuspid	5 mos. in utero	9 mos.	16 mos.	3 1/4 yrs.
First molar	5 mos. in utero	5 1/2 mos.	12 mos.	2 1/4 yrs.
Second molar	6 mos. in utero	10 mos.	20 mos.	3 yrs.
PERMANENT DENTITION				
Maxillary				
Central incisor	3–4 mos.	4–5 yrs.	7–8 yrs.	10 yrs.
Lateral incisor	10–12 mos.	4–5 yrs.	8–9 yrs.	11 yrs.
Cuspid	4–5 mos.	6–7 yrs.	11–12 yrs.	13–15 yrs.
First bicuspid	1 1/2–1 3/4 yrs.	5–6 yrs.	10–11 yrs.	12–13 yrs.
Second bicuspid	2–2 1/4 yrs.	6–7 yrs.	10–12 yrs.	12–14 yrs.
First molar	At birth	2 1/2–3 yrs.	6–7 yrs.	9–10 yrs.
Second molar	2 1/2–3 yrs.	7–8 yrs.	12–13 yrs.	14–16 yrs.
Third molar	7–9 yrs.	12–16 yrs.	17–21 yrs.	18–25 yrs.
Mandibular				
Central incisor	3–4 mos.	4–5 yrs.	6–7 yrs.	9 yrs.
Lateral incisor	3–4 mos.	4–5 yrs.	7–8 yrs.	10 yrs.
Cuspid	4–5 mos.	6–7 yrs.	9–10 yrs.	12–14 yrs.
First bicuspid	1 1/2–2 yrs.	5–6 yrs.	10–12 yrs.	12–13 yrs.
Second bicuspid	2 1/4–2 1/2 yrs.	6–7 yrs.	11–12 yrs.	13–14 yrs.
First molar	At birth	2 1/2–3 yrs.	6–7 yrs.	9–10 yrs.
Second molar	2 1/2–3 yrs.	7–8 yrs.	11–13 yrs.	14–15 yrs.
Third molar	8–10 yrs.	12–16 yrs.	17–21 yrs.	18–25 yrs.

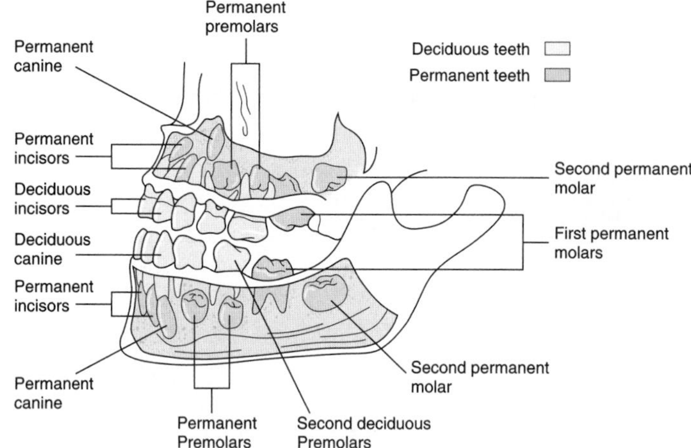

Figure 2–7 Mixed dentition

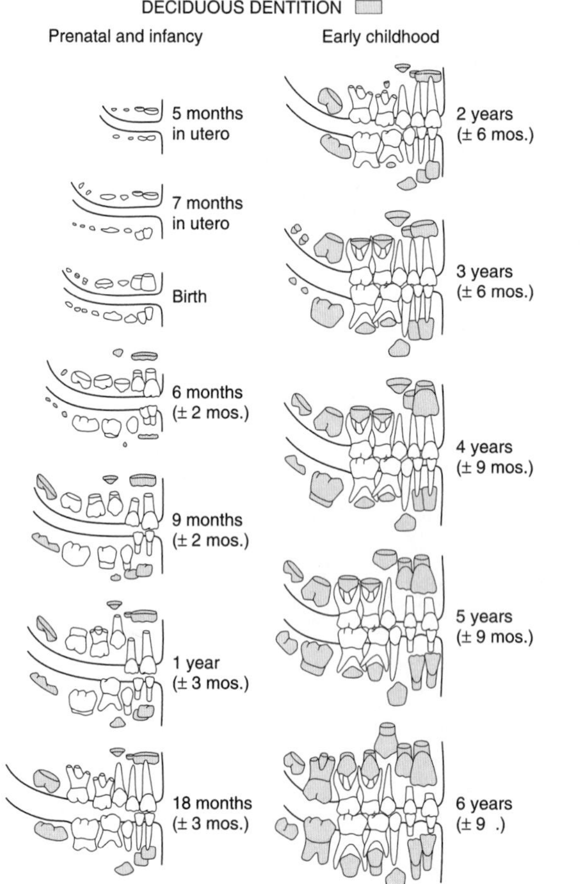

Figure 2–8 (A) Developmemt of human dentition

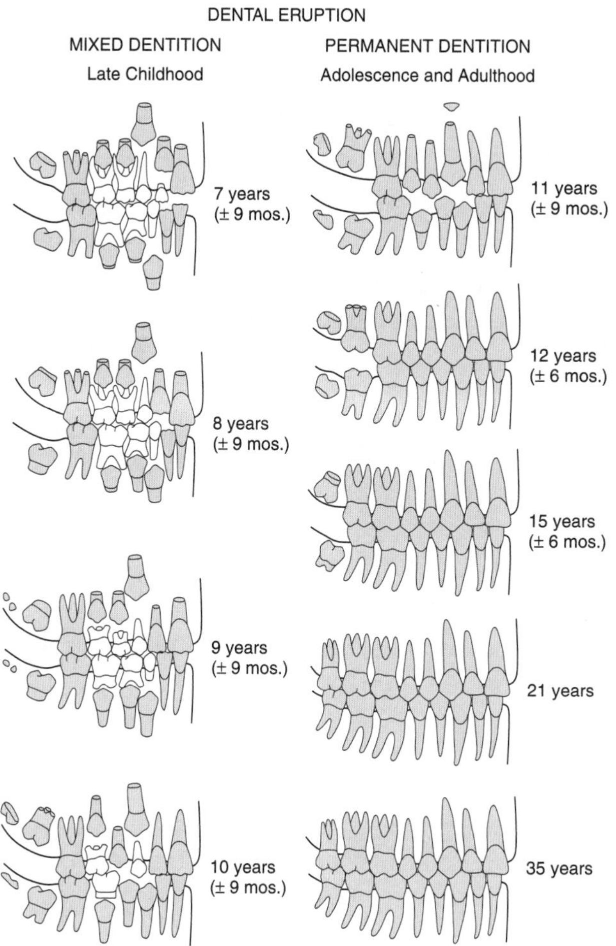

Figure 2–8 (B) Developmemt of human dentition

The enamel is completed at approximately 11 months prior to the date of **eruption** when the root formation begins and the tooth emerges within the alveolar process toward the oral cavity.

The mineralization of the permanent teeth begins at birth and continues into puberty. The deciduous teeth are shed and replaced with the permanent teeth through a process called **exfoliation**. Between the ages of 6 to 12 years the deciduous and permanent teeth co-exist together; this is known as **mixed dentition** (Figure 2–7). The development of the human dentition from prenatal through adulthood is shown in Figure 2–8A and B.

Review Questions

Multiple Choice

Directions: Select the letter of the choice that *best* answers the question.

1. The method that designates each quadrant with a symbol is the:
   a. Zsigmondy-Palmer Notation system.
   b. American Dental Association Universal/National system.
   c. International Standards Organization/Fédération Dentaire Internationale system.
   d. None of the above.
2. The method that uses "#" in front of the tooth number is the:
   a. Zsigmondy-Palmer Notation system.
   b. American Dental Association Universal/National system.
   c. International Standards Organization/Fédération Dentaire Internationale system.
   d. None of the above.
3. The method that uses the "two-digit" system to identify teeth is called the:
   a. Zsigmondy-Palmer Notation system.
   b. American Dental Association Universal/National system.
   c. International Standards Organization/Fédération Dentaire Internationale system.
   d. All of the above.
4. The permanent maxillary right first molar is designated as _____ using the Zsigmondy-Palmer Notation system.
   a. 6┘
   b. └6
   c. 3
   d. 14
5. The method that denotes deciduous teeth by uppercase letters A through E is the:
   a. Zsigmondy-Palmer Notation system.
   b. American Dental Association Universal/National system.
   c. International Standards Organization/Fédération Dentaire Internationale system.
   d. None of the above.

6. The American Dental Association Universal/National system uses _____ for the deciduous dentition.
   a. uppercase letters A through E
   b. lowercase letters a through t
   c. quadrants numbered 5 through 8
   d. uppercase letters A through T
7. The method that uses the uppercase letters A–T to designate deciduous teeth is the:
   a. Zsigmondy-Palmer Notation system.
   b. American Dental Association Universal/National system.
   c. International Standards Organization/Fédération Dentaire Internationale system.
   d. All of the above.
8. The system that uses a total of eight quadrants is the:
   a. Zsigmondy-Palmer Notation system.
   b. American Dental Association Universal/National system.
   c. International Standards Organization/Fédération Dentaire Internationale system.
   d. All of the above.
9. Using the International Standards Organization/Fédération Dentaire International system, the deciduous mandibular left canine is designated as:
   a. 33.
   b. 53.
   c. 13.
   d. 73.
10. When using the ISO/FDI system, tooth 42 is spoken as:
    a. forty-two.
    b. four-two.
    c. All of the above.
    d. None of the above.

Answers

1. **a,** 2. **b,** 3. **c,** 4. **a,** 5. **a,** 6. **d,** 7. **b,** 8. **d,** 9. **d,** 10. **b**

References

Ahlberg, J. E. (1987). We must get our numbers right. FDI *Newsletter*, 158, 8–9.

Beale, D. R. (1991). The importance of dental records for identification. *New Zealand Dental Journal*, 84, 84-87.

Clark, D. & Sainio, P. (1992). *Practical forensic odontology*. Wright: Oxford, England. 101–110.

Coppock, D. A. (1989). Keeping up-to-date with dental notation [letter]. *British Dental Journal*, 166, 108.

Cunningham, G. (1883). On a system of dental notation, being a code of symbols for the use of dentists' recording. *British Dental Journal*, 4, 456.

Cunningham, G. (1890). The international dental notation. *British Journal of Dental Science*, 33, 256–261.

Dorland's illustrated medical dictionary (28th ed.). (1994). Philadelphia: W. B. Saunders Company.

Elderton, R. J. (1989). Keeping up-to-date with tooth notation. *British Dental Journal*, 166, 55–56.

Fédération Dentaire Internationale/two-digit system of designating teeth. (1971). *International Dental Journal*, 104, 21.

Lyons, I. I. (1947). Committee adopts official method for the symbolic designation of teeth. *Journal of the American Dental Association*, 34, 647.

Palmer, C. (1870). Dental recording. *Dental Cosmos*, 12 (10), 522–524.

Palmer, C. (1891). Palmer's dental notation. *Dental Cosmos*, 33, (3), 194–198.

Peck, S. & Peck, L. (1993). A time for change of tooth numbering systems. *Journal of Dental Education*, 57.

Sandham, J. A. (1984). The FDI two-digit system of designating teeth. *International Dental Journal*, 33, 390–392.

Sharma, R. S., & Wadhwa P. (1977). Evaluation of the FDI two-digit system of designating teeth. *Quintessence International*, 10, 99–101.

Ubelaker, D. H. (1978). *Human skeletal remains: Excavation, analysis, interpretation*. Chicago: Aldine.

Villa, V. M. A., Arenal, A. A., & Gonzalez, M. A. R. (1989). Notation of numerical abnormalities by an addition to the FDI system. *Quintessence International*, 20, 299–302.

Zsigmondy, A. (1874). A practical method for rapidly noting dental observations and operations. *British Journal of Dental Science*, 17, 580–582.

CHAPTER 3

Dental Charts for Tooth Assessment

Key Terms

Anatomic Chart
Dental Charts
Dental Records
Geometric Chart
Letter Codes
Numeric Coding System Chart
Periodontal Chart
Permanent Record

Comprehensive patient **dental records** provide an accurate description and assessment of the patient's medical and dental status. The **permanent record** includes complete and accurate information based on a thorough examination that includes personal, medical, and dental histories, radiographic and clinical evaluation, diagnosis, prognosis, and treatment plan (Figure 3–1).

Dental charts for manual charting are available in several styles and include the anatomic, geometric, and numeric coding system charts. The teeth are graphically represented on anatomic and geometric charts whereas the numeric coding system uses **letter codes** rather than a visual representation. The anatomic and geometric versions are used most frequently.

Anatomic Dental Charts

Three types of **anatomic charts** are described here. Figure 3–2 is an example of a segment of an anatomic charting form representing the crowns of the teeth. This type of chart makes it difficult to accurately document periapical and other root structure conditions. Figure 3–3 shows the crowns and only a

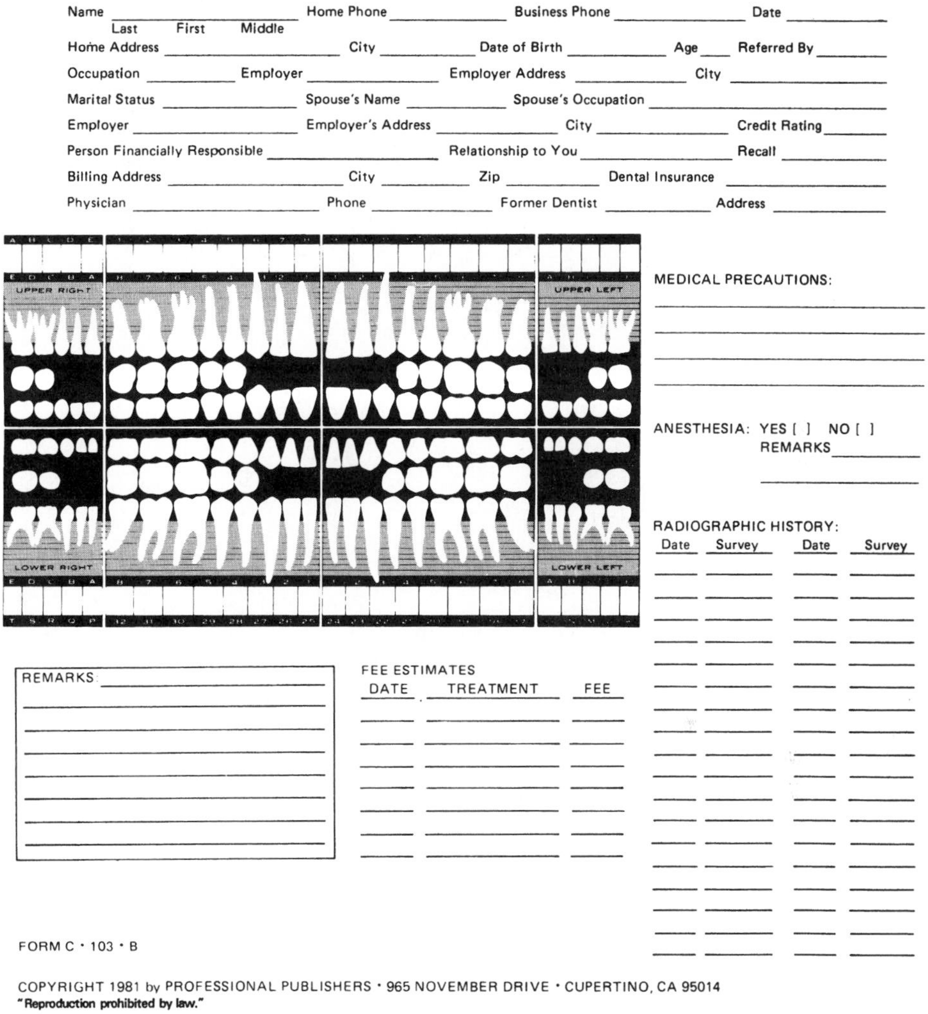

Name ______ Home Phone ______ Business Phone ______ Date ______
Last First Middle
Home Address ______ City ______ Date of Birth ______ Age ___ Referred By ______
Occupation ______ Employer ______ Employer Address ______ City ______
Marital Status ______ Spouse's Name ______ Spouse's Occupation ______
Employer ______ Employer's Address ______ City ______ Credit Rating ______
Person Financially Responsible ______ Relationship to You ______ Recall ______
Billing Address ______ City ______ Zip ______ Dental Insurance ______
Physician ______ Phone ______ Former Dentist ______ Address ______

UPPER RIGHT
UPPER LEFT
LOWER RIGHT
LOWER LEFT

MEDICAL PRECAUTIONS:

ANESTHESIA: YES [ ] NO [ ]
REMARKS ______

RADIOGRAPHIC HISTORY:

Date	Survey	Date	Survey

REMARKS: ______

FEE ESTIMATES

DATE	TREATMENT	FEE

FORM C · 103 · B

Figure 3–1 Dental chart (Courtesy Professional Publishers, Cupertino, CA. Reproduction prohibited by law)

small portion of the root. The amount of root structure shown makes it possible to indicate problems located at, and near, the CEJ.

The anatomic dental chart that provides the best representation of tooth surfaces and root structure is shown in Figure 3–4. This dental chart in Figure 3–4 allows the examiner to provide the most accurate description of the

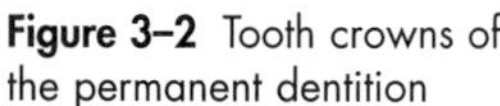

Figure 3–2 Tooth crowns of the permanent dentition

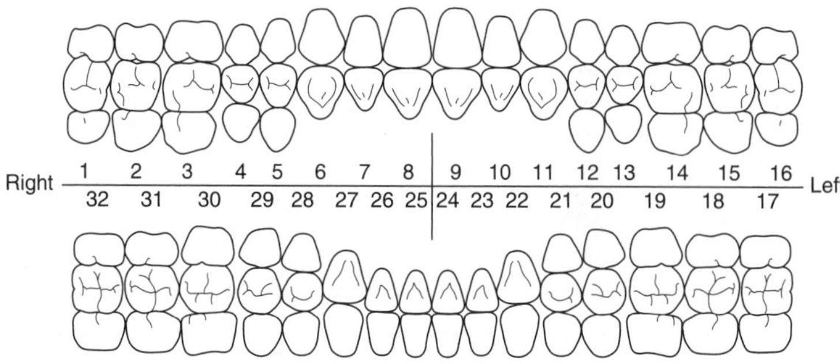

Figure 3–3 Tooth crowns and partial roots of the permanent dentition

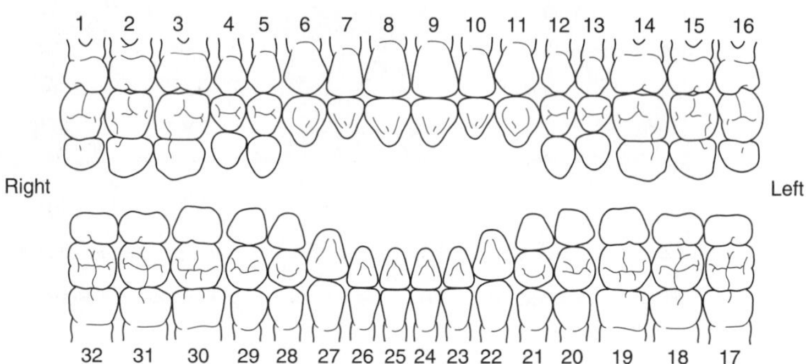

patient's dental status compared to the examples illustrated in Figures 3–2 and 3–3. Showing the Facial and Lingual root surfaces and the addition of Mesial and Distal wings on the Occlusal and Incisal tooth surface views permits the examiner to indicate a more realistic depiction of the existing conditions present in the patient's mouth.

Geometric Dental Charts

Three types of **geometric charts** are described here. Figure 3–5 is an example of a geometric charting form representing the diagrammatic stylized design of the teeth. The upper and lower rows of circles indicate the maxillary and mandibular arches. The circles numbered 1 through 32 designate the permanent teeth and the deciduous teeth are represented with uppercase letters A through T.

EXAMINATION RECORD

Last Name	First Name	Date

18	17	16	15	14	13	12	11	21	22	23	24	25	26	27	28
8	7	6	5	4	3	2	1	1	2	3	4	5	6	7	8
1	2	3	4	5	6	7	8	9	10	11	12	13	14	15	16
32	31	30	29	28	27	26	25	24	23	22	21	20	19	18	17
8	7	6	5	4	3	2	1	1	2	3	4	5	6	7	8
48	47	46	45	44	43	42	41	31	32	33	34	35	36	37	38

CLINICAL DATA

Oral Cancer Examination

55	54	53	52	51	61	62	63	64	65
E	D	C	B	A	A	B	C	D	E
A	B	C	D	E	F	G	H	I	J
T	S	R	Q	P	O	N	M	L	K
E	D	C	B	A	A	B	C	D	E
85	84	83	82	81	71	72	73	74	75

Plaque:	Slight ☐	Moderate ☐	Excessive ☐
Calculus:	Slight ☐	Moderate ☐	Excessive ☐
Stains:	Slight ☐	Moderate ☐	Excessive ☐

Clinical Examination

X-Ray Examination

Figure 3–4 Anatomic dental chart showing Facial, Occlusal, and Lingual tooth surfaces and Facial and Lingual root surfaces

The crown of the tooth is shown with two circles: an inner circle, which represents the Occlusal and Incisal surfaces, and an outer circle that indicates the Mesial, Distal, Facial (Labial and Buccal), and Lingual tooth surfaces (Figure 3–6). This type of chart requires less time to fill in because the exact

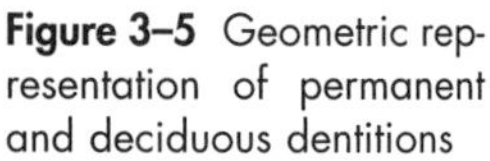

Figure 3–5 Geometric representation of permanent and deciduous dentitions

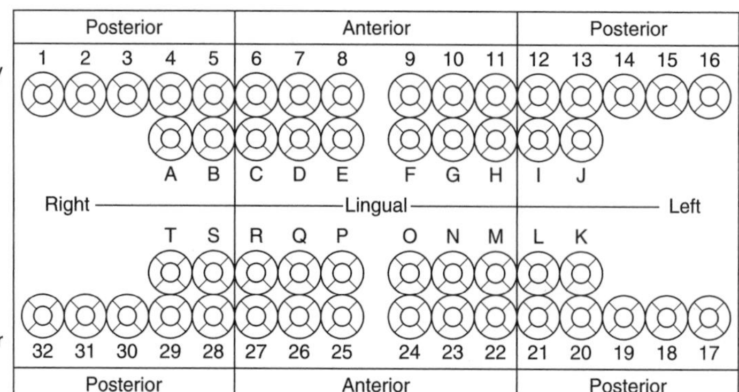

Figure 3–6 Geometric representation of Mesial, Distal, Facial, and Lingual tooth surfaces of permanent and deciduous dentitions

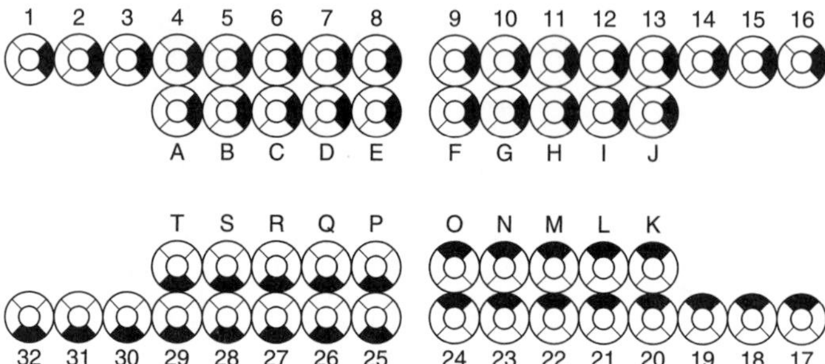

anatomic characteristics are not drawn in. The examiner must completely fill in the designated area rather than marking only a portion of it and, consequently, this does not provide an accurate depiction of some restorative treatment.

Figure 3–7 shows the geometric representation of each tooth with additional lines indicating tooth surface divisions and only a small portion of the root and Figure 3–8 shows a similar chart with complete roots.

When comparing Figure 3–5 to Figure 3–8, the addition of horizontal lines on the Buccal and Lingual tooth surfaces allow for a more accurate depiction of the restorative treatment particularly because the geometric chart requires the examiner to completely fill in the designated space. For example, tooth #30 has an amalgam restoration involving the Buccal groove so when using the chart in Figure 3–5, the entire Buccal surface of tooth #30 must be filled

EXAMINATION RECORD

Last Name	First Name	Date

18	17	16	15	14	13	12	11	21	22	23	24	25	26	27	28
8	7	6	5	4	3	2	1	1	2	3	4	5	6	7	8
1	2	3	4	5	6	7	8	9	10	11	12	13	14	15	16

32	31	30	29	28	27	26	25	24	23	22	21	20	19	18	17
8	7	6	5	4	3	2	1	1	2	3	4	5	6	7	8
48	47	46	45	44	43	42	41	31	32	33	34	35	36	37	38

CLINICAL DATA

Oral Cancer Examination

55	54	53	52	51	61	62	63	64	65
E	D	C	B	A	A	B	C	D	E
A	B	C	D	E	F	G	H	I	J

T	S	R	Q	P	O	N	M	L	K
E	D	C	B	A	A	B	C	D	E
85	84	83	82	81	71	72	73	74	75

Plaque:	Slight ☐	Moderate ☐	Excessive ☐
Calculus:	Slight ☐	Moderate ☐	Excessive ☐
Stains:	Slight ☐	Moderate ☐	Excessive ☐

Clinical Examination

X-Ray Examination

Figure 3–7 Geometric dental chart showing permanent and deciduous dentitions with lines indicating tooth surface divisions and partial roots

in. When using the chart in Figure 3–8, only the center space that indicates the Buccal tooth surface is filled in. Because the geometric charts do not require precise anatomic drawings, using the chart in Figure 3–8 provides the most accurate representation of the patient's restorations.

EXAMINATION RECORD

Last Name	First Name	Date

18	17	16	15	14	13	12	11	21	22	23	24	25	26	27	28
8	7	6	5	4	3	2	1	1	2	3	4	5	6	7	8
1	2	3	4	5	6	7	8	9	10	11	12	13	14	15	16
32	31	30	29	28	27	26	25	24	23	22	21	20	19	18	17
8	7	6	5	4	3	2	1	1	2	3	4	5	6	7	8
48	47	46	45	44	43	42	41	31	32	33	34	35	36	37	38

CLINICAL DATA

Oral Cancer Examination

55	54	53	52	51	61	62	63	64	65
E	D	C	B	A	A	B	C	D	E
A	B	C	D	E	F	G	H	I	J
T	S	R	Q	P	O	N	M	L	K
E	D	C	B	A	A	B	C	D	E
85	84	83	82	81	71	72	73	74	75

Plaque:	Slight ☐	Moderate ☐	Excessive ☐
Calculus:	Slight ☐	Moderate ☐	Excessive ☐
Stains:	Slight ☐	Moderate ☐	Excessive ☐

Clinical Examination

X-Ray Examination

Figure 3–8 Geometric dental chart showing permanent and deciduous dentitions with lines indicating tooth surface divisions and complete roots

Numeric Coding System Chart

Figure 3–9 shows a **numeric coding system chart.** This chart uses numbers, letter codes, and symbols instead of drawings to represent the conditions of the teeth. The date of the visit is entered in the left column, and

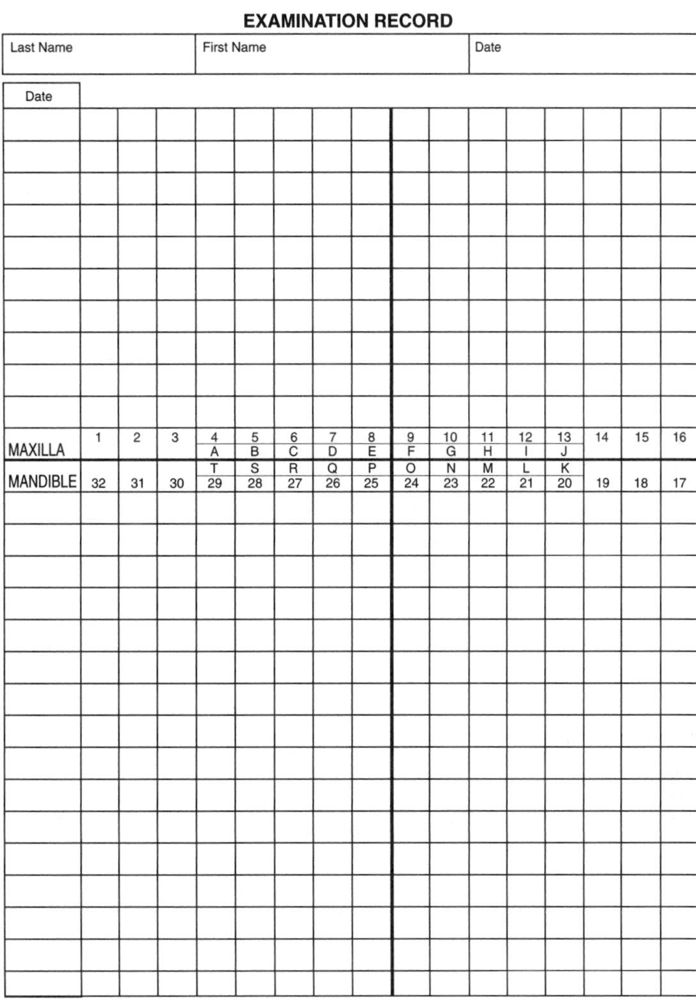

EXAMINATION RECORD

Last Name	First Name	Date

Date																
MAXILLA	1	2	3	4 A	5 B	6 C	7 D	8 E	9 F	10 G	11 H	12 I	13 J	14	15	16
MANDIBLE	32	31	30	T 29	S 28	R 27	Q 26	P 25	O 24	N 23	M 22	L 21	K 20	19	18	17

Figure 3–9 Numeric coding system chart

to the right the restorative procedures and tooth surfaces are abbreviated and entered above or below the designated tooth number to indicate the existing condition. As conditions change with subsequent visits they are noted by entering the new information above or below the preexisting information.

Periodical Chart

Figure 3–10 shows an example of a **periodontal chart**. This chart enables the examiner to document dental deposits, mobility, gingival, and periodontal conditions. A more detailed explanation of utilizing this chart is provided in Chapter 15.

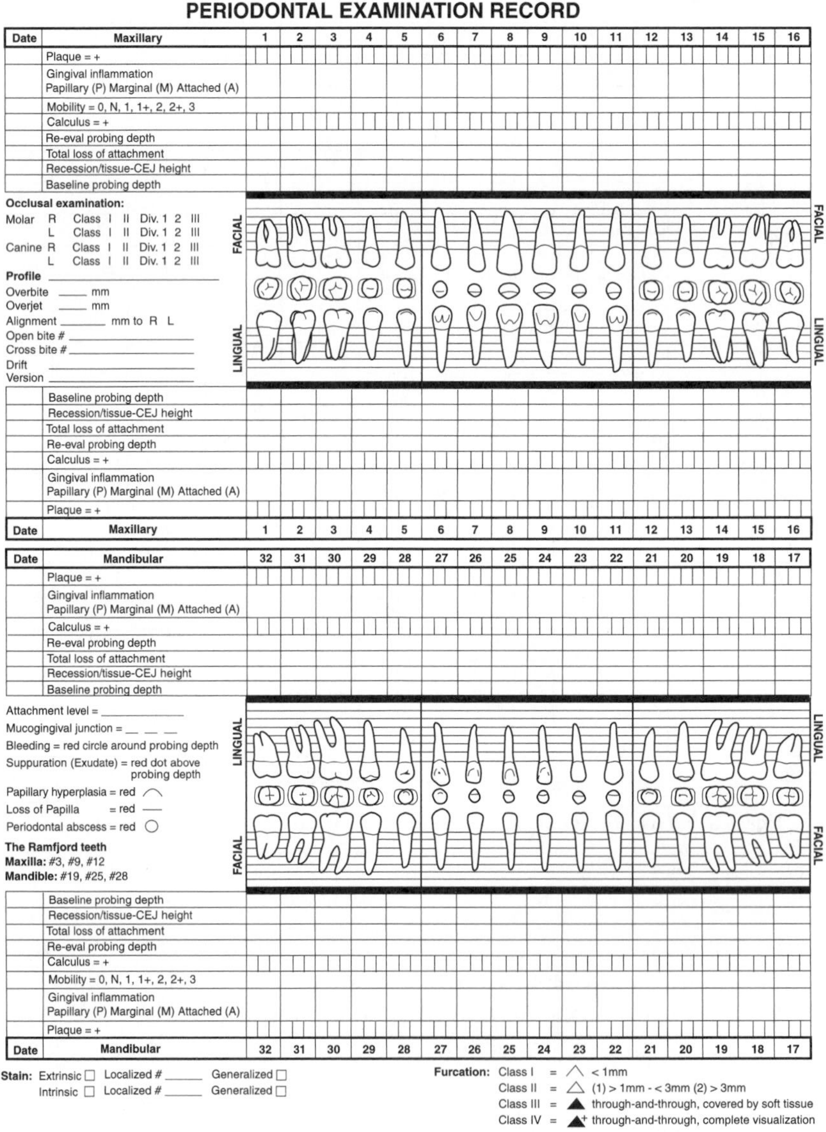

PERIODONTAL EXAMINATION RECORD

Date	Maxillary	1	2	3	4	5	6	7	8	9	10	11	12	13	14	15	16
	Plaque = +																
	Gingival inflammation Papillary (P) Marginal (M) Attached (A)																
	Mobility = 0, N, 1, 1+, 2, 2+, 3																
	Calculus = +																
	Re-eval probing depth																
	Total loss of attachment																
	Recession/tissue-CEJ height																
	Baseline probing depth																

Occlusal examination:
Molar R Class I II Div. 1 2 III
L Class I II Div. 1 2 III
Canine R Class I II Div. 1 2 III
L Class I II Div. 1 2 III
Profile ____________
Overbite ____ mm
Overjet ____ mm
Alignment ______ mm to R L
Open bite # ____________
Cross bite # ____________
Drift ____________
Version ____________

Date	Maxillary	1	2	3	4	5	6	7	8	9	10	11	12	13	14	15	16
	Baseline probing depth																
	Recession/tissue-CEJ height																
	Total loss of attachment																
	Re-eval probing depth																
	Calculus = +																
	Gingival inflammation Papillary (P) Marginal (M) Attached (A)																
	Plaque = +																

Date	Mandibular	32	31	30	29	28	27	26	25	24	23	22	21	20	19	18	17
	Plaque = +																
	Gingival inflammation Papillary (P) Marginal (M) Attached (A)																
	Calculus = +																
	Re-eval probing depth																
	Total loss of attachment																
	Recession/tissue-CEJ height																
	Baseline probing depth																

Attachment level = ____________
Mucogingival junction = __ __ __
Bleeding = red circle around probing depth
Suppuration (Exudate) = red dot above probing depth
Papillary hyperplasia = red ⌒
Loss of Papilla = red —
Periodontal abscess = red ○

The Ramfjord teeth
Maxilla: #3, #9, #12
Mandible: #19, #25, #28

Date	Mandibular	32	31	30	29	28	27	26	25	24	23	22	21	20	19	18	17
	Baseline probing depth																
	Recession/tissue-CEJ height																
	Total loss of attachment																
	Re-eval probing depth																
	Calculus = +																
	Mobility = 0, N, 1, 1+, 2, 2+, 3																
	Gingival inflammation Papillary (P) Marginal (M) Attached (A)																
	Plaque = +																

Stain: Extrinsic ☐ Localized # _____ Generalized ☐
Intrinsic ☐ Localized # _____ Generalized ☐

Furcation: Class I = △ < 1mm
Class II = △ (1) > 1mm - < 3mm (2) > 3mm
Class III = ▲ through-and-through, covered by soft tissue
Class IV = ▲+ through-and-through, complete visualization

*Record all abnormal conditions in red EXCEPT attachment level and mucogingival junction * All recorded in Arabic numerals * Mobility measurement is in millimeters

Figure 3–10 Periodontal examination record

Review Questions

Multiple Choice

Directions: Select the letter of the choice that *best* answers the question.

1. Which type of chart is used to document gingival conditions?
   a. Anatomic chart
   b. Geometric chart
   c. Numeric coding system chart
   d. Periodontal chart
2. The type of chart(s) in which existing restorations are charted is/are:
   a. anatomic chart.
   b. geometric chart.
   c. numeric coding system chart.
   d. all of the above.
3. Identify the type(s) of chart(s) that utilize(s) tooth diagrams.
   a. Anatomic
   b. Geometric
   c. Numeric coding system
   d. Periodontal

True or False

Directions: Select the letter of the choice that *best* answers the question.

1. Documenting existing conditions on an anatomic chart requires less time than using the geometric chart. T or F
2. Documenting existing restorations on an anatomic chart requires the examiner to use a coding system. T or F
3. When compared to the other types of dental charts, the geometric chart provides the most accurate description of the restoration. T or F
4. When using an anatomic chart it is necessary to replicate the exact design of the restoration. T or F
5. The numeric coding system chart uses a series of diagrams to describe a restoration. T or F

6. The geometric chart shows the anatomic crown structure as two circles. T or F
7. The numeric coding system chart always requires entering the date the procedure was performed. T or F

Answers

1. **d,** 2. **d,** 3. **a, d** 1. **F,** 2. **F,** 3. **F,** 4. **T,** 5. **F,** 6. **T,** 7. **T**

References

Anderson, P. C. & Burkard, M. R. (1995). *The dental assistant* (6th ed.). Albany: Delmar Publishers Inc.

Darby, M. L. & Walsh, M. M. (1995). *Dental hygiene theory and practice*. Philadelphia: W. B. Saunders Company.

Wilkins, E. M. (1994). *Clinical practice of the dental hygienist* (7th ed.). Baltimore: Williams and Wilkins.

Woodall, I. R. (1993). *Comprehensive dental hygiene care* (4th ed.). St. Louis: Mosby-Year Book Inc.

CHAPTER 4

Principles of Dental Charting

Key Terms

Anatomic Landmarks
Bitewing Radiograph
Dental Radiology
Extraoral Radiograph
Generalized Principles
Intraoral Radiograph
Missing
Non-restored
Panoramic Radiograph
Partially Erupted
Periapical Radiograph
Primary Code
Radiograph
Radiolucent
Radiopaque
Restored
Secondary Code
Specialized Principles
Unerupted
Virgin

To accurately describe dental restorations, it is first necessary to understand the principles of dental charting. Dental charting principles consist of two categories: generalized and specialized. **Generalized principles** of dental charting are the basic guidelines for dental charting procedures that refer to all types of dental charts. **Specialized principles** of dental charting are specific procedures that apply to individual dental charting formats, anatomic, geometric, and numeric coding systems.

Genralized Principles of Dental Charting

A **primary code** is an abbreviation for the anatomic surfaces of the teeth or existing conditions. One or more codes must always be assigned for each tooth.

- Primary code abbreviations for the anatomic surfaces of the teeth (CAPMI4, AFIP, and WinID©):
  - Mesial = M
  - Occlusal = O (Teeth #1–#5, #12–#16, #17–#21, #28–#32)
  - Incisal = I (Teeth #6–#11, #22–#27)
  - Distal = D
  - Buccal = B (Teeth #1–#5, #12–#16, #17–#21, #28–#32)
  - Facial = F (Teeth #6–#11, #22–#27) (CAPM14, F= teeth, #1–#32)
  - Lingual = L

- Primary code abbreviation for existing conditions (CAPMI4, AFIP, and WinID©):
  - Crown = C
  - Unerupted = U
  - Virgin (non-restored tooth) = V
  - Missing/Extracted = X
  - No Data = /

- Record all existing restorations in blue.
- Begin with the maxillary right permanent third molar (#1, 8⌋, or 18) through the maxillary left permanent third molar (#16, ⌊8, or 28); descend to the mandibular left permanent third molar (#17, ⌈8, or 38) through the mandibular right permanent third molar (#32, 8⌉, or 48). For the primary dentition, proceed through the four quadrants sequentially beginning with the maxillary right second primary molar and ending with the mandibular right second primary molar.
- When read, the tooth number or letter should be voiced first followed by the existing condition.
- A tooth that is present but not restored and unaffected by clinical pathology is considered a **non-restored** tooth indicated as a **Virgin** "V." Assign Virgin "V" when there is either a question regarding a characteristic or there is not any information available for an individual tooth from the antemortem dental records received for missing persons.
- No Data "/" code is utilized primarily in the CAPMI4 system for dental records received on unidentified persons. Assign No Data "/" for jaw fragment missing, nonrecognizable, fractured crown, traumatic avulsion, and when information is unknown for missing teeth postmortem.
- A tooth that is present and **restored**; the existing restoration is identified first by the anatomic location and followed by the restorative material (#2 DO-S).

- Anatomic location is abbreviated and read and written according to the following guidelines:
  - Mesial "M" is always first if present (MI, MO, or MD).
  - Occlusal "O" applies to the chewing surfaces of posterior teeth, and Incisal "I" applies to Incisal edges of the anterior teeth. These are first only when Mesial or Distal are not involved (OB, IF, OL, or IL,) and will only be second if Mesial and Distal are involved (MO, DO, MI, DI, MOD, MID, DIB, or DOB).
  - Distal "D" is first to all tooth surfaces when Mesial is not present (DO, DI, or DB), in third position when Mesial is present (MOD), and second if just Mesial is present (MD).
  - Facial "F" applies to the exterior surfaces of both anterior and posterior teeth and Buccal "B" applies only to the surfaces of posterior teeth. To be as specific as possible, Facial should only be used to describe the anterior surfaces of teeth #6 through #11 and #22 through #27 unless using the CAPMI4 computerized system, then "F" is designated for all anterior tooth surfaces. Facial or Buccal when read and written is first when it stands alone (F or B) and always follows Mesial, Occlusal or Incisal, and Distal (MODB, MIDF, MIF, or MOB), and is always prior to Lingual (BL).
  - Lingual "L" applies to all surfaces facing the tongue, and is always read and written last (ML, MODBL, MOL, and MIL) when referring to tooth surfaces.
- Existing restorations are abbreviated and read and written according to the following guidelines:
  - Crown "C" is always read and written first when referring to all full cast Gold and Non-precious alloys.
  - Missing/Extracted "X" and Unerupted "U" teeth are the existing conditions that are always charted first.

A **secondary code** is an abbreviation for existing conditions. Zero or more codes are assigned to each tooth. The primary code precedes the secondary code and is separated from the secondary code with a hyphen (-).

- Secondary code abbreviation for existing conditions are charted in blue (CAPMI4, AFIP, and WinID©).
  - Anomaly = A
  - Deciduous = B
  - Carious = C (use Z for the computerized system CAPMI4)
  - Resin = E
  - Gold = G

- Porcelain = H
- Missing Postmortem = J
- Non-precious =N
- Pontic = P
- Pontic Implant = Pi (use P for the computerized system CAPMI4)
- Retention Post/Pin = •p
- Three-Quarter = Q (a type of Crown that does not involve the Facial, Labial, or Buccal tooth surface)
- Root Canal = R
- Silver Amalgam = S
- Denture = T
- Temporary Restoration = Z

• The primary code is always separated from the secondary code with a hyphen (-). A Silver Amalgam restoration involving the Mesial and Occlusal tooth surfaces is written as MO-S.
• Two separate restorations or conditions are written with the symbol (•) separating the two restorations. DO-S • B-S and are spoken as Disto-Occlusal Silver Amalgam "and also" a Buccal Silver Amalgam.
• The symbol (•) will precede the secondary code "p" to reference a Retention Post/Pin.
• Deciduous dentition is always charted on the designated charting area for Deciduous teeth on the anatomic and geometric charts.
• Mixed dentition is always charted on the designated charting area for permanent teeth on the anatomic and geometric charts.
• Primary and secondary code abbreviations for abnormal conditions are charted in red.
  - Carious (Clinical and Radiographic) = C
  - Carious Watch (Incipient)= C^W
  - Carious Recurrent = C^R
  - Food Impaction = ↑ and ↓
  - Fracture (for Crown and Root) = FX
  - Overhanging Margin = ▲
  - Open Margin = △
  - Deficient Margin = ∧
  - Fistula = Ⓐ
  - Periapical Radiolucency = Ⓐ
  - Root Tip = RT
  - Supernumerary = ◇SU◇

Automated Dental Charting Systems

In addition to manual charting methods, an automated form of charting exists using a personal computer. Computerized systems can be practice management programs that integrate dental office tasks such as appointments, medical histories, reports, and general office management, to increase efficiency. Some programs utilize voice activation and are voice-operated or mouse-controlled systems to aid in the prevention of cross-contamination. Yet another system, the intraoral photographic imaging system, uses a fiber-optic camera. When the wand is placed into the oral cavity, the existing dental conditions and abnormalities are projected onto a monitor for the patient and dentist to view. The recorded image can also be printed out as a photograph.

In an effort to determine the characteristics of computer-based dental management systems and propose guidelines for standards of development, the American Dental Association convened a volunteer committee called the ASC MD 156 Working Group I. This working group formulated the Proposed ANSI/ADA Technical Report No. 1004 *Computer Software Performance for Dental Practice Software*. According to the American Dental Association's working group, dental practice software is classified into the following two areas:

- Management systems:
  - Resource management
  - Schedule management
  - Financial management
- Clinical systems:
  - Acquisition of computerized patient information
  - Communication of computerized patient information
  - Presentation of computerized patient information
  - Storage of computerized patient information
  - Retrieval of computerized patient information

In addition, the Department of Dental Informatics of the American Dental Association has compiled the *Directory of Practice Management Software Vendors*.

Computer-Based Identification Programs

Two computerized systems are most commonly used for facilitating rapid identification of human remains. The Computer-Assisted Postmortem

Identification (CAPMI) system was developed by Dr. Lewis Lorton, Robert Weed, and the United States Army Institute of Dental Research (USAIDR) in 1982. This program has been modified, with the assistance of the Armed Forces Institute of Pathology (AFIP) and Robert Weed, to CAPMI Version 4.0 (CAPMI4). This system has proven to be the most effective program available and the most concise because of its long history of practical uses and success. The CAPMI4 system uses abbreviations for existing conditions called primary and secondary codes. The program is designed to compare ante- and postmortem dental records and also physical characteristics; the computer sorts through the data and provides a list of matches, possible matches, and mismatches.

The second computerized system utilized for rapid identification is WinID© developed in 1997 by Dr. James McGivney. The codes used for this program are an extension of the CAPMI4 codes. This program also sorts through the data and ranks possible matches.

The CAPMI4 and WinID© computerized systems' primary and secondary codes are used in this text to represent existing restorations and conditions.

The computer identification program referred to as CAV-ID (Computer-Aided Victim Identification) system was developed by the New York City and Philadelphia Medical Examiner offices. This DOS-based program is at the present being utilized by only a few jurisdictions and because of this has yet to prove its validity.

Computerized Program for Missing and Unidentified Persons

In 1975 the FBI established the National Crime Information Center (NCIC) Missing Person File and in 1983 instituted the Unidentified Person File. In 1984 the Washington State Patrol Missing/Unidentified Persons Unit (WSP M/UPU) was created by the Washington State legislature. Legislative action made it mandatory for investigating agencies to submit dental information on all missing and unidentified persons who have been missing for more than thirty days to the M/UPU.

In 1990 in Washington State, the M/UPU used the NCIC and Washington Crime Information System (WACIC) with the CAPMI program as a comparison system to search its missing and unidentified persons databases to aid in the identification process. The Washington State Patrol enters all dental records in NCIC and CAPMI4.

Because of the present difficulties with the NCIC system, a task force has been assembled to reevaluate and modify the existing program. The current project is identified as the NCIC 2000 system.

Specialized Principles of Dental Charting

Three types of dental charting forms are most commonly used for manual charting (described in Chapter 3) and each form requires its own unique procedure for charting existing and abnormal conditions.

Dental Charting Procedures for the Anatomic Dental Chart

Existing restorations are read and written according to the following guidelines and shown in Figure 4–1:

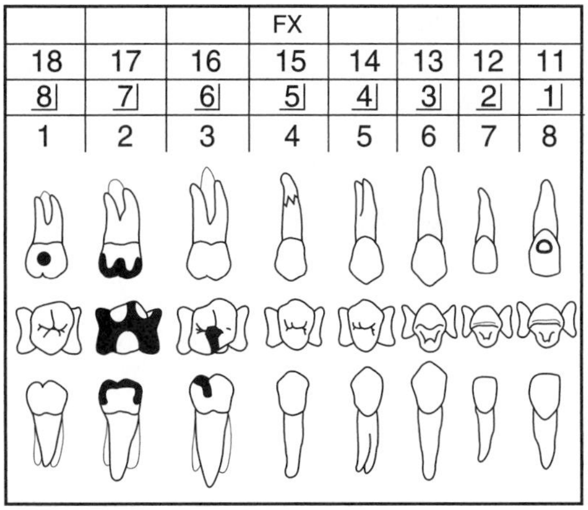

			FX				
18	17	16	15	14	13	12	11
8		7		6		5		4		3		2		1	
1	2	3	4	5	6	7	8

Figure 4–1 Anatomic examination chart showing anatomic symbols and drawings on teeth #1, #2, #3, #4, and #8

- Single-surface restorations are drawn on only one view. For example, a B-S (Buccal Silver Amalgam) is drawn on tooth #1 and a F-E (Facial Resin) is drawn on tooth #8.
- All two-, three-, four-, and five-surface restorations are charted on all three views with the exception of OB or OL. Tooth #2 shows a MODB-S (Mesio-Occluso-Disto-Buccal Silver Amalgam) and tooth #3 shows an OL-S (Occluso-Lingual Silver Amalgam).
- Only particular dental charting diagrams require an explanation that must be recorded in the designated box located above or below the tooth numbers or letters on the dental chart. This explanation is expressed as an

abbreviation or code. The abbreviations and codes for existing restorations are recorded in blue and abnormal conditions in red. For example, a tooth with a Root Fracture requires the code "FX" to be written in the box in red in addition to drawing the Fracture line in on the Facial view. Tooth #4 is shown with a Root Fracture.

- When charting on an anatomic chart it is important to replicate the restoration exactly as it appears.

Dental Charting Procedures for the Geometric Dental Chart

Existing restorations are read and written according to the following guidelines and shown in Figure 4–2:

- Include the entire outline of the designated tooth surface(s) and outline or fill the whole area in. Do not replicate the filling as it appears on the tooth. Tooth #1 is shown with a Silver Amalgam filling involving the Buccal pit (B-S), and tooth #8 has a Facial Resin (F-E).
- Particular dental charting diagrams that require an explanation are recorded in the designated box located above or below the tooth numbers or letters on the dental chart and include the graphic description. For example, tooth #2 has a Mesial Root Fracture indicated in red as "FX" and an irregular line drawn on the Mesial root.
- Figure 4–3 is an example of a geometric chart without stylized root anatomy and shows the three previously mentioned examples charted.

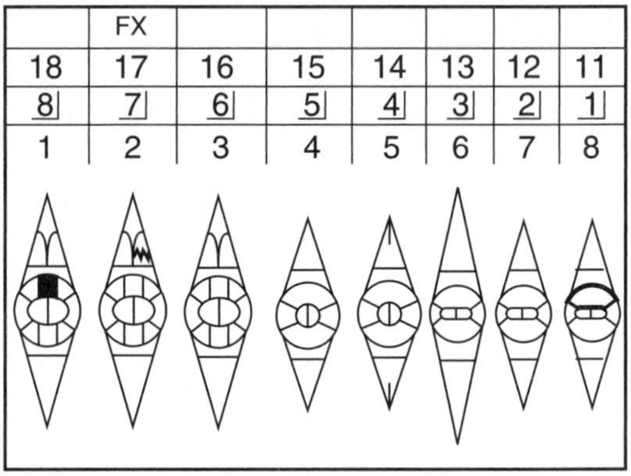

	FX						
18	17	16	15	14	13	12	11
8⌋	7⌋	6⌋	5⌋	4⌋	3⌋	2⌋	1⌋
1	2	3	4	5	6	7	8

Figure 4–2 Geometric examination chart with stylized root anatomy showing existing restorations and conditions charted on teeth #1, #2, and #8

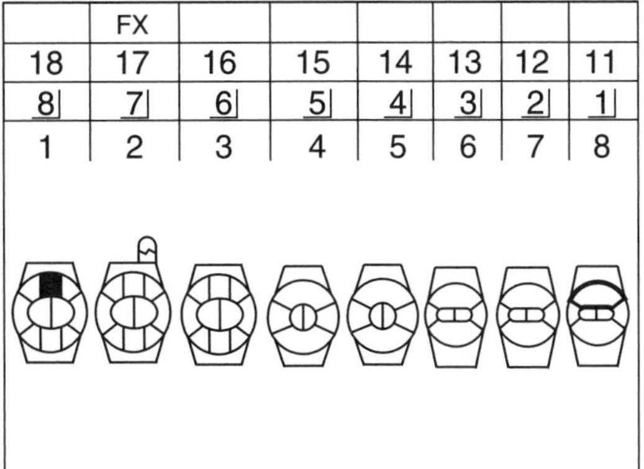

Figure 4–3 Geometric examination chart without stylized root anatomy showing existing restorations and conditions charted on teeth #1, #2, and #8

Dental Charting Procedures for the Numeric Coding System Dental Chart

Existing restorations are read and written according to the following guidelines and shown in Figure 4–4:

- The date is entered above or below each dental arch for each appointment. The date lines are in the same row of boxes as the teeth being recorded and treated.
- With each new appointment as conditions change, the new date and codes are entered in the next row of boxes above (indicating the maxillary teeth) and below (indicating the mandibular teeth).

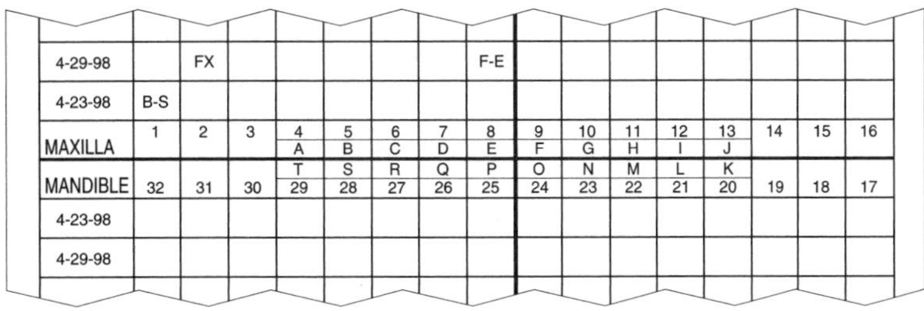

Figure 4–4 Numeric coding system chart with charting symbols entered into the boxes indicating teeth #1, #2, and #8

Dental Maxillofacial Imaging

The branch of dental science that deals with the study of radiant energy (x-rays) and radioactive materials is called **dental radiology**. Wilhelm Conrad Roentgen discovered x-rays in 1895, and in 1896 Dr. Otto Walkhoff, a dentist, made the first dental use of x-rays. The film on which dental images are produced due to exposure to x-rays is referred to as a **radiograph**.

Two terms that describe the location of film used inside or outside the mouth are **intraoral** and **extraoral radiograph.** Intraoral radiographs include: periapical, bitewing (interproximal), and occlusal. Extraoral radiographs include: lateral oblique projection (mandible), lateral skull projection, posteroanterior projection, posteroanterior projection of the sinuses (Waters'), transcranial projection, panoramic, and computerized digital radiology.

Intraoral Radiographic Survey

The full-mouth survey consists of periapical and bitewing radiograph films and is the intraoral radiographic procedure of choice most often utilized in conjunction with the clinical dental examination to aid oral diagnosis and treatment planning. Occlusal radiography is a supplementary intraoral procedure used to show the entire maxillary or mandibular arch each on a single film.

A complete full-mouth survey usually consists of fourteen to sixteen periapical and four bitewing radiographs. A **periapical radiograph** shows the crown, root, and apex of a tooth, including the surrounding supporting tissues. A **bitewing radiograph** shows the crowns of teeth of the opposing arches, the root portions near or above the junction of the cervical and middle thirds, and includes the surrounding supporting tissues (Figure 4–5).

Figure 4–6 shows a schematic diagram of a full-mouth survey, which consists of fourteen periapical radiographs and four bitewing radiographs.

Periapical Radiographic Imaging

Periapical radiograph films are used to detect diseases of the pulp, tooth, and periodontal supporting structures. The number of periapical films and

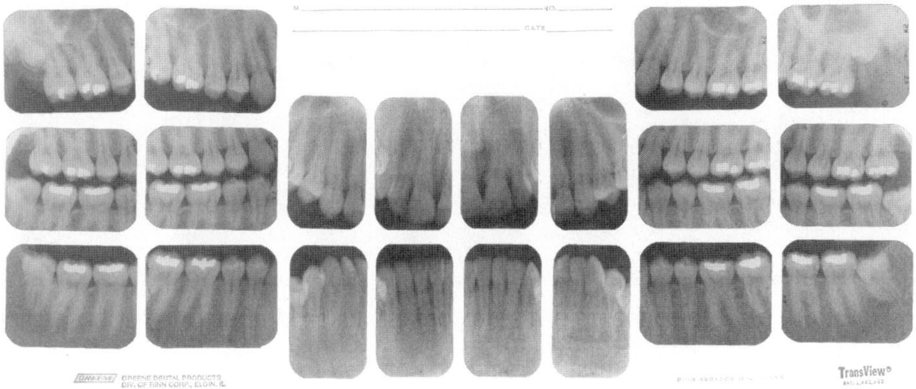

Figure 4–5 Full-mouth intraoral radiographic survey with sixteen periapical and four bitewing films (Reprinted courtesy of Eastman Kodak Company)

frequency varies between adult (complete dentition or edentulous) and pediatric patients. Figure 4–7 shows periapical radiograph films of an edentulous mouth. The number of films used is based on individual patient evaluation. A child between the ages of 6 to 9 years with a mixed dentition may require periapical films to assess tooth development and eruption.

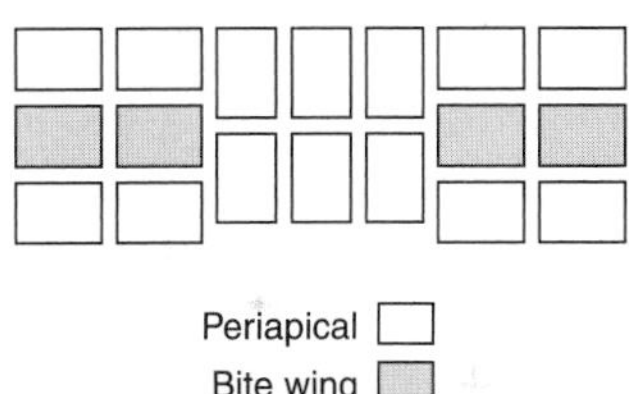

Figure 4–6 Schematic drawing of a full-mouth survey with fourteen periapical and four bitewing films

Bitewing Radiographic Imaging

Bitewing radiograph films can be placed in three different positions: horizontal, vertical, and reverse. When normal horizontal bitewing placement does not show the desired structures, vertical bitewings are utilized.

Vertical Bitewings

Vertical bitewings would be indicated for evaluating caries and bone loss and are used for anterior and posterior regions. The film is placed into the oral cavity with the long side of the film positioned vertically.

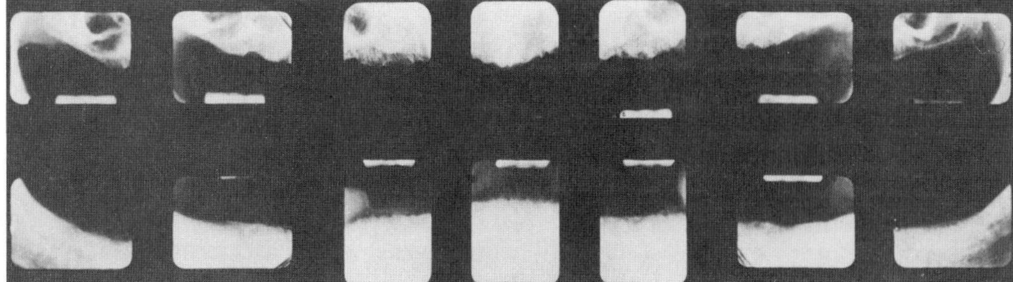

Figure 4–7 Full-mouth edentulous intraoral radiographic survey with fourteen periapical films (Reprinted courtesy of Eastman Kodak Company)

Reverse Bitewings

Reverse bitewings are indicated when children disrupt proper horizontal film placement with their tongue, which results in an unacceptable film. In this technique, the bitewing tab is attached to the film packet and the film is positioned horizontally into the buccal vestibule. The teeth are drawn together to hold the film in place. The central x-ray is directed from the opposite side of the mandible (lateral oblique projection) toward the teeth adjacent to the film. Due to the increased Focal-Film Distance (FFD) the exposure time must be increased by a factor of 4 or 5. A reverse bitewing radiograph will provide less detail than a bitewing radiograph placed in the normal horizontal position.

Adult and child patient bitewing radiograph films are taken depending on the individual patient evaluation and the clinician's preference. The Department of Health and Human Services recommends a child who is asymptomatic with closed posterior contacts have only two bitewing films taken and no radiographs should be taken if there are open posterior contacts.

Occlusal Radiographic Imaging

The occlusal film is used to expose larger areas of the dental arch. The film is placed on the occlusal surfaces of either the maxillary (Figure 4–8A and B) or mandibular teeth (Figure 4–8C). The occlusal radiograph provides the ability to view salivary ducts, impacted teeth, supernumerary teeth, bone fractures, and pathological lesions.

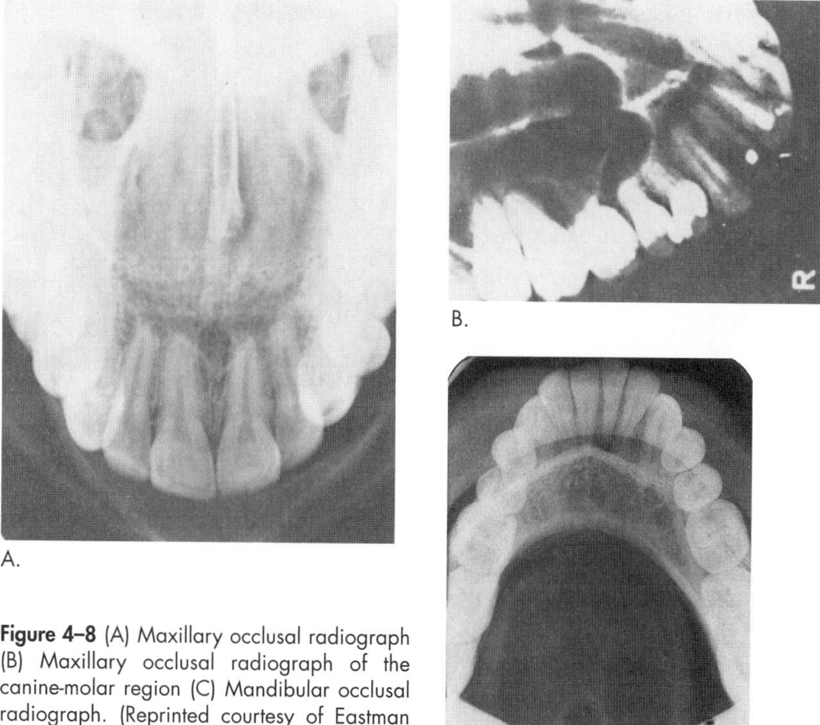

A.

B.

C.

Figure 4–8 (A) Maxillary occlusal radiograph (B) Maxillary occlusal radiograph of the canine-molar region (C) Mandibular occlusal radiograph. (Reprinted courtesy of Eastman Kodak Company)

Intraoral Film Sizes

There are five sizes of intraoral films and each film is named according to the type of radiographic technique utilized.

Periapical Film Sizes

There are four sizes of periapical films. No. 3 film is extra long, $2^{1}/_{8}$" × $1^{1}/_{16}$". No. 2 film is standard size, $1^{5}/_{8}$" × $1^{1}/_{4}$", and designed to be used in all regions of the adult mouth. No. 1 film is used for the anterior region of the adult mouth and it is $1^{5}/_{16}$" × $1^{5}/_{16}$". No. 0 film is used in all regions of a child's mouth and it is $^{7}/_{8}$" × $1^{1}/_{8}$" (Figure 4–9).

Bitewing Film Sizes

There are four sizes of bitewing film. No. 3 film is extra long, $2^1/_8$" × $1^1/_{16}$". No. 2 film is standard size, $1^5/_8$" × $1^1/_4$". No. 1 film is used for the anterior region of the adult mouth, $^{15}/_{16}$" × $1^5/_{16}$". No. 0 film is used in a child's mouth, $^7/_8$" × $1^1/_8$" (see Figure 4–9).

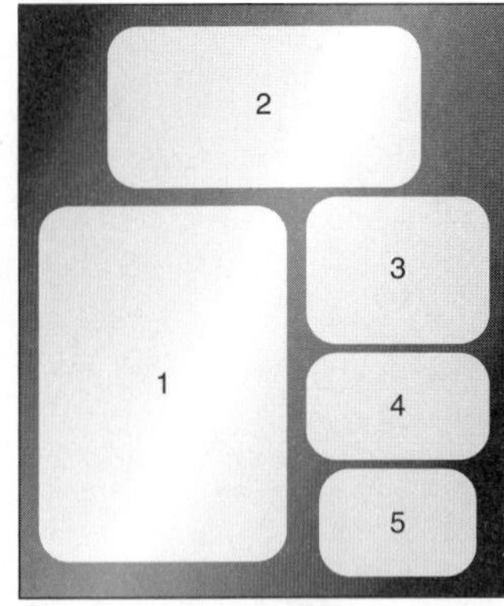

Figure 4–9 Intraoral dental film in varying sizes: (1) occlusal film (2) No. 3 film (3) No. 2 film (4) No. 1 film (5) No. 0 film

Occlusal Film

Occlusal film is a large piece of intraoral film, $2^1/_4$" × 3", that is placed on either the maxillary or mandibular teeth occlusal surfaces (see Figure 4–9).

Extraoral Radiographic Survey

To supplement information obtained from intraoral periapical, bitewing, and occlusal radiograph films, extraoral radiographs are beneficial in examination of areas of the maxilla, mandible, and orofacial complex that cannot be seen on intraoral radiographs. Extraoral radiographs consist of the following projections: lateral oblique, lateral skull, which also includes the posteroanterior and posteroanterior sinus view, and transcranial. Additional forms of maxillofacial imaging included are panoramic radiograph, computerized digital radiology, computerized tomography, and magnetic resonance imaging.

Lateral Oblique Radiographic Imaging

The lateral oblique projection is valuable for assessing anatomic structures that are distal to the canine and include the posterior body, angle, coronoid process, and condyle of the mandible (Figure 4–10). The use of either a 5 × 7 or an 8 × 10-inch cassette is supported by a holding device on the side of the patient's mandible that is to be radiographed.

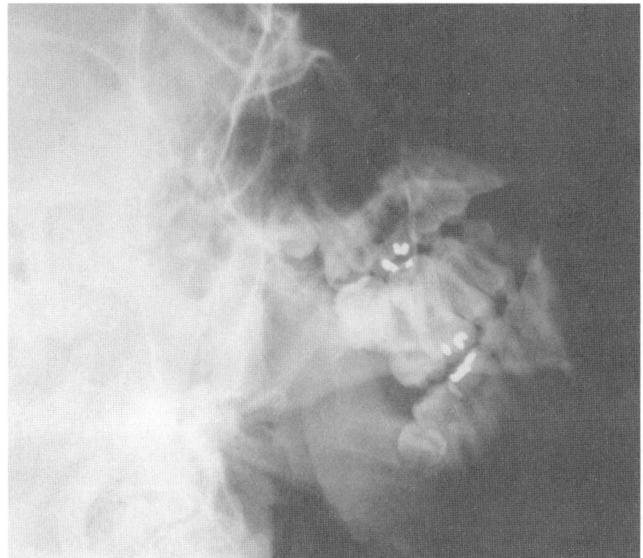

Figure 4–10 Lateral oblique projection

Lateral Skull Radiographic Imaging

The lateral skull projection superimposes the right and left sides of the skull on each other and provides a view of the entire cranium. This projection is used to detect pathologic conditions and fractures (Figure 4–11A).

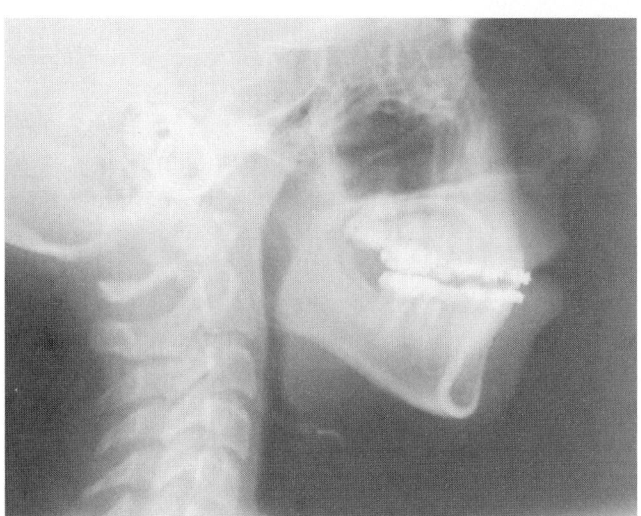

Figure 4–11 (A) Lateral skull projection showing the anatomic landmarks (Courtesy Donald L. Storm, DDS, MS)

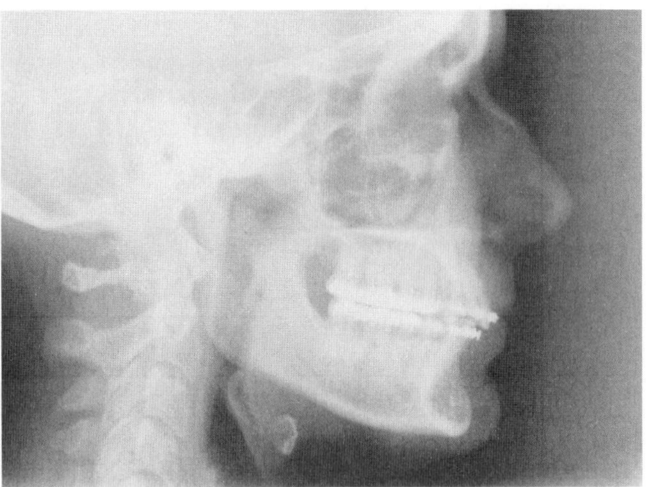

Figure 4–11 (B) Lateral skull projection showing the soft-tissue profile and anatomical landmarks (Courtesy Donald L. Storm, DDS, MS)

In orthodontics, the lateral skull projection is utilized for cephalometric analysis to measure and determine facial relationships and developmental patterns. The radiograph shows the anatomic structures and soft-tissue profile (Figure 4–11B). This radiograph is used for cephalometric tracings, which determine angular and dimensional relationships from the base of the cranium to the facial structures and to compare the initial and final phases of treatment. To obtain lateral skull radiographs that can be compared, a device called a cephalostat is used to position and secure the patient's head adjacent to an 8 × 10-inch cassette in a predetermined relationship of the central x-ray beam to the Frankfort horizontal plane.

Posteroanterior Skull Radiographic Imaging

The posteroanterior projection is used to identify fractures and pathologic conditions of the cranium. The patient is positioned with the nose and forehead placed against an 8 × 10-inch cassette and the central x-ray beam is directed above the base of the cranium, through the external occipital protuberance (Figure 4–12).

The posteroanterior projection radiograph does not provide an adequate view of the maxillary sinuses. The Waters' projection is a modification of the posteroanterior projection and produces a radiograph that clearly defines the sinus and middle region of the face. In this projection, the patient's head is repositioned so that the chin and nose are placed against the cassette and the mouth is kept open. The direction of the central ray remains unchanged.

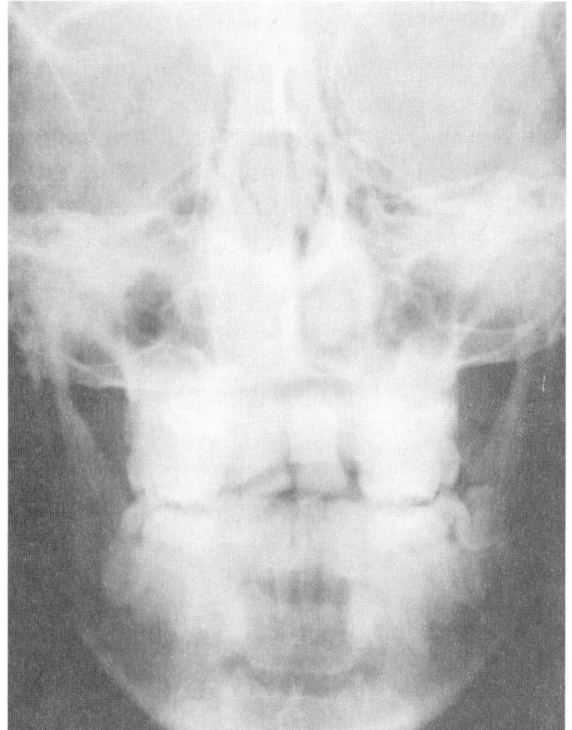

Figure 4–12 Posteroanterior projection

Transcranial Radiographic Imaging

The transcranial projection is used to detect and evaluate conditions associated with the temporomandibular joint (TMJ). The use of an 8 × 10-inch cassette allows for two exposures each to be taken of both the right and left temporomandibular joints while in the open and closed positions on a single film (Figure 4–13).

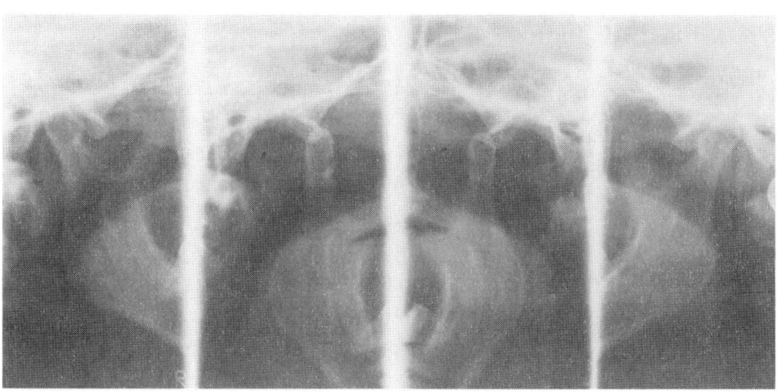

Figure 4–13 Transcranial projection of the temporomandibular joint (Courtesy Damian O. Fennig, DDS)

Panoramic Radiographic Imaging

Panoramic radiographic imaging produces a **panoramic radiograph** (also referred to as pantomograph) that shows the maxillary and mandibular arches and their supporting structures (Figure 4–14). Figure 4–15 shows a schematic drawing of a panoramic radiograph illustrating the specific anatomic landmarks.

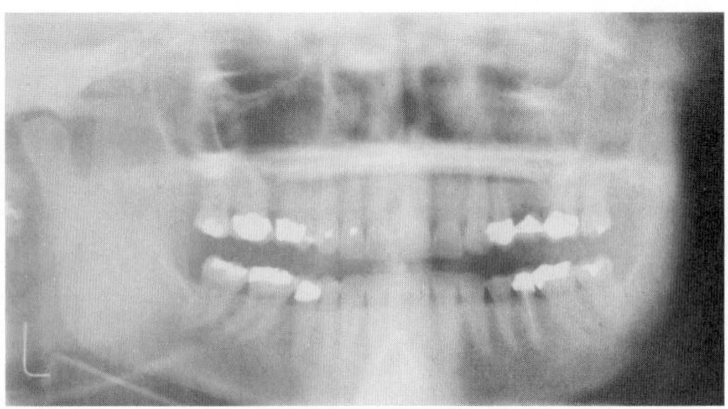

Figure 4–14 Panoramic radiograph

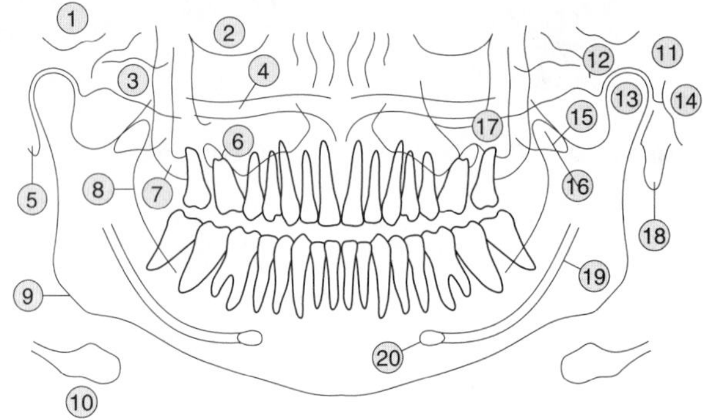

Figure 4–15 Schematic diagram of a panoramic radiograph showing numbered anatomic landmarks (Courtesy Dentsply-Gendex, Des Plaines, IL)

1. Middle cranial fossa
2. Orbit
3. Zygomatic arch
4. Palate
5. Styloid process
6. Septa in maxillary sinus
7. Maxillary tuberosity
8. External oblique line
9. Angle of mandible
10. Hyoid bone
11. Glenoid fossa
12. Articular eminence
13. Mandibular condyle
14. Temporal bone
15. Coronoid process
16. Pterygoid plates
17. Maxillary sinus
18. Ear lobe
19. Mandibular canal
20. Mental foramen

Computerized Digital Radiographic Imaging

Digital imaging uses a computer with a photo-stimulated phosphor imaging plate that is placed into the patient's mouth. The image is captured by the imaging plate then scanned by the DenOptix laser scanner. It is then stored in the computer and displayed onto the monitor and the information can either be stored or printed out on hard copy. The advantages of digital imaging over using conventional intraoral film are decreased exposure to radiation, the image is produced faster, and the size and contrast can be modified (Figure 4–16).

Computerized Tomography (CT) and Magnetic Resonance Imaging (MRI)

Computerized tomography (CT) involves the use of x-rays and unlike ordinary radiographic techniques, it can produce a three-dimensional image and show differences in soft-tissue densities (Figure 4–17).

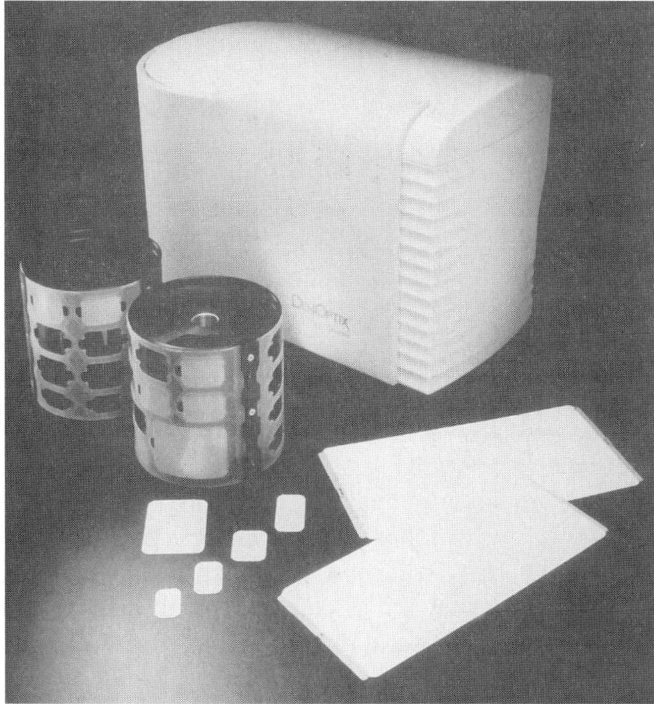

Figure 4–16 Intraoral digital imaging computer system (Courtesy Dentsply-Gendex, Des Plaines, IL)

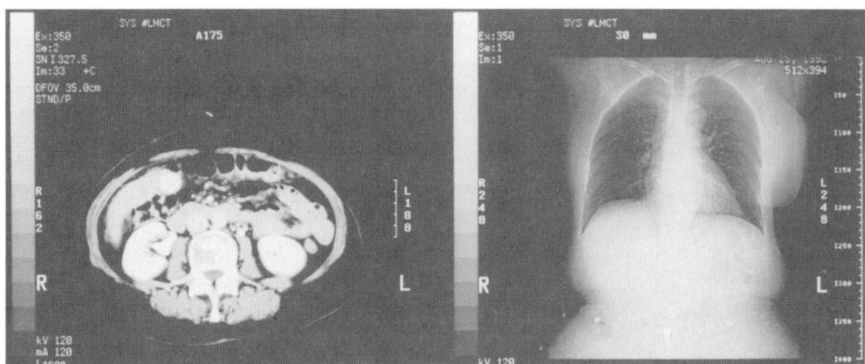

Figure 4–17 CT scan of the chest

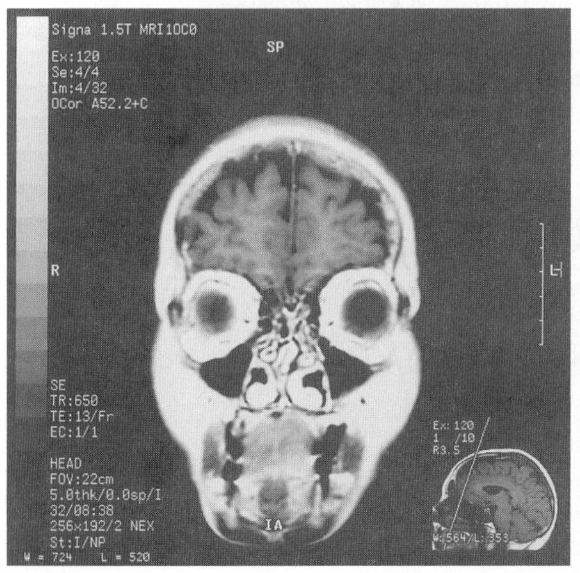

A.

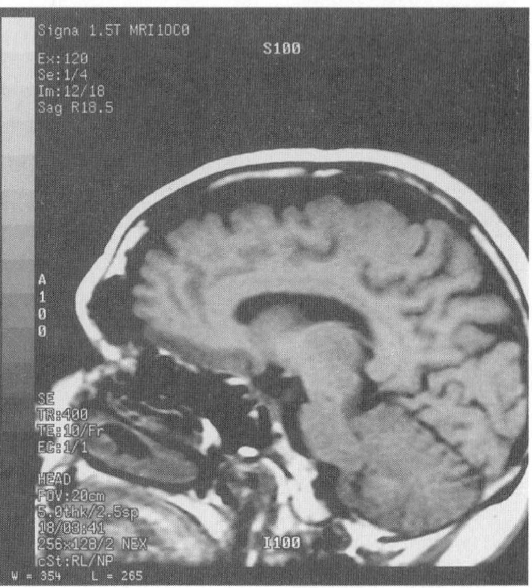

B.

Figure 4–18 MRI image of the human skull and brain: (A) Frontal view (B) Sagittal view

The procedure called magnetic resonance imaging (MRI) uses a magnetic field and radio waves to generate and amplify a signal, which is processed by a computer to create a sectional image. MRI is useful for visualizing and evaluating anatomical structures, soft tissue, and distinguishes between normal and diseased tissue (Figure 4–18A and B).

Film Position and Mounting of Intraoral Radiographs

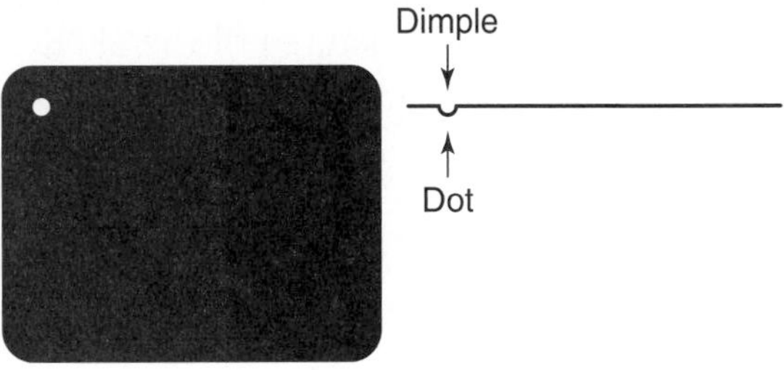

Figure 4–19 Schematic diagram of an intraoral radiograph indicating the raised dot and dimple

Intraoral radiographic film is manufactured with a raised dot (convex) and when the film is positioned in the mouth, the dot faces the tube head from which the central x-ray beam is directed (Figure 4–19). The raised dot is positioned near the incisal or occlusal surfaces. This is done so that when the film is viewed, the dot does not interfere with the evaluation of the anatomic structures on the radiograph. Radiographs can be mounted either with the raised dot facing out, which indicates the patient's right side is on the operator's left side, or with the raised dot facing in i.e., dimple (concave); the patient's right side would be on the operator's right side. The American Dental Association recommends mounting radiographs with the dot facing toward the operator.

Radiopaque and Radiolucent Structures

When viewing a radiograph of the teeth and supporting structures the densest tissues, such as enamel and bone, appear as white areas. Because the tissue is more dense, it allows less radiation to penetrate the structures and reach the film creating lighter areas referred to as **radiopaque**. In contrast, the dark areas are referred to as **radiolucent** because they are less dense structures that permit greater penetration and absorption of most of the x-ray beam. Because of the variation in densities of the oral structures and restorative materials, there will be graduations from white to black on the radiograph.

Anatomic Structures of the Skull

Knowledge of facial and cranial anatomy benefits dental personnel in positioning, exposing, mounting, and interpreting dental radiographs. The anatomical structures of the skull are identified by numbers in the legend included in Figure 4–20A, B, and C.

Radiographic Landmarks of the Maxillary Arch

The structures routinely seen on maxillary dental radiographs are referred to as **anatomic landmarks**. These structures vary in density and will appear radiopaque and radiolucent.

Radiographic Appearance of the Teeth and Supporting Structures

The radiopaque structures that make up the tooth are the enamel, dentin, and cementum. The area where the cementum meets the dentin is difficult to discern on the dental radiograph because the densities of the two tissues are somewhat similar. The internal structures of the tooth are the pulp chamber and canal and appear radiolucent as shown in Figure 4–21.

The supporting structures of the teeth appear radiopaque with the exception of the periodontal membrane, which appears radiolucent on a dental radiograph. The alveolar bone consists of cancellous and compact bone connective tissue (described in Chapter 1). The lamina dura consists of compact bone tissue that lines the tooth socket and provides attachment for the periodontal membrane. This area appears as a radiopaque line (see Figure 4–21).

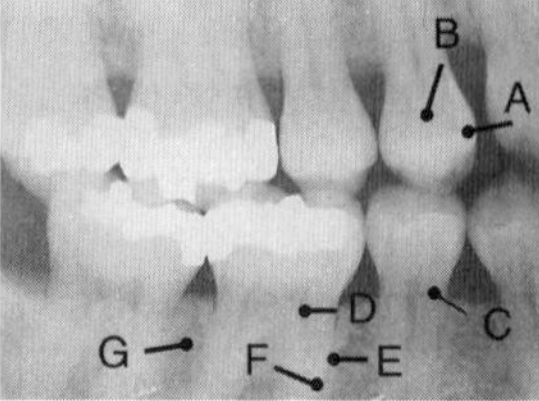

Figure 4–21 A radiograph of the teeth and the supporting structures: (A) Enamel (B) Dentin (C) Cementum (D) Pulp chamber and canal (E) Lamina dura (F) Periodontal membrane (G) Alveolar bone

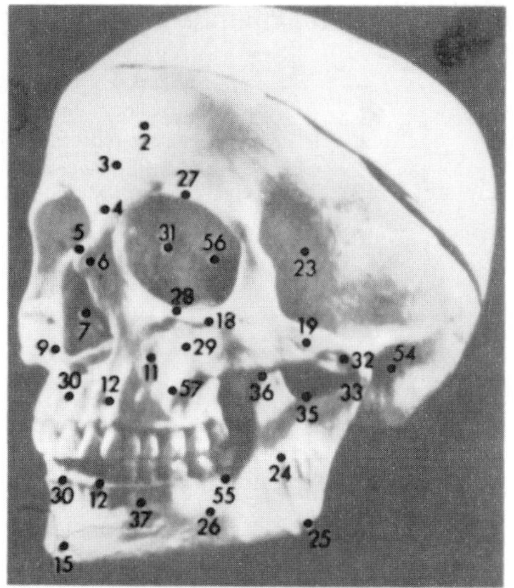

A. Facial Bones

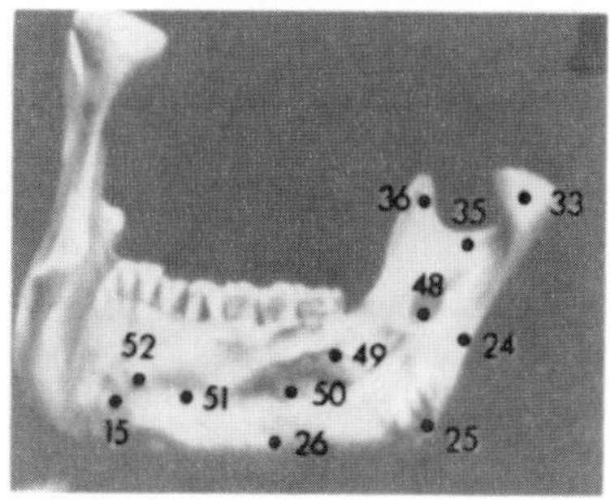

B. Medial Aspect of Mandible

LEGEND

1 Forehead
2 Frontal bone
3 Glabella
4 Frontonasal suture (nasion)
5 Bridge of nose
6 Nasal bone
7 Nasal cavity
8 Nostrils
9 Anterior nasal spine
10 Ala of nose
11 Canine fossa
12 Alveolar ridges
13 Labial commissure
14 Chin
15 Symphysis menti
16 Inner canthus of eye
17 Outer canthus of eye
18 Cheekbone (zygomatic bone)
19 Zygomatic arch
20 Temporomandibular articulation
21 Tragus
22 Auricle
23 A. Temple
B. Temporal fossa
24 Ramus of mandible
25 Angle of mandible
26 Body of mandible
27 Supraorbital ridge
28 Infraorbital ridge
29 Zygomatic process of maxilla
30 Alveolar process
31 Orbit
32 Articular eminence
33 Mandibular condyle
34 Glenoid fossa
35 Mandibular notch
36 Coronoid process
37 Mental foramen
38 Median palatine suture
39 Palatine bone
40 Transverse palatine suture
41 Greater palatine foramen
42 Incisive foramen
43 Nasal septum
44 Posterior nasal spine
45 Vomer
46 Lateral pterygoid plate
47 Medial pterygoid plate
48 Mandibular foramen and lingula
49 Mylohyoid ridge
50 Submaxillary depression
51 Sublingual depression
52 Genial tubercles
53 Styloid process
54 External auditory meatus
55 External oblique ridge
56 Optic foramen
57 Maxilla

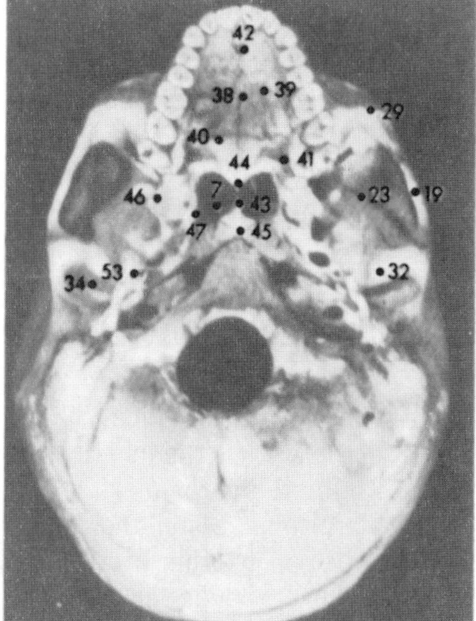

C. Hard Palate and Adjoining Structures.

Figure 4–20 Anatomic structures of the skull: (A) Human skull (B) Medial aspect of the mandible (C) Inferior aspect of the skull

Landmarks of the Maxillary Central and Lateral Incisor Region

The radiolucent area located near the apices of the central incisors is referred to as the incisive foramen. The radiopaque area located superior to the foramen is the median palatine suture, which divides the palatine process of the maxilla (hard palate) into right and left halves. The area superior to this process, which appears radiopaque, is the nasal septum and the bilateral radiolucent areas adjacent to this area are the nasal fossa (Figure 4–22).

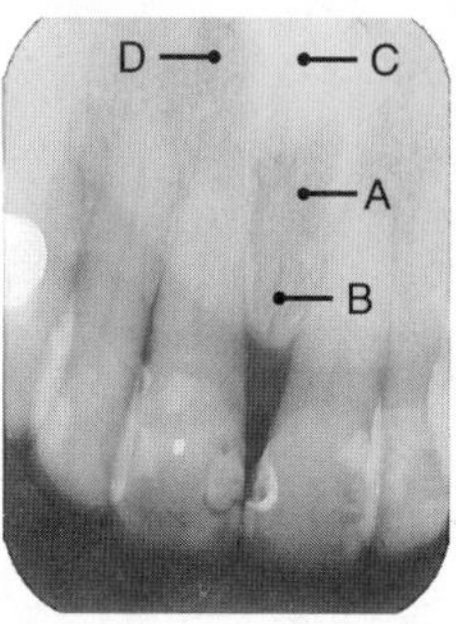

Figure 4–22 Radiograph of the maxillary central and lateral incisor region: (A) Incisive foramen (B) Median palatine suture (C) Nasal septum (D) Nasal fossa

Landmarks of the Maxillary Canine Region

The appearance of two radiopaque lines that form an inverted "Y" are produced by the inferior border of the nasal fossa and the medial and inferior borders of the maxillary sinus (Figure 4–23).

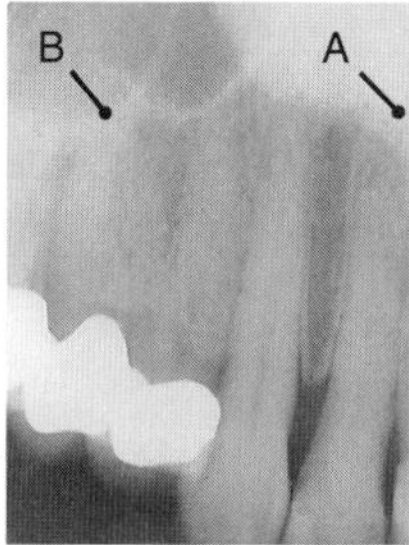

Figure 4–23 Radiograph of the maxillary canine region: (A) Nasal fossa (B) Maxillary sinus

Landmarks of the Maxillary Premolar Region

The radiopaque line superior to the apices of the teeth is the inferior border of the maxillary sinus. Distal and superior to the first molar is a radiopaque area that is referred to as the zygomatic process of the maxilla (Figure 4–24).

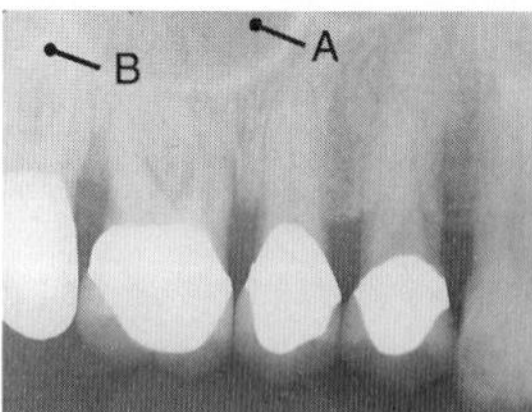

Figure 4–24 Radiograph of the maxillary premolar region: (A) Maxillary sinus (B) Zygomatic process of the maxilla

Landmarks of the Maxillary Molar Region

The radiopaque line that extends posteriorly and distal to the third molar is the inferior border of the maxillary sinus. The "U" shaped radiopaque area that is located superior to the apices of the first and second molar teeth is referred to as the zygomatic bone.

Located distal to the third molar is the alveolar process, which has an extended ridge of bone referred to as the maxillary tuberosity. Another radiopaque image that appears distal to the tuberosity is the process of the medial pterygoid plate referred to as the hamular process. A large radiopaque image located inferior to the third molar occlusal plane and the maxillary tuberosity is the coronoid process of the mandible. The coronoid process is visible on a periapical radiograph that is taken of the molar area when the mouth is opened. Otherwise, radiographs taken with the mouth in the closed position would show the ramus of the mandible instead (Figure 4–25).

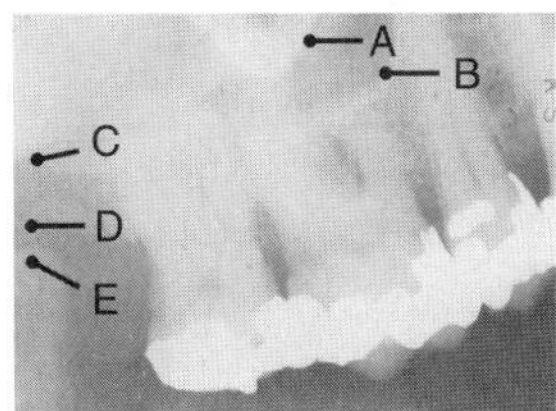

Figure 4–25 Radiograph of the maxillary molar region: (A) Zygomatic bone (B) Maxillary sinus (C) Maxillary tuberosity (D) Hamular process (E) Coronoid process

Radiographic Landmarks of the Mandibular Arch

The teeth and supporting structures of the mandible have the same radiographic characteristics as those of the maxilla. The landmarks of the mandibular arch are slightly more difficult to detect than those of the maxillary arch.

Landmarks of the Mandibular Central and Lateral Incisor Region

The radiopaque image shown on a mandibular central and lateral incisor radiograph that is located inferior to the apices of the central incisors and superior to the inferior border of the mandible is referred to as the genial tubercles. These structures are small bony eminences projecting from the bone, which serve as attachment sites of tendons. Located in the center of the tubercles is a small radiolucent area referred to as the lingual foramen.

The radiopaque area adjacent to the symphysis of the mandible and inferior to the central and lateral incisors is a ridge of bone referred to as the mental ridge. The ridge of bone that begins posterior and inferior to the mental ridge and extends posteriorly to the molar region is a radiopaque area called the mylohyoid ridge (Figure 4–26).

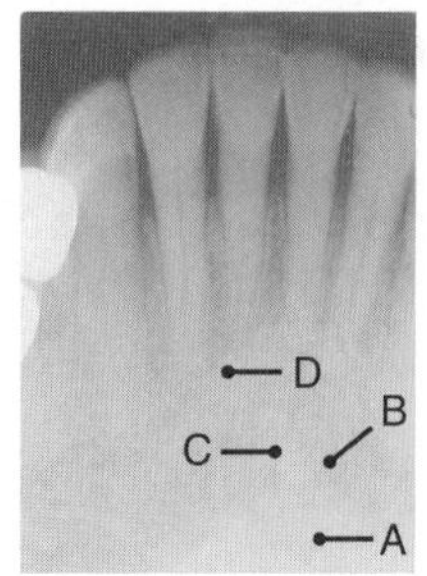

Figure 4–26 Radiograph of the mandibular central and later incisor region: (A) Inferior border of the mandible (B) Genial tubercles (C) Lingual foramen. (D) Mental process

Landmarks of the Mandibular Canine Region

The landmarks that are present on the mandibular canine radiograph that appear radiopaque are the inferior border of the mandible, internal oblique ridge, and the posterior region of the mental ridge. The radiolucent area inferior to the internal oblique ridge is referred to as the submandibular fossa (Figure 4–27).

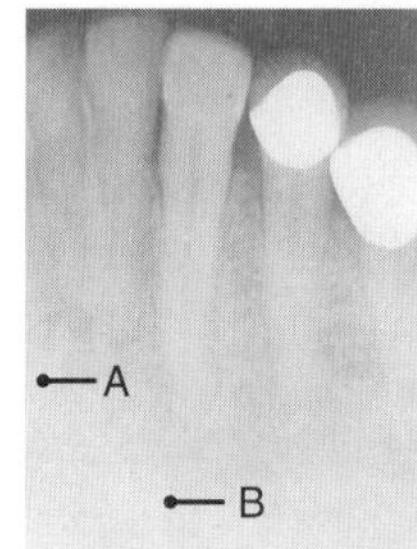

Figure 4–27 Radiograph of the mandibular canine region: (A) Mental ridge (B) Inferior border of the mandible

Landmarks of the Mandibular Premolar Region

The radiolucent area on the mandibular premolar radiograph that is located inferior to the apices of the first and second premolar teeth is the mental foramen. The radiolucent area that extends toward the foramen is the mandibular canal and is not always apparent on some radiographs (Figure 4–28).

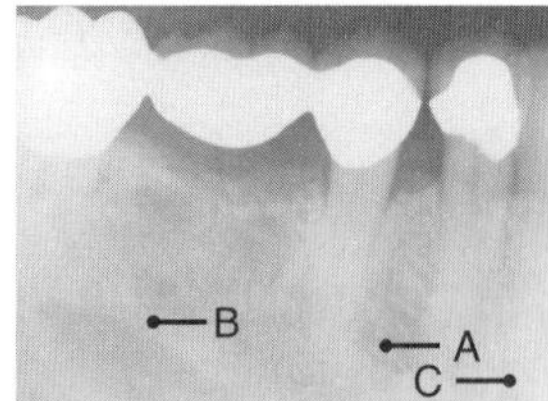

Figure 4–28 Radiograph of the mandibular premolar region: (A) Mental foramen (B) Mylohyoid ridge (internal oblique ridge) (C) Inferior border of the mandible

Landmarks of the Mandibular Molar Region

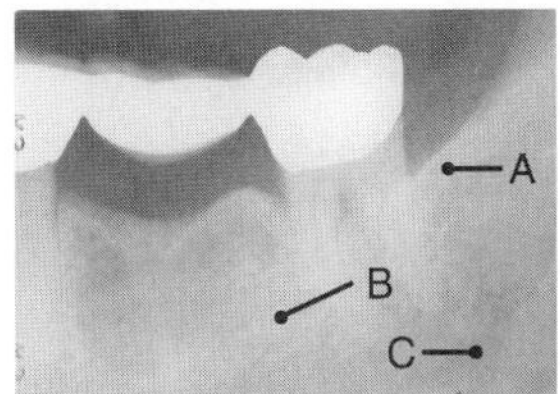

Figure 4–29 Radiograph of the mandibular molar region: (A) External oblique ridge (B) Mylohyoid ridge (internal oblique ridge) (C) Mandibular canal

The mandibular radiograph shows two radiopaque lines that extend from the ramus of the mandible. The external oblique ridge extends downward and past the first and second molar teeth. The mylohyoid or internal oblique ridge begins at the ramus on the medial aspect of the mandible and crosses over the middle and apical third regions of the root surfaces of the molar teeth and extends anteriorly toward the mandibular symphysis. The mandibular canal appears as a radiolucent line located inferior to this ridge. The large radiolucent area located superior to the border of the mandible is the submandibular fossa (Figure 4–29).

Missing, Unerupted, Partially Erupted, and Impacted Teeth

Clinical data alone cannot determine if a tooth is **Missing**, To Be Extracted, Impacted, or **Unerupted**. Evaluation of a radiographic survey and patient dental history in addition to clinical data can provide the necessary information to assess the situation. Missing teeth occur for the following reasons: a lack of tooth bud formation, failure to erupt due to space constraints, the tooth has yet to erupt, or it was extracted.

Charting Missing Teeth on an Anatomic Chart

Based on clinical observation, teeth #17 and #19 are not present in Figure 4–30; the mandibular molar periapical radiograph indicates these two teeth are Missing.

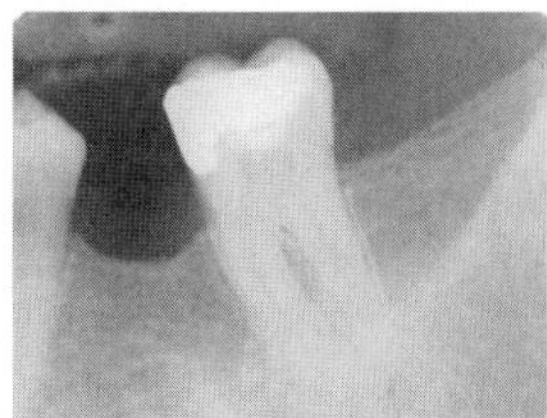

Universal System
#20 #18

Palmer System
|5 |7

ISO/FDI System
35 37

Figure 4–30 Mandibular left periapical radiograph shown with teeth #17 and #19 as Missing

Figure 4–31 represents an anatomic chart with teeth #17 and #19 charted as Missing. To chart Missing teeth on an anatomic chart, use a blue pencil and on the appropriate tooth number, draw a large "X" that extends over all three views.

In a mixed dentition, if the permanent tooth is Missing and the primary tooth is present, use a blue pencil and mark an "X" over the tooth notation number or letter that indicates the Missing permanent tooth. The reason for crossing out the tooth notation number instead of the tooth diagram is to allow the tooth diagram to be utilized to chart an existing restoration or abnormal condition on the remaining tooth.

Figure 4–31 Anatomic chart illustrating Missing, Unerupted, Partially Erupted, and Impacted teeth

U	U		U		U					-B(H)					
18	17	16	15	14	13	12	11	21	22	23	24	25	26	27	28
8	7	6	5	4	3	2	1	1	2	IMP	4	5	6	7	8
1	2	3	4	5	6	7	8	9	10	11	12	13	14	15	16

32	31	30	29	28	27	26	25	24	23	22	21	20	19	18	17
8	7	6	5	4	3	2	1	1	2	3	4	5	6	7	8
48	47	46	45	44	43	42	41	31	32	33	34	35	36	37	38
U	PE		U						-B(N)						

In the box below the tooth print a hyphen (-), which separates a primary code from a secondary code, followed by an uppercase letter "B"—the secondary code indicating a Deciduous tooth is present and erupted. After the letter "B" use parentheses and indicate which uppercase letter specifies the Deciduous tooth that is present. Figure 4–31 shows tooth #23 is Missing, tooth letter "N" is present and unrestored, and it is written as -B(N).

Charting Missing Teeth on a Geometric Chart

Figure 4–32 represents a geometric chart with teeth #17 and #19 charted as Missing. To chart on a geometric chart, use a blue pencil and draw a large "X" over the stylized diagram. Regardless of whether the diagram is shown with or without roots, always draw the "X" so that it covers the entire diagram.

Figure 4–32 represents a geometric chart shown with permanent tooth #23 as Missing with the retained Deciduous tooth "N" present and unrestored. Mixed dentitions with Missing permanent teeth and retained Deciduous teeth are charted on the geometric chart the same way as on an anatomic chart.

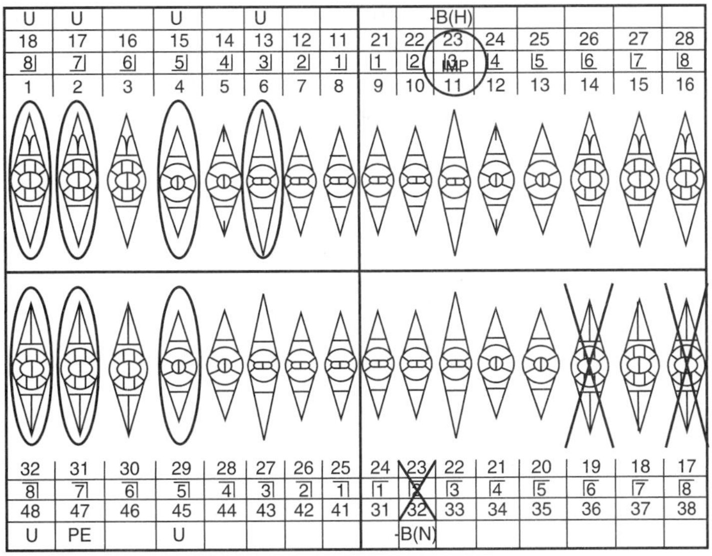

Figure 4–32 Geometric chart illustrating Missing, Unerupted, Partially Erupted, and Impacted teeth

Charting Missing Teeth on a Numeric Coding System Chart

To chart Missing teeth on a numeric coding system chart, use a black pen to enter the date in the appropriate column and with a blue pencil below teeth #17 and #19, mark the entire box with a large "X." In Figure 4–33 teeth #17 and #19 are indicated as Missing.

To chart a Missing permanent tooth with a retained Deciduous tooth on the numeric coding system chart, enter the date in black ink, and with a blue pencil cross out the tooth notation number indicating the Missing permanent tooth. Enter the secondary code for Deciduous "-B" and the tooth notation letter "N" in parentheses in the box (-B(N)). When read, this chart indicates that permanent tooth #23 is Missing and Deciduous tooth letter "N" is present and unrestored.

Charting Unerupted and Partially Erupted Teeth on an Anatomic Chart

Teeth that are not clinically apparent in the mouth and are not Impacted, but can be viewed on the dental radiograph and have enough space to erupt are referred to as Unerupted. Figure 4–34 is a panoramic radiograph that shows teeth #1, #2, #4, #6, #29, and #32 as Unerupted.

4-8-97											-B(H)					
3-4-97	(U)	(U)		(U)		(U)										
1-5-96																
MAXILLA	1	2	3	4 A	5 B	6 C	7 D	8 E	9 F	10 G	(IMP) ~~H~~	12 I	13 J	14	15	16
MANDIBLE	32	31	30	T 29	S 28	R 27	Q 26	P 25	O 24	N ~~23~~	M 22	L 21	K 20	19	18	17
1-5-96										-B(N)				X		X
3-4-97	(U)	(PE)		(U)												
4-8-97																

Figure 4–33 Numeric coding system chart illustrating Missing, Unerupted, Partially Erupted, and Impacted teeth

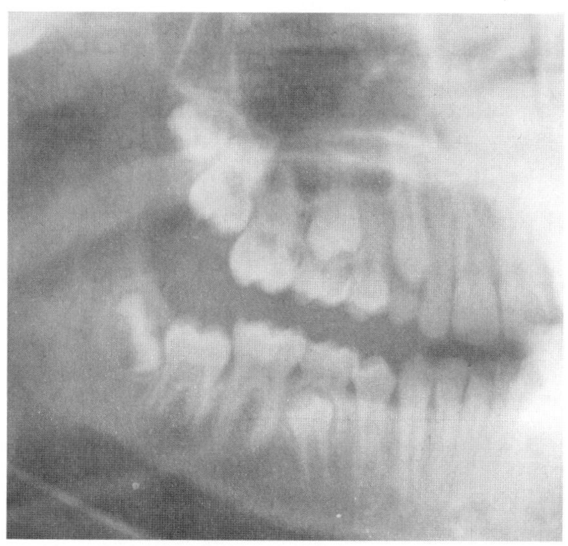

Universal System

			#4		#6		
#1	#2	#3	A	#5	C	#7	#8
#32	#31	#30	T	#28	#27	#26	#25
			#29				

Palmer System

			5⌋		3⌋		
8⌋	7⌋	6⌋	E⌋	4⌋	C⌋	2⌋	1⌋
8⌉	7⌉	6⌉	E⌉	4⌉	3⌉	2⌉	1⌉
			5⌉				

ISO/FDI System

			15		13		
18	17	16	55	14	53	12	11
48	47	46	85	44	43	42	41
			45				

Figure 4–34 Panoramic radiograph of maxillary and mandibular right side

To indicate a tooth is Unerupted on an anatomic dental chart, use a blue pencil to draw a circle around the tooth including all three views. In the box located above or below the tooth number or letter, place the primary code "U." This indicates the tooth is Unerupted. The anatomic chart in Figure 4–31 shows teeth #1, #2, #4, #6, #29, and #32 charted as Unerupted teeth.

When the clinical Crown of a tooth emerges into the oral cavity and has yet to establish alignment with the Occlusal plane, the tooth is referred to as **Partially Erupted**. Figure 4–34 shows tooth #31 as being Partially Erupted.

To chart a Partially Erupted tooth on an anatomic chart, use a blue pencil and draw a circle around all three views. In the box located above or below the tooth notation number or letter, print the uppercase letters "PE" (see Figure 4–31).

Charting Unerupted and Partially Erupted Teeth on a Geometric Chart

Figure 4–34 is a panoramic radiograph that shows teeth #1, #2, #4, #6, #29, and #32 as Unerupted. To chart Unerupted teeth on a geometric chart, draw a circle around the entire tooth diagram with a blue pencil. Print the primary code "U" in the box located above or below the designated tooth notation numbers or letters as shown in Figure 4–32.

As indicated in Figure 4–34, tooth #31 is Partially Erupted. To chart this condition on a geometric chart, use a blue pencil and draw a circle around the tooth diagram and label it with the uppercase letters "PE" (see Figure 4–32).

Charting Unerupted and Partially Erupted Teeth on a Numeric Coding System Chart

To indicate an Unerupted tooth on a numeric coding system chart, record the date in the designated area using black ink. In the box located above or below the designated tooth notation number or letter located on the same line as the date, draw a circle in blue pencil and label the inside with the primary code "U." Figure 4–34 is a panoramic radiograph that shows teeth #1, #2, #4, #6, #29, and #32 as Unerupted. These Unerupted teeth are shown charted on the numeric coding system chart (see Figure 4–33).

To indicate the presence of a Partially Erupted tooth on a numeric coding system chart, follow the same procedure indicated for charting an Unerupted tooth and label the designated circle with the letters "PE" instead of "U." Figure 4-33 shows tooth #31 is Partially Erupted.

Charting Impacted Teeth on an Anatomic, Geometric, and Numeric Coding System Charts

A tooth that remains embedded in the bone or soft tissue and is incapable of erupting is referred to as Impacted. Figure 4–35 is a periapical radiograph, which shows permanent tooth #11 is Impacted and Deciduous tooth letter "H" is present and clinically apparent.

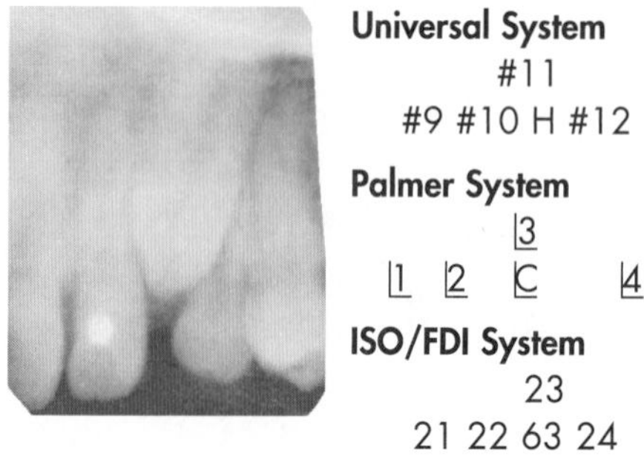

Figure 4–35 Maxillary left periapical radiograph

On an anatomic and geometric chart, to indicate tooth letter "H" is present and unrestored and tooth #11 is Impacted, use a blue pencil to draw a circle around the tooth notation number and within the circle enter the uppercase letters "IMP." In the box located above the tooth notation numbers, enter "-B(H)," which is read as Deciduous tooth "H" is present. Because the diagram below tooth letter "H" does not indicate the presence of any restorative work, the chart is also read as not restored (see Figures 4–31 and 4–32). Figure 4–33 shows the impacted permanent tooth #11 charted on the numeric coding system chart.

Review Questions

Multiple Choice

Directions: Select the letter of the choice that *best* answers the question.

1. An image that appears black on a dental radiograph is referred to as:
   a. translucent. b. radiopaque.
   c. transparent. d. radiolucent.
2. Which type of radiograph shows the soft tissue profile?
   a. Panoramic b. Lateral skull
   c. Lateral oblique d. Periapical
3. Which type of radiograph is used to detect pathology around a root tip?
   a. Panoramic b. Lateral skull
   c. Lateral oblique d. Periapical
4. Which type of radiograph is used to detect caries?
   a. Panoramic b. Lateral skull
   c. Lateral oblique d. Bitewing
5. Which type of radiograph uses an 8 × 10-inch cassette to detect TMJ problems?
   a. Panoramic b. Lateral skull
   c. Lateral oblique d. Transcranial
6. The anatomic landmark that appears as a radiopaque line above the root apices is referred to as the/a:
   a. coronoid process. b. maxillary sinus.
   c. hamulus. d. none of the above.

7. The anatomic landmark that appears as a radiolucent image between the maxillary central incisors is referred to as the:
   a. incisive process. b. incisive fossa.
   c. incisive foramen. d. incisive sinus.
8. The area distal to the maxillary third molar is called the:
   a. maxillary tuberosity. b. coronoid process.
   c. maxillary sinus. d. median palatine suture.
9. The "U" shaped radiopaque area is usually seen on the maxillary _________ radiograph.
   a. central and incisor b. canine
   c. premolar d. molar
10. The mental foramen is usually seen on the mandibular _________ radiograph.
   a. central and incisor b. canine
   c. premolar d. molar

Answers

1. **d,** 2. **b,** 3. **d,** 4. **d,** 5. **d,** 6. **b,** 7. **c,** 8. **a,** 9. **d,** 10. **c**

References

Adriaens, P. A., De Boever, J., & Vande Velde, F. (1982). Comparison of intraoral long-cone paralleling radiographic surveys and orthopantomographs with special reference to the bone height. *Journal of Oral Rehabilitation*, 9, 355–365.

Akesson, L., Rohlin, M., & Hakansson, J. (1989). Marginal bone in periodontal disease: An evaluation of image quality in panoramic and intra-oral radiography. *Dentomaxillofacial Radiology*, 72–76.

American Academy of Dental Radiology. (1983) Recommendations for quality assurance in dental radiography. *Oral Surgery*, 55, 421–426.

American Dental Association, Council on Dental Materials, Instruments, and Equipment. (January 1989). Recommendations in radiographic practices: An Update. *Journal of the American Dental Association*, 118, 115–117.

Bell, G. L. (1993). Testing of the National Crime Information Center Missing/Unidentified Persons computer comparison routine. *Journal of Forensic Sciences*, 38 (1), 13–22.

Benn, D. K. (1992). Frequent, low-dose, improved-contrast radiographic images with the use of narrow x-ray beams. *Oral Surgery, Oral Medicine, and Oral Pathology*, 74.

Fédération Dentaire Internationale, Commision on Dental Products. (1989). Recommendations on radiographic procedures. *International Dental Journal*, 39, 147–148.

Goren, A. D., Sciubba, J. J., Friedman, R., & Malamud, H. (1989). Survey of radiologic practices among dental practitioners. *Oral Surgery, Oral Medicine, and Oral Pathology*, 67.

Gornbein, J. A. (1990). Prediction of efficacy of bitewing radiographs for caries detection. *Oral Surgery, Oral Medicine, and Oral Pathology*, 69.

Hamada, M. O. (1989). Implantology: Radiographic resources. *Journal of the California Dental Association*, 17, 20-31.

Herzog, A. (1988). Dental radiography: A review for dental hygiene practitioners. *Journal of Dental Hygiene*, 62, 242–249.

Hintze, H., & Wenzel, A. (1990). Accuracy of clinical diagnosis for the detection of dentoalveolar anomalies with panoramic radiography as validating criterion. *Journal of Dentistry for Children*, 57.

Kantor, M. L., & Slome, B. A. (1989). Efficacy of panoramic radiography in dental diagnosis and treatment planning. *Journal of Dental Research*, 68.

Kidd, E. A. M., & Pitts, N. B. (1990). A reappraisal of the value of the bitewing radiograph in the diagnosis of posterior approximal caries. *British Dental Journal*, 169, 195–200.

Lew, K. K. K. (1992). The prediction of eruption-sequence from panoramic radiographs. *Journal of Dentistry for Children*, 59, 346–349.

Lorton, L., & Langley, W. H. (1984). Postmortem identification: A computer-assisted system. (Research report.) Washington, DC: U.S. Army Institute of Dental Research, Walter Reed Army Medical Center.

Lorton, L., & Langley, W. H. (1986). Decision-making concepts in postmortem identification. *Journal of Forensic Sciences*, 31 (1), 190–196.

Lorton, L., Rethman, M., & Friedman, R. (1988). The computer-assisted postmortem identification (CAPMI) system: A computer-based identification program. *Journal of Forensic Sciences*, JFSCA, 33 (4), 977–984.

Lorton, L., Rethman, M., & Friedman, R. (1989). The Computer-assisted postmortem identification (CAPMI) system: Sorting algorithm improvements. *Journal of Forensic Sciences*, JFSCA, 34 (4) 996–1002.

Lyman, S., & Boucher, L. J. (1990). Radiographic examination of edentulous mouths. *Journal of Prosthetic Dentistry*, 64, 180–182.

Matteson, S. R., Phillips, C., Kantor, M. L., & Leinedecker, T. (1989). The effect of lesion sixe, restorative material, and film speed on the detection of recurrent caries. *Oral Surgery, Oral Medicine, and Oral Pathology*, 68.

Monsour, P. A. J., Kruger, B. J., Barnes, A., & MacLeod, A. G. (1988). A survey of dental radiography. *Australian Dental Journal*, 33, 9–13.

Rohlin, M., Akesson, L., Hadansson, J., Hakansson, H., & Nasstrom, K. (1989). Comparison between panoramic and periapical radiography in the diagnosis of periodontal bone loss. *Dentomaxillofacial Radiology*, 18, 72–76.

Seals, R. R., Williams, E. O., & Jones, J. D. (1992). Panoramic radiographs: necessary for edentulous patients? *Journal of the American Dental Association*, 123.

Sidi, A. D., & Naylor, M. N. (1988). A comparison of bitewing radiography and interdental transillumination as adjuncts to the clinical identification of approximal caries in posterior teeth. *British Dental Journal*, 164, 15–18.

Ubelaker, D. H., & Donnell, G. O. (1992). Computer-Assisted facial reproduction. *Journal of Forensic Sciences*, JFSCA, 37, (1), 155–162.

White, S. C., Gratt, B. M., & Bauer, J. G. (1988). A clinical comparison of xeroradiography film radiography for the detection of proxima. *Oral Surgery, Oral Medicine, and Oral Pathology*, 65.

CHAPTER 5

Charting Silver Amalgam Restorations

Key Terms

- Alloy
- Cavity Classification
- Dental Caries
- Dental Caries
- Radiograph
- Radiopaque
- Restoration
- Retention Pin
- Silver Amalgam
- Single-Surface

PRIMARY CODE	SECONDARY CODE
M = Mesial	-S = Silver Amalgam (Solid Blue)
I = Incisal (#6–#11 & #22–#27)	• = and also
O = Occlusal (#1–#5, #12–#16, #17–#21, & #27–#32)	•p = Retention Pin
D = Distal	
F = Facial (#6–#11 & #22–#27)	
B = Buccal (#1–#5, #12–#16, #17–#21, & #27–#32)	
L = Lingual	

Introduction

One of the most frequently used restorative materials is **Silver Amalgam**. Amalgam is an **alloy** (a solid mixture of two or more metals) composed of a minimum of 65% silver, and a maximum of 29% tin, 6% copper, 2% zinc, and 3% mercury. Some Silver Amalgam alloys are zinc-free. The formula, which is free of zinc, is intended to reduce the amount of expansion of the restorative material if the alloy comes in contact with moisture. Dr. G. V. Black developed the system of classifying **dental caries** according to their location on the surfaces of the teeth referred to as Black's **Cavity Classification** (summarized in Chapter 13, Figure 13–1) and shown in Figure 5–1. This standard method for classifying dental caries is a reference used for charting dental restorations.

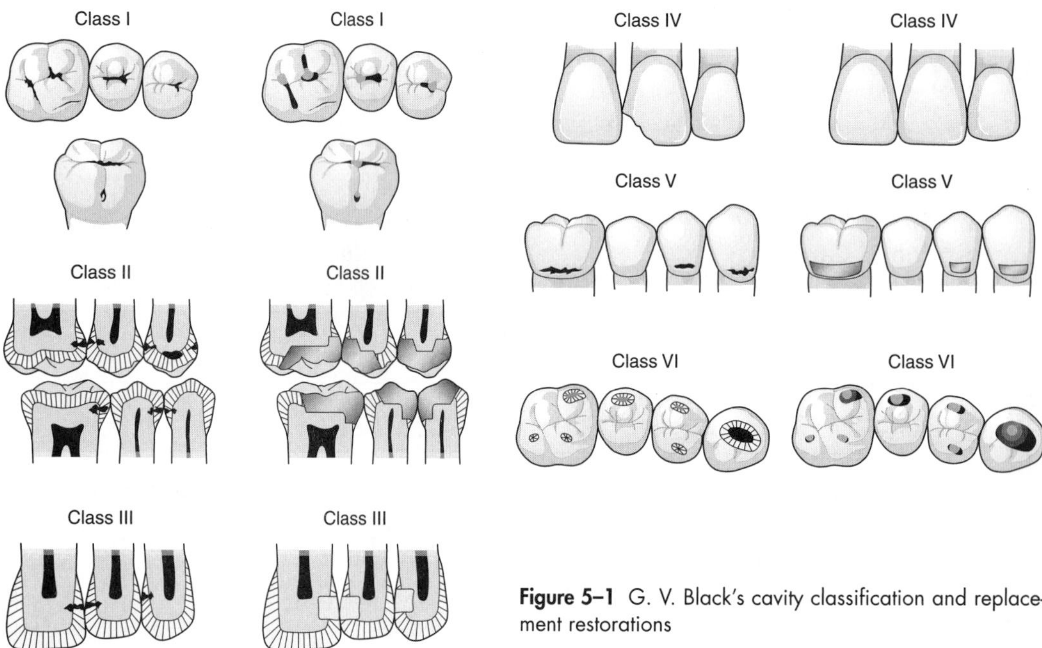

Figure 5–1 G. V. Black's cavity classification and replacement restorations

Single-Surface Silver Amalgam Restoration

A **single-surface** Silver Amalgam **restoration** generally involves Class I, V, and VI caries. Dental caries can begin on the pits and fissures of the Occlusal surfaces and Buccal grooves of posterior teeth. As indicated in the photograph in Figure 5–2, it is not unusual for the pit on the Lingual surface of the maxillary incisors above the cingulum to develop dental caries that require restoration.

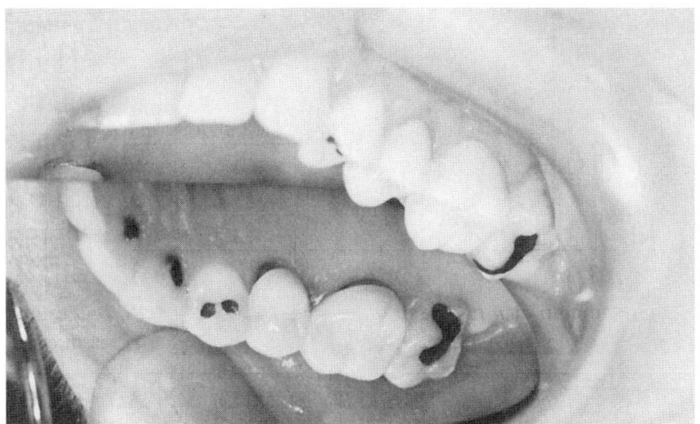

Universal System
#10 #11 #12 #13 #14

Palmer System
|2 |3 |4 |5 |6

ISO/FDI System
22 23 24 25 26

Figure 5–2 Maxillary left quadrant

In Figure 5–2 teeth #10 and #11 represent single-surface Silver Amalgam restorations located on the Lingual surface. The anterior periapical **radiograph** shows the Silver Amalgam restoration on tooth #10 as a **radiopaque** image (described in Chapter 4) as shown in Figure 5–3. Tooth #10 in Figure 5–2 clearly indicates that the restoration is located on the Lingual surface. When viewing the radiograph, it could be assumed that the restoration may also involve the Facial surface. It is highly unlikely that a Silver Amalgam restoration would be placed on an anterior tooth's Facial surface. Therefore, when viewing an anterior periapical radiograph with a single-surface Silver Amalgam restoration, it can only be assumed to exist on the Lingual surface. Currently, the anterior teeth are only restored using composite Resin restorative materials.

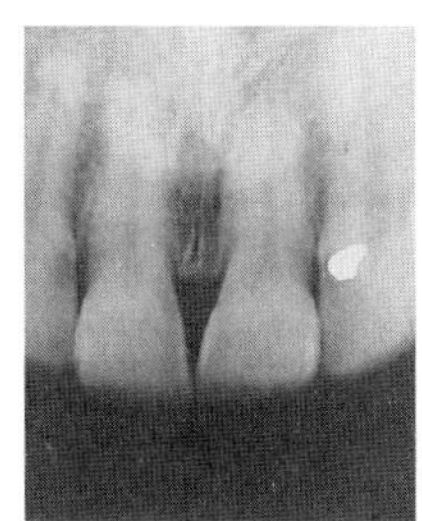

Universal System
#7 #8 #9 #10

Palmer System
2| 1| |1 |2

ISO/FDI System
12 11 21 22

Figure 5–3 Anterior periapical radiograph

Maxillary and mandibular molars have grooves or fissures in the region of the Occlusal and middle third on the Buccal and Lingual tooth surfaces. The Lingual groove on a mandibular molar is less likely to decay due to the self-cleansing action of the tongue. As indicated in the photograph, teeth #30 and #31 show Class I and Class II restorations with single-surface Silver Amalgam restorations located on the Buccal teeth surface (Figure 5–4).

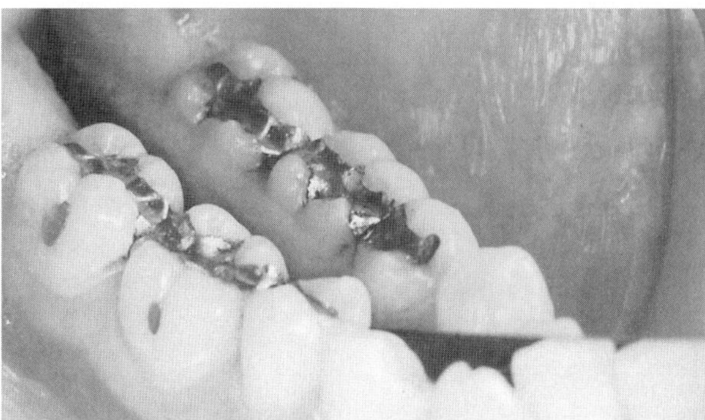

Universal System
#31 #30 #29 #28

Palmer System
7┐ 6┐ 5┐ 4┐

ISO/FDI System
47 46 45 44

Figure 5–4 Mandibular right quadrant

The bitewing radiograph shows the Silver Amalgam restorations on teeth #30 and #31 as radiopaque images (Figure 5–5). When viewing the radiograph, it appears that the single-surface Silver Amalgam restoration may be present on either the Buccal, Lingual, or both tooth surfaces. A radiograph of a Class V restoration would also present this situation.

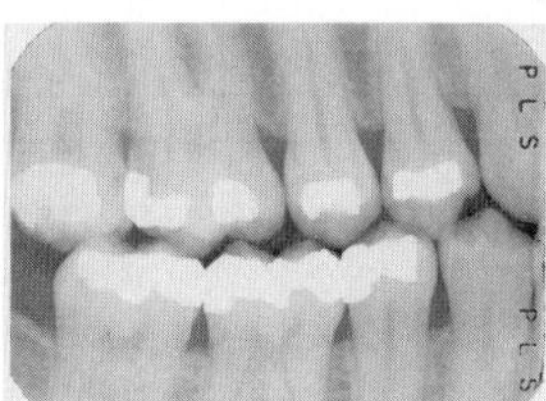

Universal System
#2 #3 #4 #5
#31 #30 #29 #28

Palmer System
7┘ 6┘ 5┘ 4┘
7┐ 6┐ 5┐ 4┐

ISO/FDI System
17 16 15 14
47 46 45 44

Figure 5–5 Maxillary and mandibular right bitewing radiograph

Charting a Single-Surface Silver Amalgam Restoration on an Anatomic Chart

Figure 5–6 represents an anatomic chart with single-surface Silver Amalgam restorations charted on teeth #10, #11, #30, and #31.

To chart single-surface Silver Amalgam restorations on an anatomic chart, it is important to remember the rules of dental charting (described in Chapter 4) and draw the restoration on only one view. With a blue pencil, on the appropriate tooth number, draw the contour of the restoration in the exact

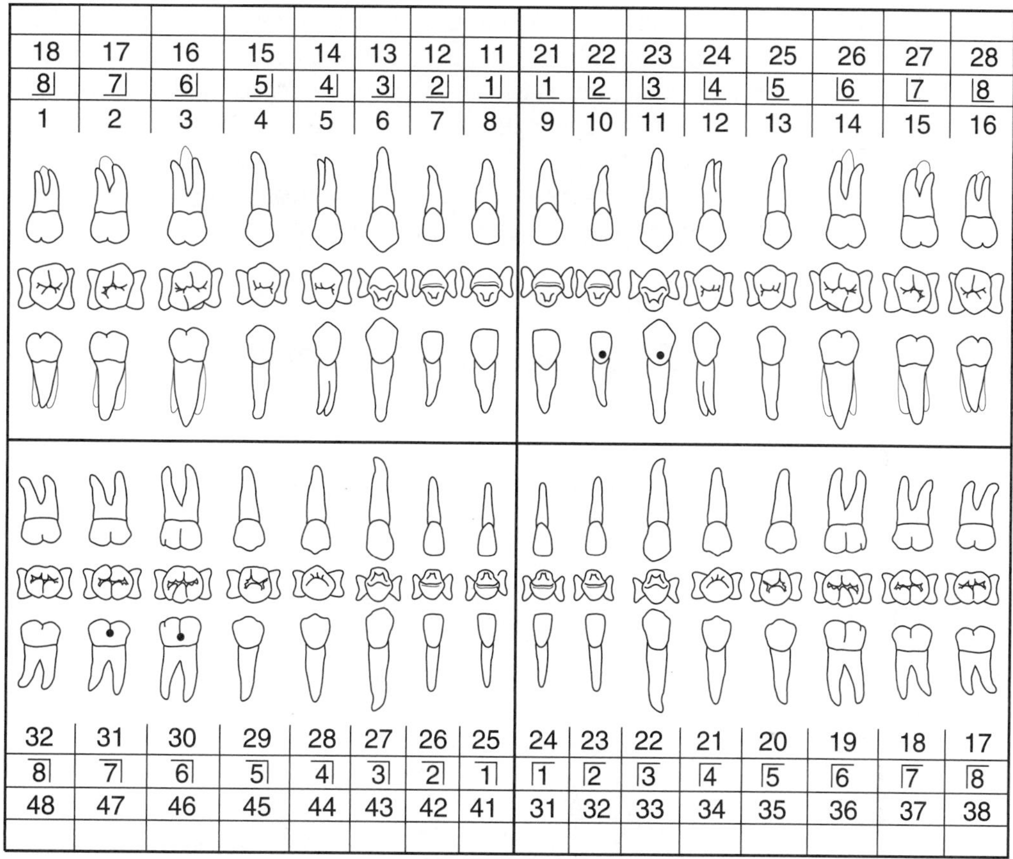

Figure 5-6 Anatomic chart illustrating single-surface Silver Amalgam restorations charted on teeth #10, #11, #30, and #31

location on the dental chart and fill it in. In Figure 5–6, teeth #10 and #11 show Silver Amalgam restorations placed on the Lingual tooth surfaces and teeth #30 and #31 show the restorations placed on the Buccal tooth surfaces. When comparing the restorations drawn on the dental chart (see Figure 5–6) to the actual photographs (see Figures 5–2 and 5–4), they appear similar.

The Silver Amalgam restorations located on the Lingual tooth surfaces are designated with the primary code "L" followed by a hyphen (-) and the secondary code "S" on the anatomic dental chart and referred to as Lingual Silver

Amalgam (L-S). The Silver Amalgam restorations involving the Buccal tooth surfaces use the primary code "B" and the secondary code "S" and are referred to as Buccal Silver Amalgam (B-S). It is not necessary to mark this abbreviation above the tooth drawing because the solid blue color appearing on a designated tooth surface indicates a Silver Amalgam restoration on that surface. Some practitioners may prefer to write the abbreviation above the tooth number in the space provided or to include it in the examination progress notes.

Charting a Single-Surface Silver Amalgam Restoration on a Geometric Chart

Figure 5–7 represents a geometric chart with a single-surface Silver Amalgam restoration charted on teeth #10, #11, #30, and #31.

To chart single-surface Silver Amalgam restorations on a geometric chart, it is important to remember to fill in the restoration on only one surface. With a blue pencil, on the appropriate tooth number, the designated surface area

Figure 5–7 Geometric chart showing single-surface Silver Amalgam restorations charted on teeth #10, #11, #30, and #31

<table>
<tr><td>18</td><td>17</td><td>16</td><td>15</td><td>14</td><td>13</td><td>12</td><td>11</td><td>21</td><td>22</td><td>23</td><td>24</td><td>25</td><td>26</td><td>27</td><td>28</td></tr>
<tr><td>8|</td><td>7|</td><td>6|</td><td>5|</td><td>4|</td><td>3|</td><td>2|</td><td>1|</td><td>|1</td><td>|2</td><td>|3</td><td>|4</td><td>|5</td><td>|6</td><td>|7</td><td>|8</td></tr>
<tr><td>1</td><td>2</td><td>3</td><td>4</td><td>5</td><td>6</td><td>7</td><td>8</td><td>9</td><td>10</td><td>11</td><td>12</td><td>13</td><td>14</td><td>15</td><td>16</td></tr>
<tr><td>32</td><td>31</td><td>30</td><td>29</td><td>28</td><td>27</td><td>26</td><td>25</td><td>24</td><td>23</td><td>22</td><td>21</td><td>20</td><td>19</td><td>18</td><td>17</td></tr>
<tr><td>8|</td><td>7|</td><td>6|</td><td>5|</td><td>4|</td><td>3|</td><td>2|</td><td>1|</td><td>|1</td><td>|2</td><td>|3</td><td>|4</td><td>|5</td><td>|6</td><td>|7</td><td>|8</td></tr>
<tr><td>48</td><td>47</td><td>46</td><td>45</td><td>44</td><td>43</td><td>42</td><td>41</td><td>31</td><td>32</td><td>33</td><td>34</td><td>35</td><td>36</td><td>37</td><td>38</td></tr>
</table>

is filled in completely. In Figure 5–7 teeth #10 and #11 show Silver Amalgam restorations placed on the Lingual tooth surfaces and teeth #30 and #31 show the restorations placed on the Buccal tooth surfaces.

The Silver Amalgam restorations on the Lingual tooth surfaces designated on the geometric chart are referred to as Lingual Silver Amalgam (L-S) and the Silver Amalgam restorations involving the Buccal tooth surfaces are referred to as Buccal Silver Amalgam (B-S). It is not necessary to mark this abbreviation above the tooth drawing because the solid blue color appearing on a designated tooth surface indicates a Silver Amalgam restoration on that surface. Some practitioners may prefer to write the abbreviation on the chart above the tooth number or to include it in the examination progress notes.

Charting a Single-Surface Silver Amalgam Restoration on a Numeric Coding System Chart

Figure 5–8 represents a numeric coding system chart with a single-surface Silver Amalgam restoration described above teeth #10 and #11, and below teeth #30 and #31.

The numeric coding system utilizes primary and secondary letter codes rather than diagrams to indicate the conditions of the teeth (presented in Chapters 3 and 4), therefore, fewer charts are used through time. Use a black ink pen to enter the date, then with a blue pencil, above or below the appropriate tooth number, the designated primary and secondary letter codes for each restoration are written in. In Figure 5–8 teeth #10 and #11 show Silver Amalgam

2-10-97										L-S	L-S					
MAXILLA	1	2	3	4	5	6	7	8	9	10	11	12	13	14	15	16
				A	B	C	D	E	F	G	H	I	J			
				T	S	R	Q	P	O	N	M	L	K			
MANDIBLE	32	31	30	29	28	27	26	25	24	23	22	21	20	19	18	17
2-10-97		B-S	B-S													

Figure 5–8 Numeric coding system chart showing single-surface Silver Amalgam restorations charted on teeth #10, #11, #30, and #31

restorations placed on the Lingual tooth surfaces and teeth #30 and #31 show the restorations placed on the Buccal tooth surfaces.

The primary and secondary letter codes used to identify the Silver Amalgam restorations on the Lingual tooth surfaces are L-S and are referred to as Lingual Silver Amalgam. The letter codes used to describe Silver Amalgam restorations involving the Buccal tooth surfaces are B-S and are referred to as Buccal Silver Amalgam shown in Figure 5–8.

Two-Surface Silver Amalgam Restorations

A two-surface Silver Amalgam restoration generally involves Class II and VI caries (summarized in Chapter 13). To repair Carious lesions located on the proximal surfaces of premolars and molars, it is necessary to enter the tooth through the Occlusal surface. As indicated in the photograph (Figure 5–9), there are two, two-surface Silver Amalgam restorations: tooth #29 presents involvement on the Distal and Occlusal tooth surfaces and tooth #31 involves the Mesial and Occlusal tooth surfaces.

The posterior bitewing radiograph shown in Figure 5–10 displays the Silver Amalgam restorations on teeth #29 and #31 as radiopaque images. The enamel tooth structure also appears radiopaque but to a lesser degree (described in Chapter 4). As shown in the radiograph, the proximal surface is involved when the contour of restoration extends around the side and down toward the middle and cervical thirds of the tooth. The restoration does not

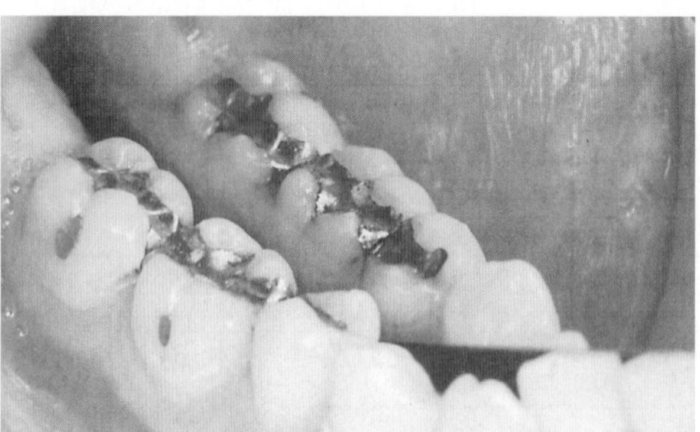

Universal System
#31 #30 #29 #28

Palmer System
7⏌ 6⏌ 5⏌ 4⏌

ISO/FDI System
47 46 45 44

Figure 5–9 Mandibular right quadrant

involve the proximal surface if the dentinoenamel junction (DEJ) is clearly visible.

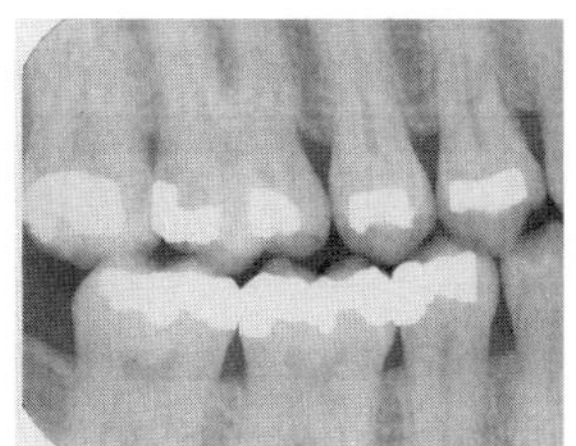

Universal System
#2 #3 #4 #5
#31 #30 #29 #28

Palmer System
7| 6| 5| 4|
7| 6| 5| 4|

ISO/FDI System
17 16 15 14
47 46 45 44

Figure 5–10 Maxillary and mandibular right bitewing radiograph

Charting a Two-Surface Silver Amalgam Restoration on an Anatomic Chart

Figure 5–11 represents an anatomic chart with four, two-surface Silver Amalgam restorations charted on teeth #29, #30, #31, and #32.

To chart two-surface Silver Amalgam restorations on an anatomic chart, draw the restoration on all three views. With a blue pencil, on the appropriate tooth number, the contour of the restoration is drawn in on the exact location on the dental chart and filled in. In Figure 5–11 tooth #29 shows a Silver Amalgam restoration placed on the Distal and Occlusal tooth surfaces and tooth #31 shows the restoration placed on the Mesial and Occlusal tooth surfaces.

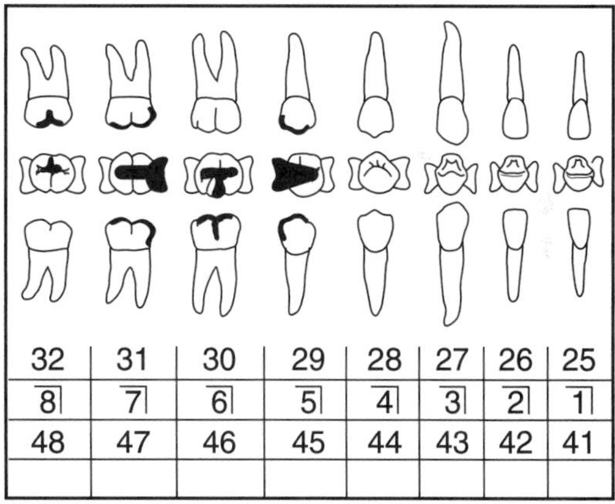

Figure 5–11 Anatomic chart illustrating two, two-surface Silver Amalgam restorations charted on teeth #29, #30, #31, and #32

When comparing the restorations drawn on the dental chart (see Figure 5–11) to the actual photograph (see Figure 5–9), they are similar. The bitewing radiograph shown in Figure 5–10 indicates the depth of the Silver Amalgam restoration. When charting dental restorations on an anatomic chart while examining dental radiographs, it is important not to duplicate the appearance of the restoration on the chart as it appears on the radiograph. Drawing the margins extended onto the Buccal and Lingual tooth surface views would imply that the Buccal and Lingual tooth surfaces are involved.

The Silver Amalgam restoration on tooth #29 involving the Distal and Occlusal tooth surfaces will use the primary codes "D" and "O" followed by the secondary code "S" and is written as DO-S and referred to as Disto-Occlusal Silver Amalgam. The Silver Amalgam restoration that involves the Mesial and Occlusal tooth surfaces will use the primary codes "M" and "O" and the secondary code "S" and is written as MO-S and referred to as Mesio-Occlusal Silver Amalgam.

It is not necessary to mark this abbreviation above the tooth drawing because the appearance of the solid blue color on a designated tooth surface indicates a Silver Amalgam restoration. Some practitioners may prefer to write the abbreviation above the tooth number in the space provided or to include it in the examination progress notes.

Charting a Two-Surface Silver Amalgam Restoration on a Geometric Chart

Figure 5–12 represents a geometric chart with four, two-surface Silver Amalgam restorations charted on teeth #29, #30, #31, and #32.

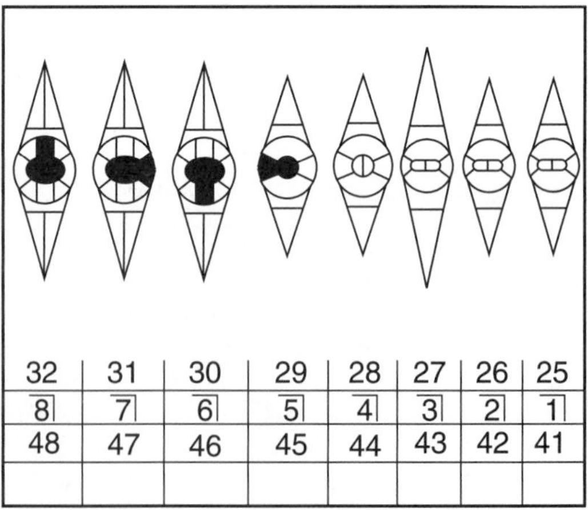

Figure 5–12 Geometric chart illustrating two, two-surface Silver Amalgam restorations charted on teeth #29, #30, #31, and #32

To chart two-surface Silver Amalgam restorations on a geometric chart, use a blue pencil to outline the designated tooth surfaces and completely fill in the areas. In Figure 5–12 tooth #29 shows a Silver Amalgam restoration placed on the Distal and Occlusal tooth surfaces and tooth #31 shows the restoration is placed on the Mesial and Occlusal tooth surfaces. On the geometric chart, the two-surface Silver Amalgam restorations on tooth #29 and tooth #31 are abbreviated as previously indicated on the anatomic chart.

It is not necessary to mark the abbreviation above the tooth diagram because the appearance of the solid blue color on the designated tooth surfaces indicate a Silver Amalgam restoration. Some practitioners may prefer to write the abbreviation on the chart or to include it in the examination progress notes.

Charting a Two-Surface Silver Amalgam Restoration on a Numeric Coding System Chart

Figure 5–13 represents a numeric coding system chart with a two-surface Silver Amalgam restoration described beneath teeth #29, #30, #31, and #32.

Because the numeric coding system utilizes primary and secondary letter codes rather than diagrams to indicate the conditions of the teeth, fewer charts are used (presented in Chapters 3 and 4). Use a black ink pen to enter the date and with a blue pencil, the designated letter codes for each restoration are written in above or below the appropriate tooth number. Beneath tooth #29, Figure 5–13 describes a two-surface Silver Amalgam restoration placed on the Distal and Occlusal tooth surfaces and the letter codes below tooth #31 indicate the restoration involves the Mesial and Occlusal tooth surfaces.

The primary and secondary letter codes used to identify the Silver Amalgam restoration involving the Distal and Occlusal tooth surfaces on tooth #29 are DO-S and is referred to as Disto-Occlusal Silver Amalgam. The letter codes used to describe the Silver Amalgam restoration on tooth #31 involving the

1-5-96																
MAXILLA	1	2	3	4 A	5 B	6 C	7 D	8 E	9 F	10 G	11 H	12 I	13 J	14	15	16
MANDIBLE	32	31	30	T 29	S 28	R 27	Q 26	P 25	O 24	N 23	M 22	L 21	K 20	19	18	17
1-5-96	OL-S	MO-S	OB-S	DO-S												

Figure 5–13 Numeric coding system chart showing two, two-surface Silver Amalgam restorations involving teeth #29, #30, #31, and #32

Mesial and Occlusal tooth surfaces are MO-S and is referred to as Mesio-Occlusal Silver Amalgam (see Figure 5–13).

The Buccal and Lingual tooth surfaces of the maxillary and mandibular molars are predisposed to developing dental caries because of the presence of deep grooves. For this reason, it is not uncommon for the dentist to extend an Occlusal surface restoration to include either the Buccal or Lingual tooth surface; this is referred to as "extension for prevention." Figures 5–11, 5–12, and 5–13 are dental charts showing examples of two, two-surface Silver Amalgam restorations involving the Occlusal and Buccal tooth surfaces on tooth #30 and the Occlusal and Lingual tooth surfaces on tooth #32.

Three-Surface Silver Amalgam Restorations

A three-surface Silver Amalgam restoration generally involves Class II caries (described in Chapter 13). To repair Carious lesions located on the proximal surfaces of premolars and molars, it is necessary to enter the tooth through the Occlusal surface. As indicated in the photograph (see Figure 5–9), there is a three-surface Silver Amalgam restoration on tooth #30, which presents the Mesial, Distal, and Occlusal tooth surfaces as having been restored.

The posterior bitewing radiograph shown in Figure 5–10 displays the Silver Amalgam restoration on tooth #30 as a radiopaque image. The enamel tooth structure also appears radiopaque but to a lesser degree (described in Chapter 4). As shown in the radiograph, the Mesial and Distal proximal tooth surfaces are involved. The contour of restoration extends around each side and down toward the middle and cervical thirds of the tooth (Figure 5–10).

Charting a Three-Surface Silver Amalgam Restoration on an Anatomic Chart

Figure 5–14 represents an anatomic chart with a three-surface Silver Amalgam restoration charted on tooth #30.

Draw three-surface Silver Amalgam restorations on an anatomic chart utilizing all three views. With a blue pencil, on the appropriate tooth diagram, the contour of the restoration is drawn in on the exact location and filled in. In Figure 5–9, tooth #30 shows a Silver Amalgam restoration placed on the Mesial, Distal, and Occlusal tooth surfaces.

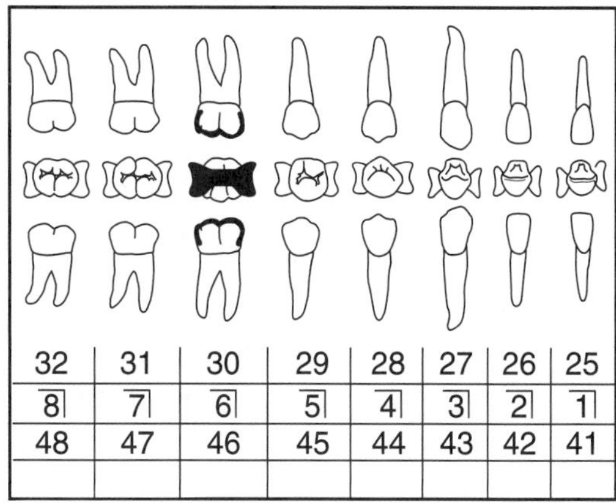

Figure 5–14 Anatomic chart illustrating a three-surface Silver Amalgam restoration charted on tooth #30

When comparing the restoration drawn on the dental chart (see Figure 5–14) to the actual photograph (see Figure 5–9), they are similar. The bitewing radiograph shown in Figure 5–10 indicates the depth of the Silver Amalgam restoration. When charting dental restorations on an anatomic chart while examining dental radiographs, it is important not to duplicate the appearance of the restoration on the chart as it appears on the radiograph. Drawing the margins extended onto the Buccal and Lingual tooth surface views implies that the Buccal and Lingual tooth surfaces are involved.

The Silver Amalgam restoration on tooth #30 involving the Mesial, Distal, and Occlusal tooth surfaces is abbreviated with the primary codes "M," "D," and "O," separated by a hyphen (-), and followed by the secondary code "S"; it is written as MOD-S and referred to as Mesio-Occluso-Distal Silver Amalgam.

It is not necessary to mark this abbreviation above the tooth drawing because the appearance of the solid blue color on a designated tooth surface indicates a Silver Amalgam restoration. Some practitioners may prefer to write the abbreviation above the tooth number in the space provided or to include it in the examination progress notes.

Charting a Three-Surface Silver Amalgam Restoration on a Geometric Chart

Figure 5–15 represents a geometric chart with a three-surface Silver Amalgam restoration charted on tooth #30.

To chart three-surface Silver Amalgam restorations on a geometric chart, use a blue pencil to outline the designated tooth surfaces and completely fill in the areas. In Figure 5–15 tooth #30 shows a Silver Amalgam restoration placed on the Mesial, Distal, and Occlusal tooth surfaces. On the geometric chart, the three-surface Silver Amalgam restoration on tooth #30 is abbreviated as previously indicated on the anatomic chart. Some practitioners may prefer to write the abbreviation on the chart or to include it in the examination progress notes.

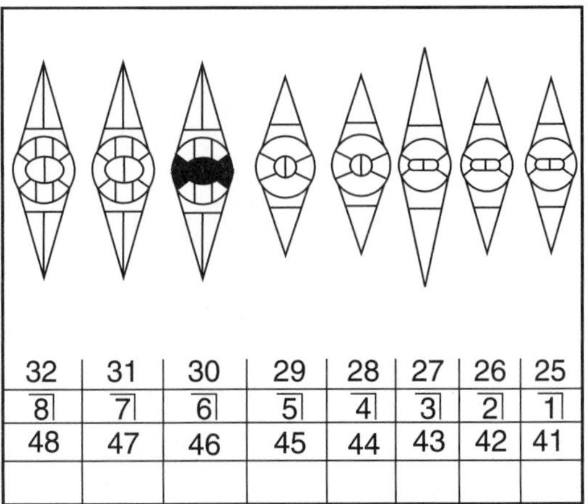

Figure 5–15 Geometric chart showing a three-surface Silver Amalgam restoration charted on tooth #30

Charting a Three-Surface Silver Amalgam Restoration on a Numeric Coding System Chart

Figure 5–16 represents a numeric coding system chart with a three-surface Silver Amalgam restoration recorded beneath tooth #30.

A black ink pen is used to enter the date and with a blue pencil, the designated primary and secondary codes are entered for each restoration above or below the appropriate tooth number.

5-16-97																
MAXILLA	1	2	3	4	5	6	7	8	9	10	11	12	13	14	15	16
				A	B	C	D	E	F	G	H	I	J			
				T	S	R	Q	P	O	N	M	L	K			
MANDIBLE	32	31	30	29	28	27	26	25	24	23	22	21	20	19	18	17
5-16-97			MOD-S													

Figure 5–16 Numeric coding system chart illustrating a three-surface Silver Amalgam restoration on tooth #30

Beneath tooth #30, Figure 5–16 describes a three-surface Silver Amalgam restoration placed on the Mesial, Distal, and Occlusal tooth surfaces. The primary codes "M," "D," and "O" entered below tooth #30 indicate the involved tooth surfaces and the secondary code "S" represents the Silver Amalgam restorative material. The restoration on tooth #30 is written as MOD-S and referred to as Mesio-Occluso-Distal Silver Amalgam.

Four-Surface Silver Amalgam Restorations

A four-surface Silver Amalgam restoration generally involves Class I and II caries (described in Chapter 13). To repair Carious lesions located on the proximal surfaces of premolars and molars, it is necessary to enter the tooth through the Occlusal surface.

The maxillary and mandibular molars have grooves or fissures in the region of the Occlusal and middle third on the Buccal and Lingual tooth surfaces and either one or both surfaces can be involved in a four-surface Silver Amalgam restoration. The Lingual groove on a mandibular molar is less likely to decay due to the self-cleansing action of the tongue. However, the maxillary molar tooth surface is susceptible to developing dental caries because of the deep groove on the Lingual tooth surface and the cleansing action of the tongue is limited in this area.

Figure 5–17 shows a four-surface Silver Amalgam restoration on tooth #3 that presents the Mesial, Distal, Occlusal, and Lingual tooth surfaces as having been repaired.

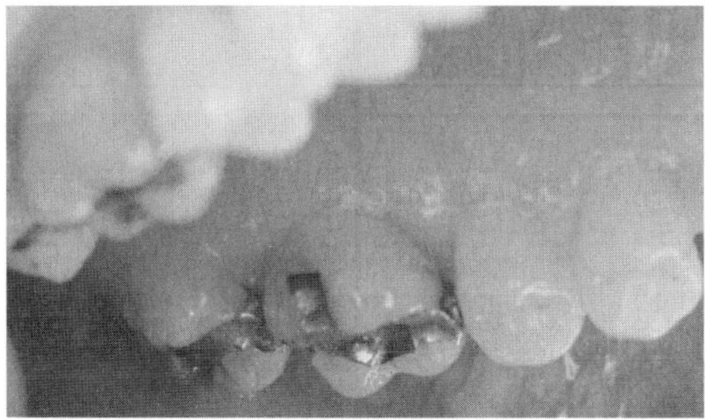

Universal System
#3 #4 #5 #6

Palmer System
6| 5| 4| 3|

ISO/FDI System
16 15 14 13

Figure 5–17 Maxillary right quadrant

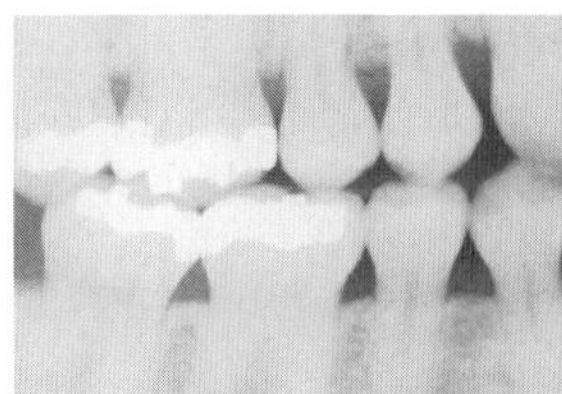

Universal System
#2 #3 #4 #5 #6
#31 #30 #29 #28

Palmer System
7| 6| 5| 4| 3|
7| 6| 5| 4|

ISO/FDI System
17 16 15 14 13
47 46 45 44

Figure 5–18 Maxillary and mandibular right bitewing radio-graph

The posterior bitewing radiograph as shown in Figure 5–18 displays the Silver Amalgam restoration on tooth #3 as a radiopaque image. The enamel tooth structure also appears radiopaque but to a lesser degree (described in Chapter 4). As shown in the radiograph, the Mesial and Distal proximal tooth surfaces are involved. The contour of restoration extends around each side and down toward the middle and cervical thirds of the tooth.

When viewing the radiograph of tooth #3 in Figure 5–18, it appears that the restoration may involve the Facial, Lingual, or both tooth surfaces. Whether or not one or both of these tooth surfaces are involved can only be ascertained through direct visual examination of the tooth or by viewing an intraoral photograph of the area.

Charting a Four-Surface Silver Amalgam Restoration on an Anatomic Chart

Figure 5–19 represents an anatomic chart with a four-surface Silver Amalgam restoration charted on tooth #3.

On an anatomic chart, draw the restoration on all three views to record a four-surface Silver Amalgam restoration. With a blue pencil, on the appropriate tooth number, the contour of the restoration is drawn in on the exact location on the dental chart and filled in. In Figure 5–19, tooth #3 shows a Silver Amalgam restoration placed on the Mesial, Distal, Occlusal, and Lingual tooth surfaces.

When comparing the restoration drawn on the dental chart (see Figure 5–19) to the actual photograph (see Figure 5–17), they are similar. The bitewing radiograph shown in Figure 5–18 indicates the depth of the Silver Amalgam restoration. When charting dental restorations on an anatomic chart while examining dental radiographs, do not duplicate the appearance of the restoration on the chart as it appears on the radiograph.

The Silver Amalgam restoration on tooth #3 is designated by the primary codes "M," "D," "L," and "O," followed by the secondary code "S," and written as MODL-S; it is referred to as Mesio-Occluso-Disto-Lingual Silver Amalgam.

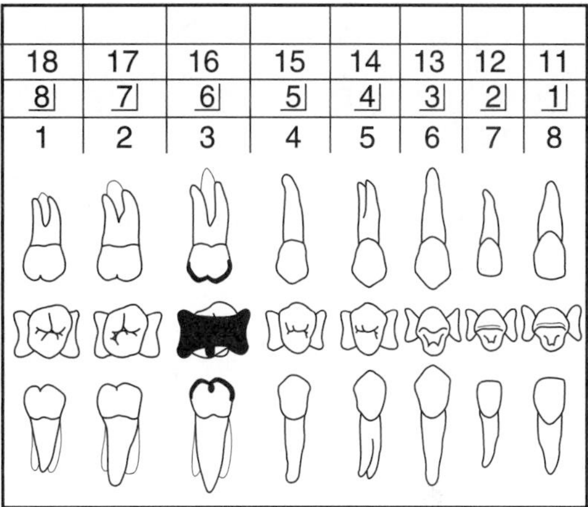

Figure 5–19 Anatomic chart illustrating a four-surface Silver Amalgam restoration charted on tooth #3

It is not necessary to mark this abbreviation above the tooth drawing because the appearance of the solid blue color on a designated tooth surface indicates a Silver Amalgam restoration involving that surface.

Charting a Four-Surface Silver Amalgam Restoration on a Geometric Chart

Figure 5–20 represents a geometric chart with a four-surface Silver Amalgam restoration charted on tooth #3.

To chart a four-surface Silver Amalgam restoration on a geometric chart, use a blue pencil to outline the designated tooth surfaces and completely fill in the areas. In Figure 5–20, tooth #3 shows a Silver Amalgam restoration placed on the Mesial, Distal, Occlusal, and Lingual tooth surfaces. The four-surface Silver Amalgam restoration on tooth #3 is abbreviated as previously indicated on an anatomic chart.

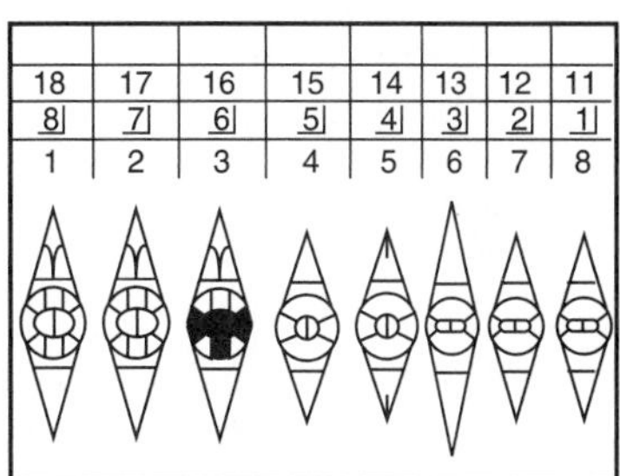

Figure 5–20 Geometric chart illustrating a four-surface Silver Amalgam restoration charted on tooth #3

Charting a Four-Surface Silver Amalgam Restoration on a Numeric Coding System Chart

Figure 5–21 represents a numeric coding system chart with a four-surface Silver Amalgam restoration described above tooth #3.

To indicate the restoration on tooth #3 on a numeric coding system chart, use a black ink pen to enter the date, and with a blue pencil record the designated primary and secondary codes.

Above tooth #3, Figure 5–21 describes a four-surface Silver Amalgam restoration placed on the Mesial, Distal, Occlusal, and Lingual tooth surfaces. The primary and secondary codes used to identify the Silver Amalgam restoration on tooth #3 are MODL-S and is referred to as Mesio-Occluso-Disto-Lingual Silver Amalgam.

Five-Surface Silver Amalgam Restorations

A five-surface Silver Amalgam restoration generally involves Class I and II caries (described in Chapter 13). To repair Carious lesions located on the proximal surfaces of premolars and molars, it is necessary to enter the tooth through the Occlusal surface.

The maxillary and mandibular molars have grooves or fissures in the region of the Occlusal and middle third on the Buccal and Lingual tooth surfaces, and both surfaces, are involved in a five-surface Silver Amalgam restoration.

As indicated in the photograph (Figure 5–22), there are three, five-surface Silver Amalgam restorations on teeth #28, #29, and #30, which present the Mesial, Distal, Occlusal, Buccal, and Lingual tooth surfaces as having been

7-15-96			MODL-S													
MAXILLA	1	2	3	4 A	5 B	6 C	7 D	8 E	9 F	10 G	11 H	12 I	13 J	14	15	16
MANDIBLE	32	31	30	T 29	S 28	R 27	Q 26	P 25	O 24	N 23	M 22	L 21	K 20	19	18	17
7-15-96																

Figure 5–21 Numeric coding system chart illustrating a four-surface Silver Amalgam restoration on tooth #3

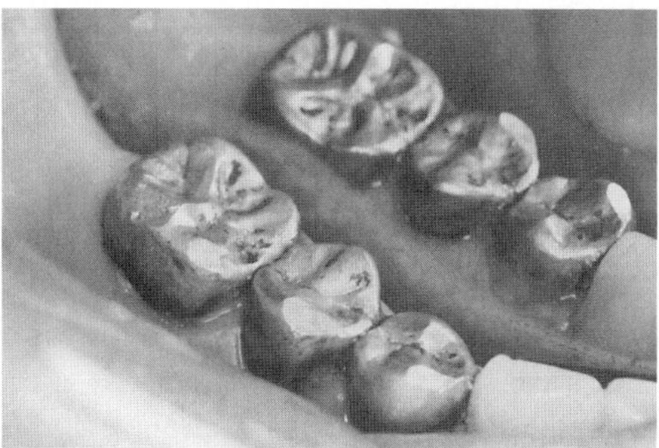

Universal System
#30 #29 #28 #27

Palmer System
6⏋ 5⏋ 4⏋ 3⏋

ISO/FDI System
46 45 44 43

Figure 5–22 Mandibular right quadrant

repaired. In general, three-, four-, and five-surface Silver Amalgam restorations show repair, which comprise one- to two-thirds of each involved tooth surface. Figure 5–22 shows the Silver Amalgam restorative material completely covering all of the tooth surfaces including the cusps. This is an example of Cusp Protecting Alloy (CPA) and it is primarily used in public health and government settings.

The posterior bitewing radiograph (Figure 5–23) shows the Silver Amalgam restorations on teeth #28, #29, and #30 as radiopaque images. A radiograph of a complete Gold Crown and a full cast Crown also appears radiopaque (described in Chapter 8) and can only be ascertained through direct visual examination of the tooth or by viewing an intraoral photograph of the area.

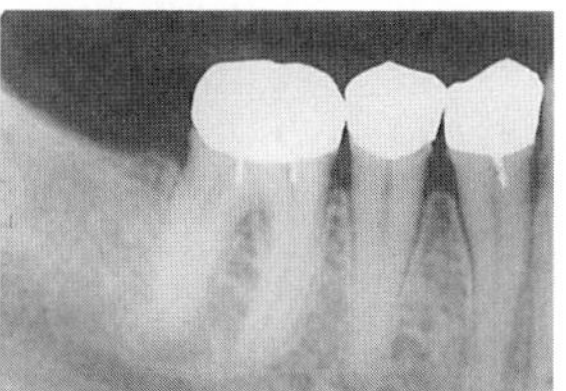

Universal System
#30 #29 #28

Palmer System
6⏋ 5⏋ 4⏋

ISO/FDI System
46 45 44

Figure 5–23 Mandibular right periapical radiograph

As shown in the periapical radiograph, the Mesial and Distal proximal tooth surfaces are involved. The contour of each restoration extends around each side and down to the cervical third of the teeth.

When viewing the radiograph of teeth #28, #29, and #30 in Figure 5–23, it appears that the restoration may involve the Facial, Lingual, or both tooth surfaces. Whether or not one or both of these tooth surfaces are involved can only be established through direct visual examination of the tooth or by viewing an intraoral photograph of the area.

Charting a Five-Surface Silver Amalgam Restoration on an Anatomic Chart

Figure 5–24 represents an anatomic chart with three, five-surface Silver Amalgam restorations charted on teeth #28, #29, and #30.

With a blue pencil, on the appropriate tooth number, draw the contour of the restoration on the exact location on the tooth diagram and completely fill it in. In Figure 5–24 the Mesial, Distal, Occlusal, Lingual, and Buccal tooth surfaces are shown completely covered.

When comparing the restoration drawn on the dental chart (see Figure 5–24) to the actual photograph (see Figure 5–23), they are similar. When recording

18	17	16	15	14	13	12	11	21	22	23	24	25	26	27	28
8	7	6	5	4	3	2	1	1	2	3	4	5	6	7	8
1	2	3	4	5	6	7	8	9	10	11	12	13	14	15	16

32	31	30	29	28	27	26	25	24	23	22	21	20	19	18	17
8	7	6	5	4	3	2	1	1	2	3	4	5	6	7	8
48	47	46	45	44	43	42	41	31	32	33	34	35	36	37	38

Figure 5–24 Anatomic chart illustrating three, five-surface Silver Amalgam restorations charted on teeth #28, #29, and #30

dental restorations on an anatomic chart while examining dental radiographs, do not duplicate the appearance of the restoration on the chart as it appears on the radiograph.

The Silver Amalgam restorations on teeth #28, #29, and #30 utilize the primary codes "M," "D," "O," "B," and "L," followed by the secondary code "S," and are written as MODBL-S; they are referred to as Mesio-Occluso-Disto-Bucco-Lingual Silver Amalgam.

Charting a Five-Surface Silver Amalgam Restoration on a Geometric Chart

Figure 5–25 represents a geometric chart with three, five-surface Silver Amalgam restorations charted on teeth #28, #29, and #30.

With a blue pencil, on the appropriate tooth diagrams, the designated tooth surfaces are outlined and completely filled in. Figure 5–25 shows teeth #28, #29, and #30 with Silver Amalgam restorations placed on the Mesial, Distal, Occlusal, Buccal, and Lingual tooth surfaces. On a geometric chart, the three, five-surface Silver Amalgam restorations are abbreviated as previously indicated on an anatomic chart.

18	17	16	15	14	13	12	11	21	22	23	24	25	26	27	28
8	7	6	5	4	3	2	1	1	2	3	4	5	6	7	8
1	2	3	4	5	6	7	8	9	10	11	12	13	14	15	16
32	31	30	29	28	27	26	25	24	23	22	21	20	19	18	17
8	7	6	5	4	3	2	1	1	2	3	4	5	6	7	8
48	47	46	45	44	43	42	41	31	32	33	34	35	36	37	38

Figure 5–25 Geometric chart illustrating three, five-surface Silver Amalgam restorations on teeth #28, #29, and #30

Charting a Five-Surface Silver Amalgam Restoration on a Numeric Coding System Chart

Figure 5–26 represents a numeric coding system chart with three, five-surface Silver Amalgam restorations described beneath teeth #28, #29, and #30.

Use a black ink pen to enter the date and with a blue pencil, the designated primary and secondary codes for each restoration are written in beneath the appropriate tooth number.

Below teeth #28, #29, and #30, Figure 5–26 describes the three, five-surface Silver Amalgam restorations placed on the Mesial, Distal, Occlusal, Buccal, and Lingual tooth surfaces. The primary and secondary codes used to identify the Silver Amalgam restorations are written as MODBL-S and referred to as Mesio-Occluso-Disto-Bucco-Lingual Silver Amalgam.

Pin-Retained Silver Amalgam Restorations

When tooth structure has been damaged to the point where it is difficult to retain the Silver Amalgam restoration within the configuration of the existing tooth structure, **Retention Pins** are drilled into the dentin to aid in retaining the restoration. Figure 5–23 shows Retention Pins placed in teeth #28 and #30. The pins appear as two radiopaque vertical lines extending from the CEJ down toward the root surface.

6-5-95																
MAXILLA	1	2	3	4 A	5 B	6 C	7 D	8 E	9 F	10 G	11 H	12 I	13 J	14	15	16
MANDIBLE	32	31	30	T 29	S 28	R 27	Q 26	P 25	O 24	N 23	M 22	L 21	K 20	19	18	17
6-5-95			MODBL-S •p	MODBL-S	MODBL-S •p											

Figure 5–26 Numeric coding system chart illustrating three, five-surface Silver Amalgam restorations on teeth #28, #29,and #30

Charting Retention Pins on Anatomic, Geometric, and Numeric Coding System Charts

Figures 5–24 and 5–25 represent anatomic and geometric charts with two, five-surface Silver Amalgam restorations with Retention Pins charted on teeth #28 and #30. On tooth #28, one short vertical line is shown extending down from the CEJ on the Buccal tooth surface onto the root surface, and tooth #30 shows two short vertical lines. The existence of a vertical line located in this location on anatomic and geometric charts indicates the presence of Retention Pins.

To indicate the presence of Retention Pins on a numeric coding system chart, use a black pen, and above or below the appropriate tooth number, following the primary and secondary codes, enter the symbol "•" followed by the superscript symbol "$^{\bullet}$" and lowercase letter "p". In Figure 5–26, MODBL-S•$^{\bullet}$p is written below teeth #28 and #30, and referred to as Mesio-Occluso-Disto-Bucco-Lingual Silver Amalgam and also Retention Pins.

Two Separate Silver Amalgam Restorations

Charting two separate Silver Amalgam restorations requires using the same methods previously mentioned. Two separate Silver Amalgam restorations can involve Class I, II, III, V, and VI caries (described in Chapter 13).

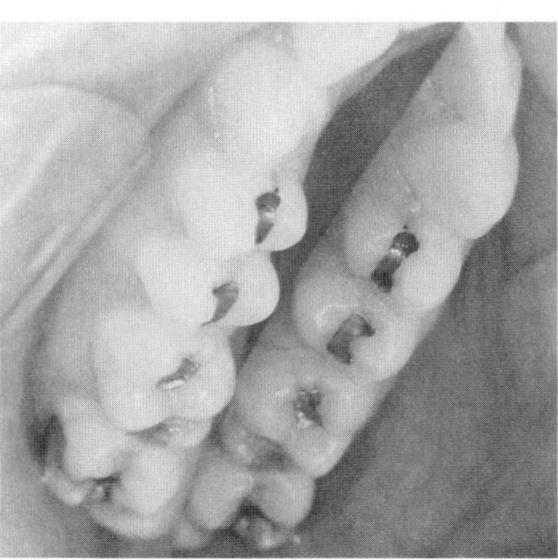

Universal System
#2 #3 #4 #5 #6

Palmer System
7| 6| 5| 4| 3|

ISO/FDI System
17 16 15 14 13

Figure 5–27 Maxillary right quadrant

As indicated in the photograph in Figure 5–27, there are two teeth shown with two separate Silver Amalgam restorations. Tooth #2 presents Silver Amalgam restorations on the Distal and Occlusal tooth surfaces and also the Buccal surface, and tooth #3 displays restorations that involve the Distal and Occlusal tooth surfaces and also the Occlusal tooth surface.

The posterior bitewing radiograph (Figure 5–28) shows the Silver Amalgam restorations on tooth #3 as two separate radiopaque images. On the radiograph, tooth #2 does not appear as two separate radiopaque areas because the two Silver Amalgam restorations are superimposed.

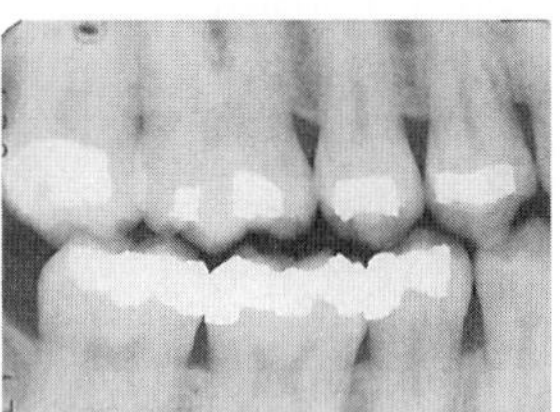

Universal System
#2 #3 #4 #5
#31 #30 #29 #28

Palmer System
7| 6| 5| 4|
7| 6| 5| 4|

ISO/FDI System
17 16 15 14
47 46 45 44

Figure 5–28 Maxillary and mandibular right bitewing radiograph

Charting Two Separate Silver Amalgam Restorations on an Anatomic Chart

Figure 5–29 represents an anatomic chart with two separate Silver Amalgam restorations charted on teeth #2 and #3.

On an anatomic chart, use all three views to chart two separate Silver Amalgam restorations that involve a single tooth. With a blue pencil, on the appropriate tooth number, the contour of the restoration is drawn in on the exact location on the tooth diagram and filled in completely.

18	17	16	15	14	13	12	11
8|	7|	6|	5|	4|	3|	2|	1|
1	2	3	4	5	6	7	8

Figure 5–29 Anatomic chart illustrating two separate Silver Amalgam restorations charted on teeth #2 and #3

In Figure 5–29 tooth #2 indicates two separate Silver Amalgam restorations. One of the two restorations shows involvement on the Distal and Occlusal tooth surfaces and the other involves the Buccal tooth surface. The part of the restoration that involves the Occlusal tooth surface only comprises the area that extends between the Distal and middle thirds of the Occlusal tooth surface.

The recorded restorations drawn on the dental chart (see Figure 5–29) when compared to the actual photograph (see Figure 5–27) will appear similar.

The Silver Amalgam restorations on tooth #2 are abbreviated as DO-S•B-S and referred to as Disto-Occlusal Silver Amalgam and also Buccal Silver Amalgam. The restorations on tooth #3 are abbreviated as DO-S•O-S and referred to as Disto-Occlusal Silver Amalgam and also Occlusal Silver Amalgam.

Charting Two Separate Silver Amalgam Restorations on a Geometric Chart

Figure 5–30 represents a geometric chart with two separate Silver Amalgam restorations charted on teeth #2 and #3.

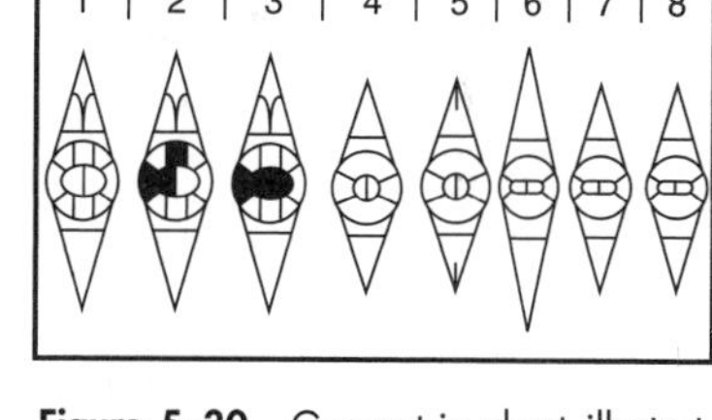

Figure 5–30 Geometric chart illustrating two separate Silver Amalgam restorations charted on teeth #2 and #3

To chart two separate Silver Amalgam restorations involving one tooth on a geometric chart, fill in the restorations on all involved tooth surfaces. On the appropriate tooth number, use a blue pencil to outline the designated tooth surfaces and completely fill the areas in.

Figure 5–30 shows tooth #2 with two separate Silver Amalgam restorations, one placed on the Distal and Occlusal tooth surfaces (DO-S), and the other located on the Buccal tooth surface (B-S). Tooth #3 also indicates two separate Silver Amalgam restorations, one placed on the Distal and Occlusal tooth surfaces (DO-S), and the other located on the Occlusal tooth surface (O-S). The geometric chart will not show these restorations recorded as two separate restorations because when a geometric chart is used, the entire area that designates a tooth surface is outlined and completely filled in. Therefore, it is necessary to mark the primary and secondary codes of the two separate restorations in the designated box above or below the tooth notation number on a geometric chart. The restorations are written and read as previously mentioned when using an anatomic chart. Some practitioners may prefer to write the abbreviation on the chart or to include it in the examination progress notes.

Charting Two Separate Silver Amalgam Restorations on a Numeric Coding System Chart

Figure 5–31 represents a numeric coding system chart with two separate Silver Amalgam restorations described above teeth #2 and #3.

Use a black pen to enter the date and with a blue pencil, the designated primary and secondary codes for each restoration are written in above the appropriate tooth numbers. In Figure 5–31, the numeric coding system chart indicates tooth #2 has two separate Silver Amalgam restorations, one placed on the Distal and Occlusal tooth surfaces, and the other located on the Buccal tooth surface. Tooth #3 shows two separate restorations, one located on the Distal and Occlusal tooth surfaces, and the other placed on the Occlusal tooth surface.

The primary and secondary codes used to describe each restoration are separated by the symbol "•," which is read as "and also." This symbol is also used to separate two or more individual restorations or other restorative conditions involving the same tooth. The restorations on teeth #2 and #3 are written and read as previously mentioned.

3-30-94		DO-S• B-S	DO-S• O-S													
MAXILLA	1	2	3	4 A	5 B	6 C	7 D	8 E	9 F	10 G	11 H	12 I	13 J	14	15	16
MANDIBLE	32	31	30	T 29	S 28	R 27	Q 26	P 25	O 24	N 23	M 22	L 21	K 20	19	18	17
3-30-94																

Figure 5–31 Numeric coding system chart indicating two separate Silver Amalgam restorations on teeth #2 and #3

Review Questions

Multiple Choice

Directions: Select the letter of the choice that *best* answers the question.

1. A single-surface Silver Amalgam would most likely not be found on the __________ surface of a tooth.
   a. Distal   b. Occlusal
   c. Lingual   d. Facial
2. Decay involving the Mesial and Distal surfaces of tooth #30 that are restored with Silver Amalgam would be charted as:
   a. MD-AM.   b. MOD-S.
   c. MD-A.   d. MOD-SA.
3. CPA stands for:
   a. Cusp Protecting Alloy.   b. Cusp Protection Alloy.
   c. Cusp Protects Alloy.   d. all of the above.

Chart the following using each of the three types of dental charts.

4. L-S on #8 and #15.
5. MODBL-S on #2.
6. MO-S on #30.
7. OBL-S on #3 and #31.
8. DO-S • O-S on #5.
9. MODL-S••p on #18.
10. DOB-S on #19.

Answers

1. **a**, 2. **b**, 3. **a**

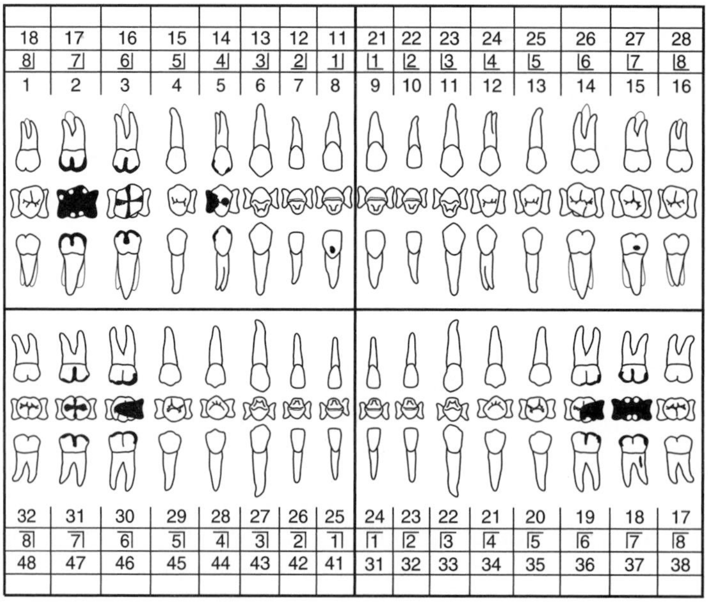

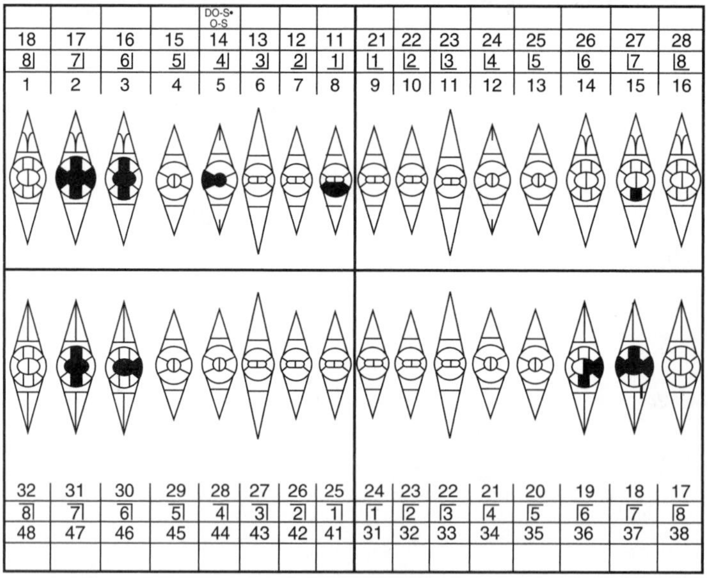

18	17	16	15	14	13	12	11	21	22	23	24	25	26	27	28
8|	7|	6|	5|	4|	3|	2|	1|	|1	|2	|3	|4	|5	|6	|7	|8
1	2	3	4	5	6	7	8	9	10	11	12	13	14	15	16

32	31	30	29	28	27	26	25	24	23	22	21	20	19	18	17
8|	7|	6|	5|	4|	3|	2|	1|	|1	|2	|3	|4	|5	|6	|7	|8
48	47	46	45	44	43	42	41	31	32	33	34	35	36	37	38

				DO-S• O-S											
18	17	16	15	14	13	12	11	21	22	23	24	25	26	27	28
8|	7|	6|	5|	4|	3|	2|	1|	|1	|2	|3	|4	|5	|6	|7	|8
1	2	3	4	5	6	7	8	9	10	11	12	13	14	15	16

32	31	30	29	28	27	26	25	24	23	22	21	20	19	18	17
8|	7|	6|	5|	4|	3|	2|	1|	|1	|2	|3	|4	|5	|6	|7	|8
48	47	46	45	44	43	42	41	31	32	33	34	35	36	37	38

2-9-98		MODBL-S	OBL-S		DO-S• O-S			L-S							L-S	
MAXILLA	1	2	3	4 A	5 B	6 C	7 D	8 E	9 F	10 G	11 H	12 I	13 J	14	15	16
MANDIBLE	32	31	30	T 29	S 28	R 27	Q 26	P 25	O 24	N 23	M 22	L 21	K 20	19	18	17
2-9-98		OBL-S	MO-S											DOB-S	MODL-S •P	

References

American Dental Association Working Group I ASC MD 156. (1997) *Computer Software Performance for Dental Practice Software* (ANSI/ADA Technical Report No. 1004). (Compiled by the American Dental Association, Department of Dental Informatics.)

Berglund, A. (1990). Estimation by a 24-hour study of the daily dose of intra-oral mercury vapor inhaled after release from dental amalgam. *Journal of Dental Research*, 146–151.

Bolewska, J., Holmstrup, P., Moller-Madsen, B., Kenrad, B., & Danscher, G. (1990). Amalgam-associated mercury accumulations in normal oral mucosa, oral mucosal lesions of lichen planus and contact lesions associated with amalgam. *Journal of Oral Pathology and Medicine*, 19, 19.

Boyer, D. B., & Edie, J. W. (1990). Composition of clinically aged amalgam restorations. *Dental Materials*, 6, 146.

Boyer, D. B., & Roth L. (1994). Fracture resistance of teeth with bonded amalgams. *American Jouranl of Dentistry*, 7, 91.

Corbin, S. B., & Kohn, W. G. (1994). The benefits and risks of dental amalgam: Current findings reviewed. *Journal of the American Dental Association*, 125, 381–388.

Craig, R. G. (1997). Restorative dental materials (10th ed.). Mosby-Year Book, Inc.

Fischer, G. M, Stewart, G. P., & Panelli, J. (1993). Amalgam retention using pins, boxes, and amalgambond. *American Journal of Dentistry*, 6, 173.

Jendresen, M. D., Allen, E. P., Bayne, S. C., Hansson, T. L., Klooster, J., & Preston, J. D. (1992). Report of the committee on scientific investigation of the american academy of restorative dentistry. *Journal of Prosthetic Dentistry*, 68 (1), 137–180.

Jokstad, A., & Mjor, I. A. (1991). Replacement reasons and service time of class-II amalgam restorations in relation to cavity design. *Acta Odontologica Scandinavia*, 49, 109–125.

Mandel, I. D. (1991). Amalgam hazards: An assessment of research. *Journal of the American Dental Association*, 122, 62.

Marek, M. (1984). Acceleration of corrosion of dental amalgam by abrasion. *Journal of Dental Research*, 63, 1010.

Mueller, H. J. & Bapna, M. S. (1990). Copper-, indium-, tin-, and calcium-fluoride admixed amalgams: Release rates and selected properties. *Dental Materials*, 6, 256.

Rogo, E. J. (1995). Overhang removal: Improving periodontal health adjacent to class II amalgam restorations. *The Journal of Practical Hygiene*, 4 (3), 15–23.

Sarkar N. K., & Park, J. R. (1988). Mechanism of improved corrosion resistance of zn-containing dental amalgams. *Journal of Dental Research*, 67, 1312.

Smales, R. J., Webster, D. A., Leppard, P. I., & Dawson, A. S. (1991). Prediction of amalgam restoration longevity. *Journal of Dentistry*, 19, 18–23.

Smales, R. J., Webster, D. A., & Leppard, P. I. (1991). Survival predictions of amalgam restorations. *Journal of Dentistry*, 19, 272–277.

Sutow, E. J., Jones, D. W., Hall, G. C., & Owen, C. G. (1991). Crevice corrosion products of dental amalgam. *Journal of Dental Research*, 70, 1082–1087.

U.S. Department of Health and Human Services, Public Health Services. (1993). Dental amalgam: A scientific review and recommended public health service strategy for research, education, and regulation. Washington, DC: Author.

Vimy, M. J., & Lorscheider, F. L. (1990). Dental amalgam mercury daily dose estimated from intra-oral vapor measurements: A predictor of mercury accumulation in human tissues. *Journal of Trace Elements and Electrolytes in Healthcare Disease*, 3, 111–123.

CHAPTER 6

Gold Inlay Restorations

Key Terms

Alloy
Copper
Gold Alloy
Gold Beating
Gold Foil
Gold Inlay
Palladium
Pure Gold
Silver
Trace Metals

PRIMARY CODE	SECONDARY CODE
M = Mesial	-G = Gold (blue diagonal lines)
I = Incisal (#6–#11 & #22–#27)	-G• = Gold Foil (blue dots)
O = Occlusal (#1–#5, #12–#16, #17–#21, & #27–#32)	• = and also
D = Distal	
F = Facial (#6–#11 & #22–#27)	
B = Buccal (#1–#5, #12–#16, #17–#21, & #27–#32)	
L = Lingual	

Introduction

Over 500 years ago **Gold Foil** was used as a restorative material to fill cavities. Gold Foil is manufactured and formed from **pure gold** in a procedure known as **gold beating**. The development of tooth-colored restorative materials that require less working time are now used in the areas of the mouth where Gold Foil restorations were placed.

An **alloy** is a metallic substance formed by the fusion of two or more metals. Restorative dental materials use alloys instead of single elements alone because the combination of metals provides more suitable properties.

A **Gold Inlay** is a restoration that is made from gold alloy contained within the boundaries of a tapered cavity preparation. **Gold alloy** consists of a combination of Gold (Au), **copper** (Cu), **silver** (Ag), **palladium** (Pd) and other **trace metals**.

Charting Single-Surface Gold Inlay and Gold Foil Restorations on an Anatomic Chart

The photograph in Plate 1 shows tooth #31 with a single-surface Gold Inlay restoration that involves the Occlusal tooth surface. This restoration appears as a radiopaque image on the dental radiograph (Figure 6–1). When the Silver Amalgam restoration on tooth #3 and the Gold restoration on tooth #31 are compared on the dental radiograph, it is difficult to determine the difference between the two restorative materials from the radiograph alone because they both appear radiopaque and show the same degree of color. When charting from a radiograph alone, the radiopaque image and presence of an undercut cavity preparation indicates a Silver Amalgam restoration and a tapered cavity preparation signifies a Gold Inlay.

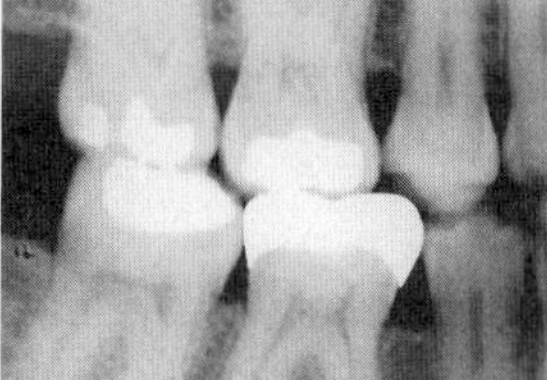

Universal System
#2 #3 #4
#31 #30 #29

Palmer System
7| 6| 5|
7| 6| 5|

ISO/FDI System
17 16 15
47 46 45

Figure 6–1 Bitewing radiograph shown with Silver Amalgam restorations on teeth #2 and #3, a Gold Onlay restoration on tooth #30, and a Gold Inlay restoration on tooth #31 that appear as radiopaque images

Figure 6–2 shows a photograph of a typodont with a Class V Gold Foil restoration on tooth #27 that would appear radiopaque on a dental radio-

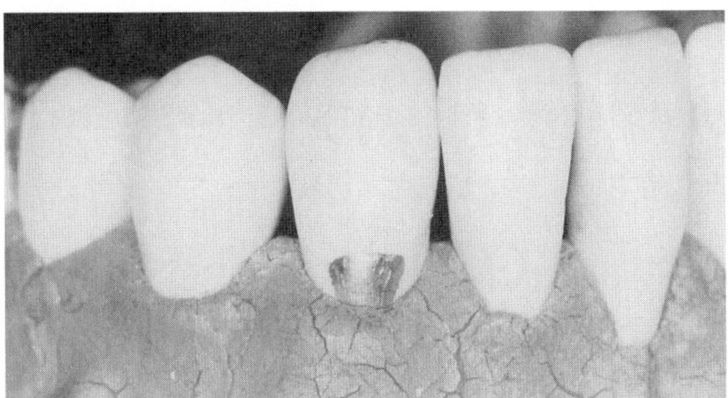

Universal System
#29 #28 #27 #26 #25

Palmer System
5| 4| 3| 2| 1|

ISO/FDI System
45 44 43 42 41

Figure 6–2 Class V Gold Foil restoration shown on tooth #27

graph. From a clinical evaluation, a Gold Foil restoration is distinguished from a Gold alloy restoration by its color. Pure gold has a rich yellow color and Gold Foil is formed from high-purity Gold and appears yellow in color. Gold-based alloys consist of >50%–75% gold (Type I gold alloy, 76% wt and Type II, 56% wt) and a combination of other metals that tend to lighten the color of the alloy, making them appear less yellow and more white in color.

To record an Occlusal Gold Inlay on tooth #31 on an anatomic chart, locate the tooth notation number and with a blue pencil on only the Occlusal surface view, outline the involved area and draw diagonal lines inside of it. An Occlusal Gold Inlay on tooth #31 is written with the primary code for the Occlusal surface "O" first followed by a hyphen (-) and then the secondary code "G" for Gold (O-G) and is read as Occlusal Gold Inlay (Figure 6–3).

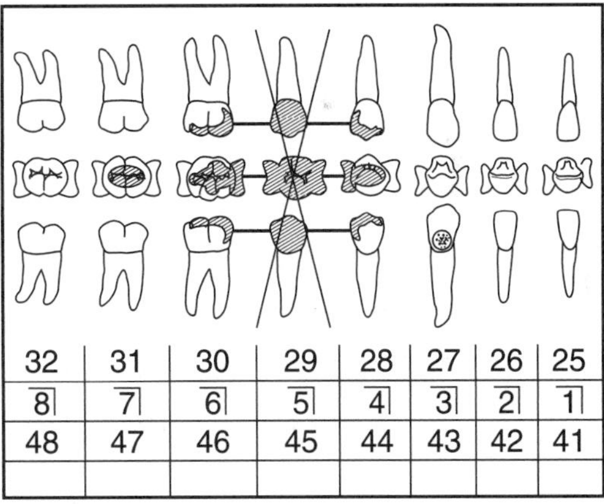

Figure 6–3 Anatomic chart shown with a Gold Foil restoration on tooth #27, abutment teeth #28 and #30 have multiple-surface Gold Inlay restorations, tooth #29 is Missing and replaced with a Gold Pontic Crown, and tooth #31 has a single-surface Gold Inlay restoration

To indicate a Gold Foil restoration is present on the Facial surface of tooth #27, follow the same procedure for charting a Gold Inlay, and instead of diagonal lines place dots within the designated area. The Gold Foil restoration in Figure 6–3 is written in the progress notes as F-G•. The primary code for Facial surface is the uppercase letter "F" and the secondary code for Gold is "G," a superscript dot "•" indicates Foil, and this is read as a Facial Gold Foil restoration.

Charting Single-Surface Gold Inlay and Gold Foil Restorations on a Geometric Chart

When using a geometric chart to indicate Gold Inlay and Gold Foil restorations, locate the tooth notation numbers and use a blue pencil to completely outline the involved tooth surfaces. Draw diagonal lines within the outlined area on tooth #31 to indicate a Gold Inlay and place dots in the outlined area on tooth #27 to represent a Gold Foil restoration (Figure 6–4). Use the same primary and secondary codes for naming these restorations on the geometric chart that were used for the anatomic chart.

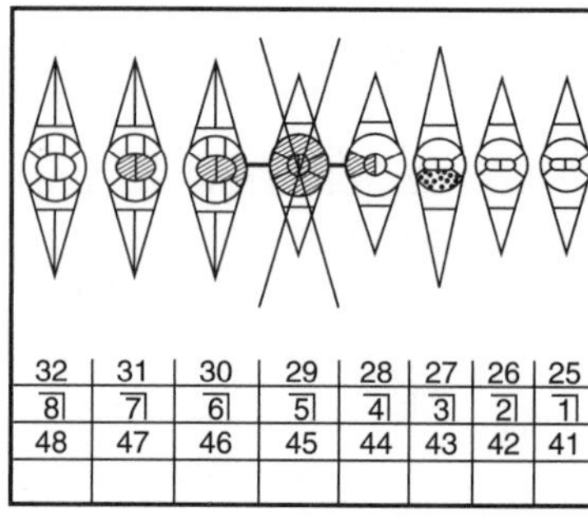

Figure 6–4 Geometric chart shown with a Gold Foil restoration on tooth #27, abutment teeth #28 and #30 have multiple-surface Gold Inlay restorations, tooth #29 is Missing and replaced with a Gold Pontic Crown, and tooth #31 has a single-surface Gold Inlay restoration

Charting Single-Surface Gold Inlay and Gold Foil Restorations on a Numeric Coding System Chart

To indicate tooth #31 has a Gold Inlay and tooth #27 has a Gold Foil restoration on a numeric coding system chart, use a black pen to enter the date in the appropriate column. In the row adjacent to the date beneath the designated tooth number, use a blue pencil to print the primary code followed by a hyphen (-) then the secondary code in uppercase letters. To indicate a Gold Foil, draw a superscript dot after the secondary code (F-G•). The numeric coding system chart in Figure 6–5 would read: on 7-21-95 tooth #31 had an Occlusal Gold Inlay and tooth #27 had a Facial Gold Foil restoration placed.

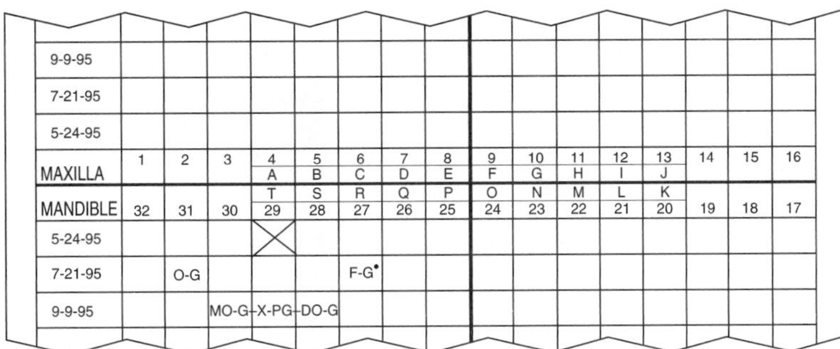

Figure 6–5 Numeric coding system chart indicates a Gold Foil restoration on tooth #27, abutment teeth #28 and #30 have multiple-surface Gold Inlay restorations, tooth #29 is Missing and replaced with a Gold Pontic Crown, and tooth #31 has a single-surface Gold Inlay restoration

Charting Multiple-Surface Gold Inlay Restorations on an Anatomic Chart

The photograph in Figure 6–6A shows two Gold Inlay restorations placed on teeth #28 and #30 that serve as the abutment teeth to support the Pontic used to replace the Missing tooth, #29. The bitewing radiograph in Figure 6–6B shows the two-surface Gold Inlay restorations and the tooth Pontic as radiopaque images.

To chart multiple-surface Gold Inlay restorations attached to a tooth Pontic on an anatomic dental chart, use a blue pencil and above tooth #29 cross out the tooth diagram to indicate the tooth is Missing. On this diagram outline

Universal System
#31 #30 #28 #27

Palmer System
7┐ 6┐ 4┐ 3┐

ISO/FDI System
47 46 44 43

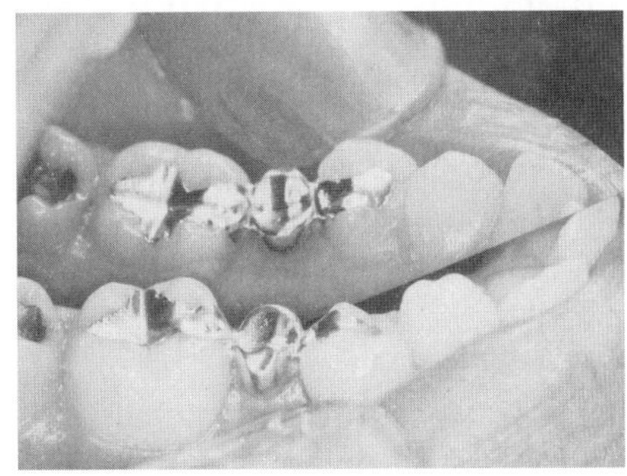

A.

Figure 6–6 (A) Photograph shown of abutment teeth #28 and #30 with Gold Inlay restorations and tooth #29 is Missing and replaced with a Gold Pontic Crown (Courtesy Olsen Dental)

all three anatomic views and fill in the areas completely with diagonal lines to indicate a Gold Crown Pontic has replaced the Missing tooth. To indicate the Pontic is fused to the adjacent abutment teeth, draw three short horizontal lines that extend out from the Mesial and Distal sides of each view of the tooth diagram and connect them to the same three views of the adjacent teeth, teeth #28 and #30. Then follow the same procedure used for charting a single-surface Gold Inlay restoration with the exception that the restorations will be drawn on all of the anatomic views instead of only one (see Figure 6–3).

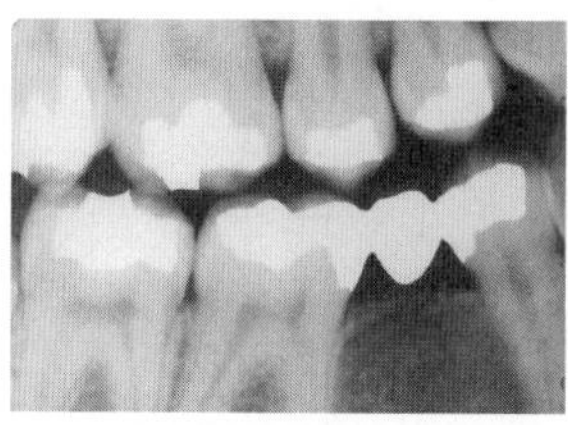

B.

Universal System
#2 #3 #4 #5
#31 #30 #28

Palmer System
7| 6| 5| 4|
7| 6| 4|

ISO/FDI System
17 16 15 14
47 46 44

Figure 6–6 (B) Bitewing radiograph showing multiple-surface Gold Inlay restorations attatched to a Pontic and all restorations appear radiopaque (Courtesy Olsen Dental)

The existing restorations are written as MO-G • X-PG • DO-G and are read as: abutment tooth #28 has a Disto-Occlusal Gold Inlay restoration, and also tooth #29 is Missing and has a Pontic made of Gold, and also abutment tooth #30 has a Mesio-Occlusal Gold Inlay restoration.

Charting Multiple-Surface Gold Inlay Restorations on a Geometric Chart

To chart the restorations shown in Figure 6–6 A on a geometric chart, locate tooth #29 and use a blue pencil to cross out the schematic diagram of the tooth. On the diagram, outline the outer circle in blue pencil and completely fill in the area with diagonal lines. Draw two short horizontal lines extended from the Mesial and Distal tooth surfaces attached to the tooth surfaces of the adjacent teeth. To chart the Gold Inlay restorations present on teeth #28 and #30, outline the involved tooth surfaces and fill in the areas with diagonal lines (see Figure 6–4). These restorations are written and read in the same manner as when using an anatomic chart.

Charting Multiple-Surface Gold Inlay Restorations on a Numeric Coding System Chart

To indicate that teeth #28 and #30 have Gold Inlay restorations and tooth #29 is Missing and has a Gold Pontic on a numeric coding system chart, enter the date, 9-9-95, using black ink in the designated column. Locate the tooth notation numbers, #28 and #30, and in the row of boxes below them use a blue pencil to print the primary codes of the involved tooth surfaces that have been restored followed by a hyphen (-), then print the secondary code. Figure 6–5 indicates that on 5-24-95 tooth #29 was marked Missing and on 9-9-95 the tooth was replaced with a Gold Pontic attached to abutment tooth #28 with a Disto-Occlusal Gold Inlay and attached to abutment tooth #30 with a Mesio-Occlusal Gold Inlay restoration.

The numeric coding system chart does not show the involved tooth surfaces outlined and filled in with diagonal lines that would help identify the restoration as a Gold Inlay. However, it can be ascertained that the restoration is a Gold Inlay and not a Gold Onlay or Crown based on the number of primary codes used to identify the tooth surfaces and the use of the secondary code "G" for Gold.

Review Questions

True or False

Directions: Select the letter of the choice that *best* answers the question.

1. Gold Foil restorations appear whiter in color than do Gold Inlay restorations. T or F
2. Gold Inlay restorations are charted using diagonal lines. T or F
3. Gold Foil restorations are used more frequently today than Gold Inlay restorations. T or F
4. Type I Gold is less than 30% wt. T or F
5. Type I and Type II alloys are used to make Gold Inlay restorations. T or F
6. All three views are used when charting an Occlusal Gold Inlay restoration on an anatomic chart. T or F

7. Gold Inlay restorations are charted on a numeric coding system chart using a black pen. T or F
8. Gold Foil restorations are outlined in blue pencil and filled in with blue dots. T or F
9. The secondary code "P" stands for Pontic. T or F
10. Gold Inlay restorations always cover the cusps of a posterior restoration. T or F

Answers

1. **F,** 2. **T,** 3. **F,** 4. **F,** 5. **T,** 6. **F,** 7. **F,** 8. **T,** 9. **T,** 10. **F**

References

Corbin, S. B., & Kohn, W. G. (1994). The benefits and risks of dental amalgam: Current findings reviewed. *Journal of the American Dental Association*, 125, 381–388.

Dorland's pocket medical dictionary (28th ed.). (1994) Philadelphia: W. B. Saunders Company.

Jendresen, M. D., Allen, E. P., Bayne, S. C., Hansson, T. L., Klooster, J., & Preston, J. D. (1992). Report of the committee on scientific investigation of the American Academy of Restorative Dentistry. *Journal of Prosthetic Dentistry*, 68 (1) 137–180.

Small, K., Goldfogel, M., & Hicks, M. (1988). Marginal finishing for cast gold restorations: Reciprocal-action instrumentation. *Journal of Prosthetic Dentistry*, 58, 632–636.

Thomas, C. L. (1997). *Taber's cyclopedic medical dictionary*. Philadelphia: F. A. Davis Company.

CHAPTER 7

Gold Onlay Restorations

Key Terms

Cusp Coverage
Cusps
Gold Onlay

PRIMARY CODE	SECONDARY CODE
M = Mesial O = Occlusal (#1–#5, #12–#16, #17–#21, & #27–#32) D = Distal B = Buccal (#1–#5, #12–#16, #17–#21, & #27–#32) L = Lingual	-G = Gold Inlay (blue diagonal lines) -G = Gold Onlay (blue diagonal lines) • = and also

Introduction

A restoration that covers the **cusps** and the Occlusal surfaces of posterior teeth is referred to as **Gold Onlay**. A modification of the design of the Gold Inlay restoration, the Gold Onlay restoration extends over the cusps on the Occlusal surface and onto the Buccal and Lingual tooth surfaces (Figure 7–1A).

Universal System
#31 #30 #29 #28
Palmer System
7| 6| 5| 4|
ISO/FDI System
47 46 45 44

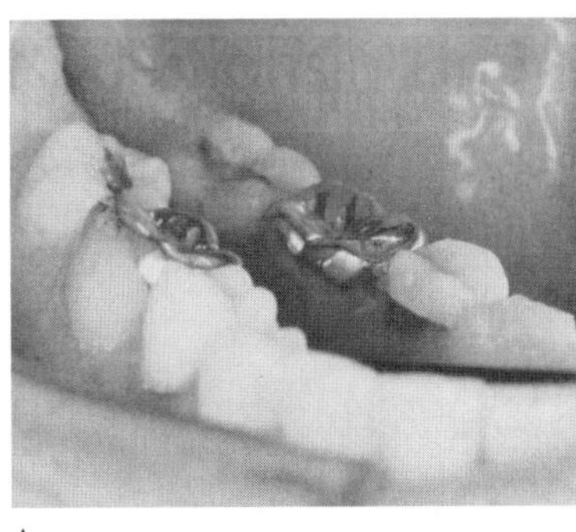

A.

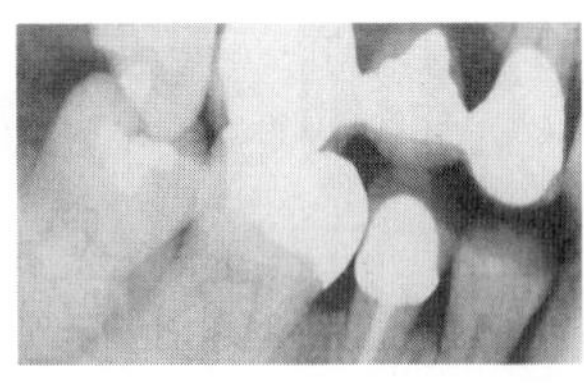

B.

Universal System
#2 #3 #5
#31 #30 #29 #28
Palmer System
7| 6| 4|
7| 6| 5| 4|
ISO/FDI System
17 16 14
47 46 45 44

Figure 7–1 (A) Photograph shown of tooth #30 with a Gold Onlay restoration (B) Bitewing radiograph showing a four-surface Gold Onlay restoration that appears radiopaque

Cusp coverage helps protect the teeth from fractures that may result due to excessive applied chewing forces. The bitewing radiograph shows that the Gold Inlay restoration covers the cusps, involves the Mesial proximal tooth surface, and it appears as a radiopaque image (Figure 7–1B).

Charting Gold Onlay Restorations on an Anatomic Chart

In Figure 7–2 and Plate 2 teeth #28 and #29 have Gold Onlay restorations that involve both Mesial and Distal proximal tooth surfaces and in Figure 7–1A and B, tooth #30 has a Gold Onlay restoration that only involves the Mesial proximal tooth surface. To chart these Gold Onlay restorations on an anatomic chart, locate the designated tooth numbers, and with a blue pencil outline the involved tooth surfaces and fill in the areas with diagonal lines and use all three views. Because the restorations extend

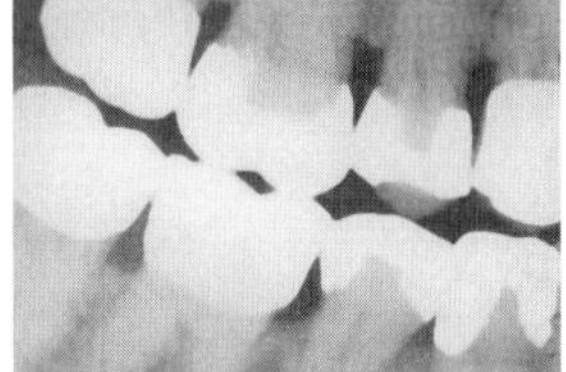

Universal System
#2 #3 #4 #5
#31 #30 #29 #28
Palmer System
7| 6| 5| 4|
7| 6| 5| 4|
ISO/FDI System
17 16 15 14
47 46 45 44

Figure 7–2 Bitewing radiograph showing the five-surface Gold Onlay restorations appear as radiopaque images

over the cusps onto the Buccal and Lingual tooth surfaces, it is necessary to include these areas and draw them just as they appear clinically (Figure 7–3).

On the Occlusal surface view of teeth #28 and #29, the Mesial and Distal tooth surfaces that face the Buccal view are only partially outlined and filled in to duplicate the way the restoration appears in the mouth. Place the secondary code "G" for Gold in the designated box above or below the tooth notation numbers.

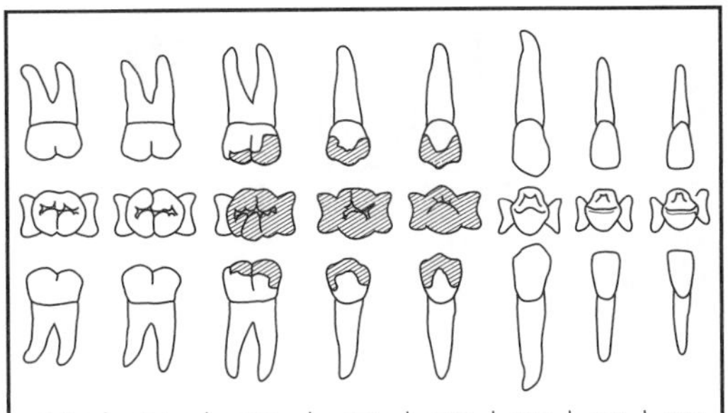

32	31	30	29	28	27	26	25
8	7	6	5	4	3	2	1
32	31	30	29	28	27	26	25
		G	G	G			

Figure 7–3 Anatomic chart shown with Gold Onlay restorations on teeth #28, #29, and #30

The restorations on teeth #28 and #29 are written with the primary codes "MOD-BL" followed by a hyphen (-), then the secondary code "G" for Gold. They are read as Mesio-Occluso-Disto-Bucco-Lingual Gold Onlay restorations. The restoration on tooth #30 is written as MOBL-G and read as Mesio-Occluso-Bucco-Lingual Gold Onlay restoration.

Charting Gold Onlay Restorations on a Geometric Chart

To chart the Gold Onlay restorations that are present on teeth #28, #29, and #30 on a geometric chart, locate the tooth designation numbers and use a blue pencil to completely outline the involved tooth surfaces; then fill in the outlined areas with diagonal lines. Place the secondary code "G" for Gold in the designated box located above or below the tooth notation numbers. The appearance of a five-surface Gold Onlay restoration when drawn on a geometric chart appears the same as a full cast Crown made of Gold so it is necessary to use the secondary code for all Gold Onlay restorations (Figure 7–4). The restorations are written and read the same as previously described for an anatomic chart.

Charting Gold Onlay Restorations on a Numeric Coding System Chart

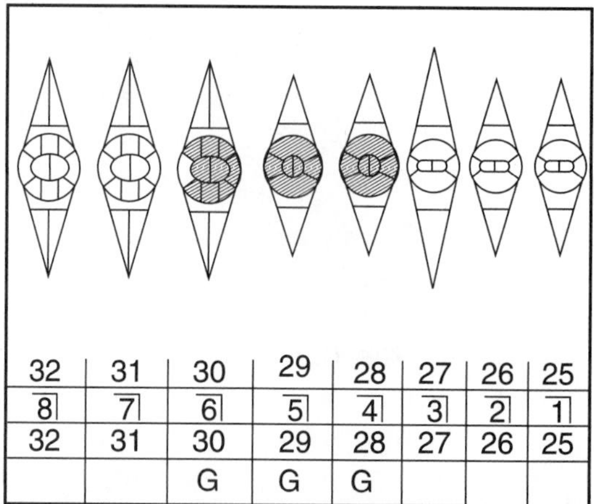

Figure 7–4 Geometric chart shown with Gold Onlay restorations on teeth #28, #29, and #30

To indicate that Gold Onlay restorations exist on teeth #28, #29, and #30, enter the date in the designated column in black ink. Locate the tooth notation numbers, and in the box below use a blue pencil to print the primary codes of the involved tooth surfaces followed by the secondary code. The numeric coding system chart indicates that on 6-12-96 teeth #28 and #29 had MODBL Gold Onlay restorations placed and tooth #30 had a MOBL Gold Onlay restoration placed (Figure 7–5).

The numeric coding system chart does not show the involved tooth surfaces outlined and filled in with diagonal lines that would help identify the restoration as a Gold Onlay. However, it can be ascertained that the restoration is a Gold Onlay and not a Gold Crown based on the number of primary codes used to identify the tooth surfaces and the use of the secondary code "G" for Gold.

6-12-96																
MAXILLA	1	2	3	4 A	5 B	6 C	7 D	8 E	9 F	10 G	11 H	12 I	13 J	14	15	16
MANDIBLE	32	31	30	T 29	S 28	R 27	Q 26	P 25	O 24	N 23	M 22	L 21	K 20	19	18	17
6-12-96			MOBL-G	MODBL-G	MODBL-G											

Figure 7–5 Numeric coding system chart shown with Gold Onlay restorations on teeth #28, #29, and #30

Review Questions

True or False

Directions: Select the letter of the choice that *best* answers the question.

1. Gold Onlay restorations always cover the cusp tips. T or F
2. The letter "g" is used as a secondary code for a Gold Onlay restoration. T or F
3. All three views are used when charting on a geometric chart. T or F
4. The secondary code for Gold to indicate a Gold Onlay restoration is always placed in the box below or above the designated tooth number. T or F
5. To indicate a Gold Onlay restoration on an anatomic chart, outline the restoration and fill it in with dots and label it "G." T or F
6. The numeric coding system chart indicates a Gold Onlay restoration with the secondary codes "GO." T or F
7. Gold Onlay restorations are made from Gold alloy. T or F
8. The cusps are covered on a Gold Onlay restoration to protect them from fracturing. T or F
9. All three views are used to chart a Gold Onlay restoration when using an anatomic chart. T or F
10. Gold Onlay restorations appear radiolucent on a dental radiograph. T or F

Answers

1. **T,** 2. **F,** 3. **F,** 4. **T,** 5. **F,** 6. **F,** 7. **T,** 8. **T,** 9. **T,** 10. **F**

References

Dorland's Pocket Medical Dictionary (28th ed.). (1994). Philadelphia: W. B. Saunders Company.

Jendresen, M. D., Allen, E. P., Bayne, S. C., Hansson, T. L., Klooster, J., & Preston, J. D. (1992). Report of the committee on scientific investigation of the American Academy of Restorative Dentistry. *The Journal of Prosthetic Dentistry*, 68 (1), 137–180.

Small, K., Goldfogel, M., & Hicks, M. (1988). Marginal finishing for cast gold restorations: Reciprocal-action instrumentation. *Journal of Prosthetic Dentistry*, 58, 632–636.

Thomas, C. L. (1997). *Taber's cyclopedic medical dictionary*. Philadelphia: F. A. Davis Company.

CHAPTER 8

Dental Crowns

Key Terms

Aluminum Shell Crowns
Crown
Full Cast Crown
Gold Crowns
Non-Precious Metal Crown
Partial Cast Crown
Pin-Pontic
Stainless Steel Crown
Steeles-Facing
Three-Quarter Crown
Tin-Silver Crown
Tru-Pontic
Veneer Crown

PRIMARY CODE	SECONDARY CODE
C = Crown	-G = Gold (blue diagonal lines)
	-H = Porcelain
	-N = Non-precious (blue cross-hatch)
	-P = Pontic
	-Q = Three-Quarter
	-Z = Temporary Restoration
	• = and also

Introduction

When a portion of the anatomic crown of a tooth is damaged or absent due to disease, chemical or mechanical impact, or fracture, an artificial covering made from Gold, Non-precious metal, or acrylic can be fabricated to replace the Missing tooth structures. A **Crown** is a restoration that covers the surfaces of the tooth normally covered with enamel.

There are three types of Crowns in common use today. The **full cast Crown** is a custom-made precision cast Crown made of precious, semi-precious, or Non-precious alloys that covers the entire anatomic crown of the tooth. The **partial cast Crown** covers three or more surfaces of the tooth and can be fabricated from the same materials as a full cast Crown. The **veneer Crown** also referred to as Porcelain-Fused-To-Metal-Crown consists of a full cast Crown covered partially or completely with a thin layer (veneer) of ceramic material (described in Chapter 9).

Type III Gold alloys are used to fabricate cast **Gold Crowns** and **Three-Quarter Crowns**. These alloys appear more yellow gold in color because they do not contain platinum (Pt), unlike the Type I and II alloys that are used to cast Gold Inlay and Gold Onlay restorations.

In Plate 2 and Figure 7–2, tooth #31 is shown with a full cast Gold Crown that appears radiopaque on the dental radiograph. It is difficult to differentiate between a full Gold Crown and a Three-Quarter Gold Crown on a dental radiograph. The Three-Quarter Gold Crown shown in Figure 11–2A is shown with all of the tooth surfaces covered in Gold except the Facial surface, which consists of natural tooth structure. On the dental radiograph in Figure 11–2B, the restoration appears as a radiopaque image and it is difficult to distinguish this restoration from a full cast Crown because it appears to have the same tooth structures covered as does the full Crown in Figure 7–2.

Another type of Gold Crown that appears similar to the Three-Quarter Crown is a full cast Gold Crown with a Porcelain or acrylic veneer facing (Figure 8–1A and B).

In this restoration, the Gold Crown has a single slot or groove on the Facial surface in which the facing is fastened to and this facing is referred to as

Universal System
#3 #6

Palmer System
6| 3|

ISO/FDI System
16 13

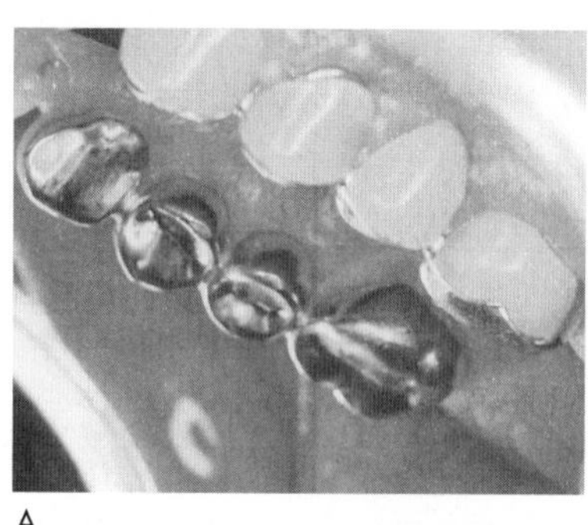

A.

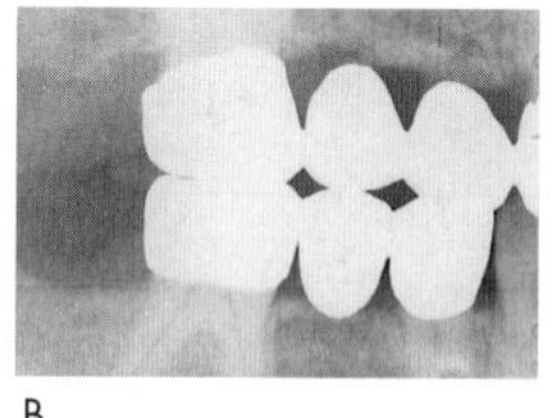

B.

Universal System
#3 #6
#30 #28 #27

Palmer System
6| 3|
6| 4| 3|

ISO/FDI System
16 13
46 44 43

Figure 8–1 (A) Photograph shown of a fixed partial denture with abutment teeth #3 and #6 with full cast Crowns made of Gold with Porcelain veneer facings (Steeles-facings) and Missing teeth #4 and #5 replaced with tru-pontics (B) Bitewing radiograph of teeth #3, #4, #5, and #6 shown as a fixed partial denture that appears as a radiopaque image

Steeles-facing. This type of veneer facing Crown system can utilize two types of artificial tooth Pontics to replace a Missing tooth, the **tru-pontic** has a single slot and the **pin-pontic** has two pins to secure the facing to.

In Figure 8–1B the bitewing radiograph shows the fixed partial denture that is made of full cast Crowns with veneer facings that appear as radiopaque images. When this radiograph is compared to the radiograph of the Three-Quarter Gold Crown in Figure 11–2B, they appear similar and it would be difficult to determine one from another from a radiograph alone.

The metals and alloys used as substitutes for Type III Gold alloys are cast nickel-chromium alloys, which are used to fabricate **Non-precious metal Crowns**. Restorations made from Non-precious alloys appear more silver in color.

The Non-precious metal Crown on tooth #30 shown in Plate 2 and Figure 7–2 appears silver in color and is radiopaque. When a comparison is made on the dental radiograph in Figure 7–2 of the full cast Gold Crown on tooth #31 and the Non-precious metal Crown on tooth #30 they both show the same degree of white.

Wrought stainless steel alloys are used to manufacture **stainless steel Crowns**. In general, **aluminum shell Crowns**, **tin-silver Crowns**, and stainless steel Crowns are preformed and not cast. These Crowns are most often used for Temporary Crown and bridge restorations and for the restoration of Deciduous teeth, which will eventually be exfoliated.

Figure 8–2A and B show tooth #3 with an aluminum shell Crown, which appears as a radiopaque image on the periapical radiograph. The Silver Amalgam restoration located on tooth #2 appears less white in color when compared to the aluminum Crown. The aluminum Crown appears whiter in color when it is compared

Universal System
#2 #3 #4 #5 #6

Palmer System
7| 6| 5| 4| 3|

ISO/FDI System
17 16 15 14 13

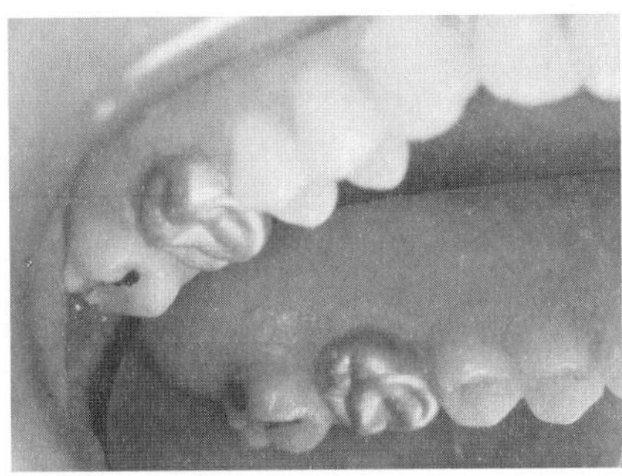

A.

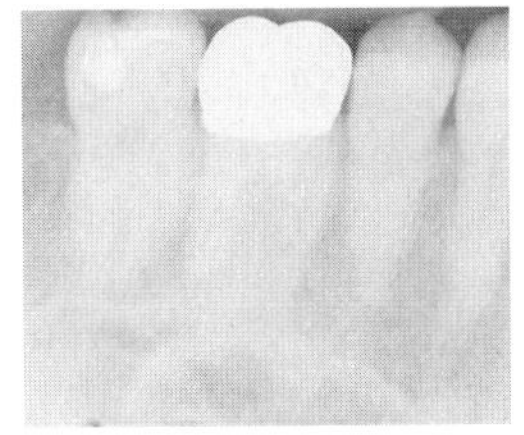

B.

Universal System
#2 #3 #4 #5

Palmer System
7| 6| 5| 4|

ISO/FDI System
17 16 15 14

Figure 8–2 (A) Photograph shown of tooth #3 with a preformed aluminum shell Crown (B) Periapical radiograph that shows the preformed Crown on tooth #3 as a radiopaque image

to the stainless steel Crown shown on the bitewing radiograph in Figure 8–3.

Because the stainless steel Crown is made of less dense material than Silver Amalgam, it allows for a greater penetration of the electromagnetic rays. The Silver Amalgam restoration underneath this Crown is not easily visualized because after the rays penetrate the stainless steel crown, the Silver Amalgam is more dense and permits little or no penetration of the x-ray beam. Because of this the stainless steel Crown is easily identified on a dental radiograph but it will be difficult to distinguish between an aluminum shell Crown and a full cast Gold or Non-precious metal Crown because they show the same degree of white.

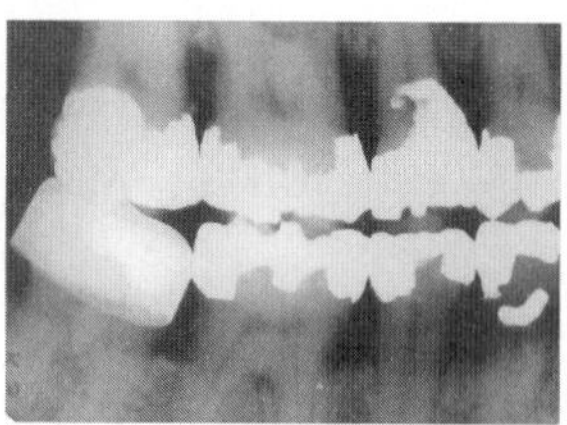

Universal System
#2 #3 #4 #5
#31 #30 #29 #28

Palmer System
7| 6| 5| 4|
7| 6| 5| 4|

ISO/FDI System
17 16 15 14
47 46 45 44

Figure 8–3 Bitewing radiograph shown of tooth #30 with a stainless steel Crown that appears as a radiopaque image

Charting Gold, Non-Precious Metal, and Preformed Metal Crowns on an Anatomic Chart

To chart the Gold Crown on tooth #31 in Plate 2 and Figure 7–2 on an anatomic chart, locate the tooth notation number and use a blue pencil to outline all of the surface views and fill in the areas with diagonal lines to indicate Gold alloy (Figure 8–4).

This restoration is written with the primary code "C" to indicate Crown followed by a hyphen (-), then the secondary code "G" to indicate Gold (C-G). This restoration is read as a Gold Crown on tooth #31.

To chart the Non-precious metal restoration on tooth #30 in Plate 2 and Figure 7–2, locate the tooth number and use a blue pencil to outline all three surface views and completely cross-hatch the area (see Figure 8–4).

This restoration is written with the primary code "C" followed by the secondary code "N" to indicate Non-precious metal (C-N). This restoration on tooth #30 is read as: a Non-precious metal Crown is present.

Aluminum shell, tin-silver, and stainless steel preformed Crowns are charted the same on an anatomic chart. To indicate tooth #3 in Figure 8–2 has a stainless steel Crown, locate the tooth designation number, and with a blue pencil outline all three views and fill in the areas completely.

The restoration is written with the primary code "C" followed by the secondary codes "N" for Non-precious metal and "Z" for Temporary (C-NZ). This restoration is read as: a Temporary Non-precious metal Crown is present on tooth #3.

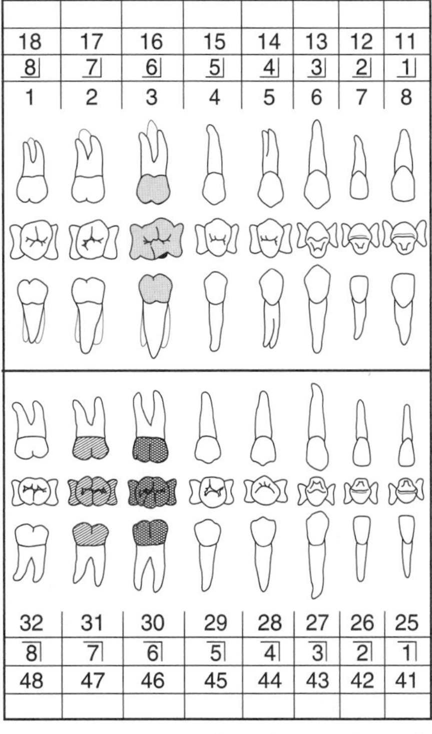

Figure 8–4 Anatomic chart shown with an aluminum shell Crown on tooth #3, a Non-precious metal Crown on tooth #30, and a Gold Crown on tooth #31

Charting Gold, Non-Precious Metal, and Preformed Metal Crowns on a Geometric Chart

To chart the Gold Crown on tooth #31 shown in Plate 2 and Figure 7–2 on a geometric chart, locate the tooth number and use a blue pencil to completely outline the outside circle of the stylized tooth diagram and fill in the area with diagonal lines (Figure 8–5). The restoration on tooth #31 is written and read as previously mentioned for the anatomic chart.

In Figure 8–2 A and B, tooth #30 is shown with a full cast Crown made of Non-precious metal. To show this on a geometric chart, follow the same steps used for the Gold Crown except cross-hatch the outlined area in blue pencil (see Figure 8–5). The restoration is written as C-N and read as: a Non-precious metal Crown is present on tooth #30.

To show the aluminum shell Crown on tooth #3 in Figure 8–2A and B on a geometric chart, follow the directions that were previously mentioned for charting Gold and Non-precious metal Crowns except completely fill in the outlined area. The primary and secondary codes used for describing this restoration are C-NZ and it is read as a Temporary Non-precious metal Crown.

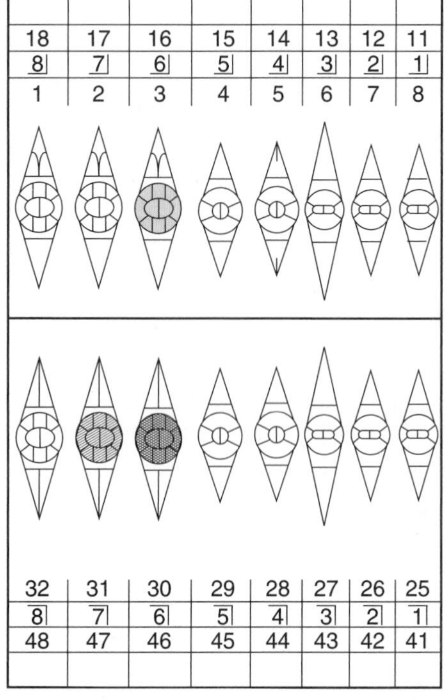

Figure 8–5 Geometric chart shown with an aluminum shell Crown on tooth #3, a Non-precious metal Crown on tooth #30, and a Gold Crown on tooth #31

Charting Gold, Non-Precious Metal, and Preformed Metal Crowns on a Numeric Coding System Chart

The numeric coding system chart in Figure 8–6 indicates a Gold Crown restoration on tooth #31 and a Non-precious Crown on tooth #30 (Plate 2). To record the restoration as a Gold Crown, enter the date in the designated column then in the box below tooth #31, enter the primary code "C" followed by the secondary code "G" (C-G). This is read as: tooth #31 has a Gold Crown (see Figure 8–6).

To indicate that tooth #30 had a Non-precious Crown placed on 6-13-94, record the date in the appropriate area and use the same primary code that was previously used, followed by the secondary code "N" (C-N). This is read as: a Non-precious Crown was placed on tooth #30 on 6-13-94.

To indicate a Temporary preformed Crown exists on tooth #3 as shown in Figure 8–2, enter the date in black ink, and above tooth #3 in blue pencil enter the primary code for Crown, uppercase letter "C," followed by the secondary codes "NZ" (C-NZ). This chart is read as: on 6-13-94 a Temporary Non-precious metal Crown was placed on tooth #3 (see Figure 8–6).

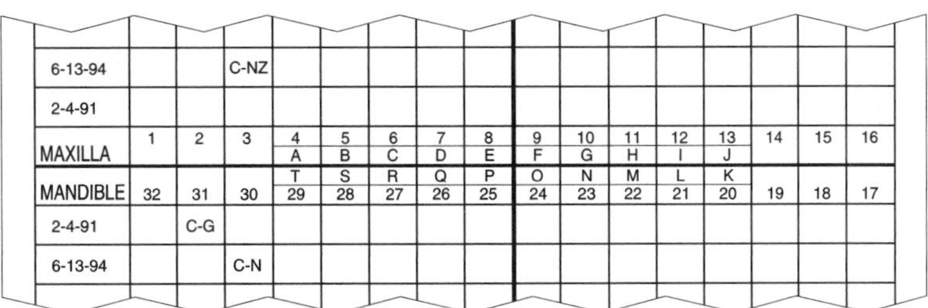

Figure 8–6 Numeric coding system chart shown with an aluminum shell Crown on tooth #3, a Non-precious metal Crown on tooth #30, and a Gold Crown on tooth #31

Review Questions

Matching

Directions: Place the uppercase letter(s) after the number to match each term with the statement that best defines it.

A Aluminum shell Crowns
B Crown
C Full cast Crown
D Gold Crown
E Non-precious metal Crown
F Partial cast Crown
G Pin-pontic
H Stainless steel Crown
I Steeles-facing
J Three-quarter Crown

1. ___ A Crown that consists of three or more tooth surfaces.
2. ___ A prefabricated Crown.
3. ___ The Facial surface consists of natural tooth structure.
4. ___ Charted with diagonal lines on all three views of an anatomic chart.
5. ___ Consists of a single slot or groove.
6. ___ The secondary codes "NZ" are used to describe this restoration.
7. ___ Consists of two pins on an artificial tooth.
8. ___ An artificial replacement that restores Missing tooth structures.
9. ___ This Crown is cast and appears silver.
10. ___ This restoration completely covers all of the tooth surfaces.

Answers

1. **F,** 2. **H** and **A,** 3. **J,** 4. **D,** 5. **I,** 6. **H,** 7. **G,** 8. **B,** 9. **E,** 10. **C**

References

Abbate, M. F., Tjan, A., & Fox, W. (1989). Comparison of the marginal fit of various ceramic crown systems. *Journal of Prosthetic Dentistry*, 61, 527–531.

Asaoka, K., Nuyayama, N., & Tesk, J. A. (1992). Influence of tempering method on residual stress in dental porcelain. *Journal of Dental Research*, 71, 1623.

Bader, J. D., Rozier, R. G., McFall, W. T., & Ramsey, D. L. (1991). Effect of crown margins on periodontal conditions in regularly attending patients. *Journal of Prosthetic Dentistry*, 65, 75–79.

Campbell, S. D. (1989). Evalutation of surface roughness and polishing techniques for new ceramic materials. *Journal of Prosthetic Dentistry*, 61, 563–568.

Castellani, D., Clauser, C., & Bernadini, U. (1994). Thermal distortion of different materials in crown construction. *Journal of Prosthetic Dentistry*, 72, 360–366.

Davis, D. R. (1988). Comparison of fit of two types of all-ceramic crowns. *Journal of Prosthetic Dentistry*, 59, 12–16.

Dorland's Pocket Medical Dictionary (28th ed.). (1994). Philadelphia: W. B. Saunders Company.

Hung, S. H., Hung, K. S., Eick, J. D., & Chappell, R. P. (1990). Marginal fit of porcelain-fused-to-metal and two types of ceramic crown. *Journal of Prosthetic Dentistry*, 63, 26–31.

Jendresen, M. D., Allen, E. P., Bayne, S. C., Hansson, T. L., Klooster, J., & Preston, J. D. (1992). Report of the committee on scientific investigation of the American Academy of Restorative Dentistry. *The Journal of Prosthetic Dentistry*, 68 (1),137–180.

Thomas, C. L. (1997). *Taber's Cyclopedic Medical Dictionary*. Philadelphia: F. A. Davis Company.

CHAPTER 9

Porcelain-Fused-to-Metal Crowns

Key Terms

Porcelain
Porcelain-Fused-To-Metal

PRIMARY CODE	SECONDARY CODE
C = Crown	-G = Gold (blue diagonal lines) -H = Porcelain -N = Non-precious (blue cross-hatch)

Introduction

Dental Crowns made from Gold and Non-precious alloys are most frequently used as posterior restorations. Generally, they are not accepted as anterior restorations because they are not esthetically pleasing. An anterior tooth that requires full coverage is more esthetic if one or more surfaces are covered with **Porcelain**, a ceramic material with a natural tooth-shaded appearance. When Porcelain is bonded to full cast Gold or Non-precious alloys, the restoration is referred to as a **Porcelain-Fused-To-Metal** Crown.

Porcelain-Fused-To-Metal Crowns are used throughout the oral cavity as single- and multiple-tooth restorations (Figure 9–1A and B).

The photograph in Figure 9–1A shows all of the restored tooth surfaces on teeth #13 and #14 covered with Porcelain. On a dental radiograph, it is easy to distinguish a full cast Crown from a Porcelain-Fused-To-Metal Crown

Universal System
#10 #11 #12 #13 #14 #15

Palmer System
|2 |3 |4 |5 |6 |7

ISO/FDI System
22 23 24 25 26 27

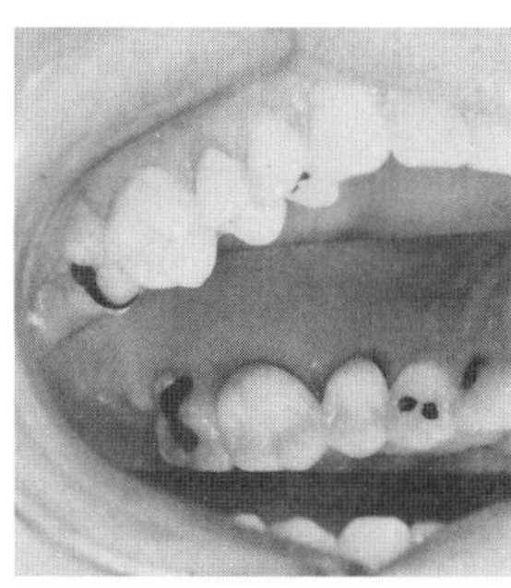

A.

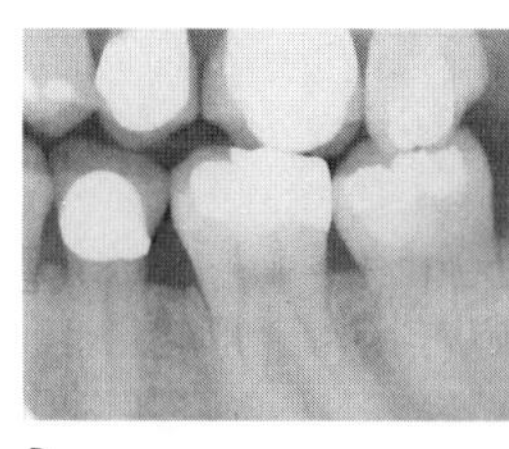

B.

Universal System
#12 #13 #14 #15
#21 #20 #19 #18

Palmer System
|4 |5 |6 |7
|4 |5 |6 |7

ISO/FDI System
24 25 26 27
34 35 36 37

Figure 9–1 (A) Photograph showing Porcelain-Fused-To-Metal Crowns on teeth #13 and #14 (B) Bitewing radiograph of teeth #13 and #14 showing the Porcelain material appears radiolucent and the Non-precious metal alloys appear as radiopaque images

because the Porcelain appears as a radiolucent area that extends away from the cast Crown. The radiograph in Figure 9–1B shows teeth #13 and #14 with Non-precious metal Crowns that appear radiopaque and the Porcelain material appears radiolucent.

Plate 3 shows a three-unit Porcelain-Fused-To-Non-precious metal fixed partial denture. A bitewing radiograph of the same area is shown in Figure 7–1B.

Charting Porcelain-Fused-to-Metal Crowns on an Anatomic Chart

To chart teeth #13 and #14 in Figure 9–1 on an anatomic chart, locate the tooth designation numbers, and with a blue pencil outline all of the tooth surface views and completely fill in the areas with cross-hatched lines. In the box located above the tooth notation number, print the secondary code "H" (Figure 9–2).

		H	H	H								H	H		
18	17	16	15	14	13	12	11	21	22	23	24	25	26	27	28
8|	7|	6|	5|	4|	3|	2|	1|	|1	|2	|3	|4	|5	|6	|7	|8
1	2	3	4	5	6	7	8	9	10	11	12	13	14	15	16

Figure 9–2 Anatomic chart shown with teeth #3, #4, and #5 charted as crowns of a Porcelain-Fused-To-Non-precious-Metal fixed partial denture and teeth #13 and #14 are Porcelain-covered Non-precious metal Crowns

The restorations are written with the primary code "C" followed by a hyphen (-) then the secondary codes "NH" (C-NH). The restorations on teeth #13 and #14 are read as Porcelain-covered Non-precious metal Crowns.

To indicate the Porcelain-covered fixed partial denture in Plate 3 on an anatomic chart, use a blue pencil to cross out tooth #4 then follow the same procedures that were previously mentioned for charting Porcelain-Fused-To-Metal Crowns (see Figure 9–2). Draw three short horizontal lines that extend from the Mesial and Distal surfaces of tooth #4 and connect them to all three surface views of the adjacent teeth #3 and #5, to indicate a fixed partial denture (described in Chapter 11).

The restorations are written as: tooth #3 C-NH, tooth #4 X-PNH, and tooth #5 C-NH. The restorations are read as: teeth #3 and #5 are abutment teeth with Porcelain Fused-To-Non-precious metal Crowns and tooth #4 is Missing and replaced with a Pontic Crown made of Porcelain-covered Non-precious metal.

Charting Porcelain-Fused-To-Metal Crowns on a Geometric Chart

To show the two Porcelain-Fused-To-Metal Crowns in Figure 9–1 and Plate 3 on a geometric chart, locate the tooth designation numbers, and with a blue pencil outline the entire outside circle on the stylized tooth diagram and completely fill in the area with cross-hatched lines. In the box located above each tooth notation number, print the secondary code "H" (Figure 9–3).

To indicate teeth #3, #4, and #5 as a Porcelain-Fused-To-Metal fixed partial denture, locate the tooth notation numbers then follow the procedures previously described for charting these restorations on an anatomic chart (see

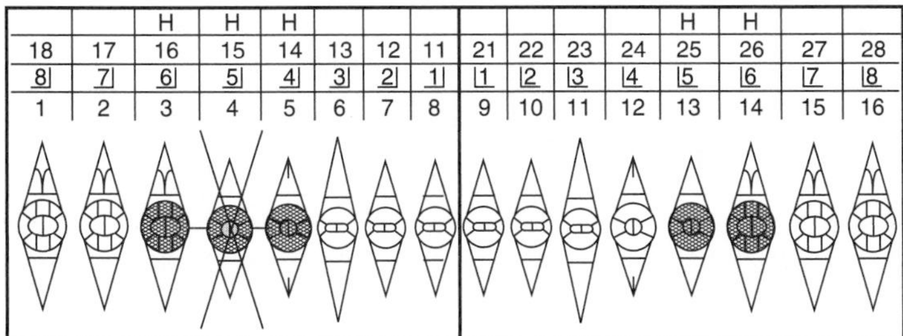

Figure 9–3 Geometric chart shown with teeth #3, #4, and #5 charted as crowns of a Porcelain-Fused-To-Non-precious-Metal fixed partial denture and teeth #13 and #14 are Porcelain-covered Non-precious metal Crowns

Figure 9–2). The restorations are written and read as previously described on the anatomic chart.

Charting Porcelain-Fused-To-Metal Crowns on a Numeric Coding System Chart

To indicate the Porcelain-Fused-To-Metal restorations on teeth #13 and #14 on a numeric coding system chart, enter the date in the designated area with a black pen and in the adjacent row locate boxes above the tooth notation numbers. With a blue pencil, print in each box the primary code "C" followed by a hyphen (-) then the secondary codes "NH" (Figure 9–4).

To show the Porcelain-covered fixed partial denture in Plate 3, follow the same procedure that was previously mentioned for designating Porcelain-Fused-To-Metal Crowns. To indicate that tooth #4 is missing, the primary code "X" is used followed by the secondary codes "PNH" (Figure 9–4). Located on each side of the box that represents tooth #4, draw a short horizontal line through each vertical line to indicate the structures are connected (described in Chapter 11).

This chart is read as: on 12-10-92 teeth #13 and #14 had Porcelain-covered Non-precious metal Crowns placed; on 7-6-95 tooth #4 is Missing and replaced with a Porcelain-Fused-To-Non-precious metal Pontic, and teeth #3 and #5 are abutment teeth with Porcelain-covered Non-precious metal Crowns.

7-6-95			C-NH-	X-PNH-	C-NH											
12-10-92													C-NH	C-NH		
MAXILLA	1	2	3	4 A	5 B	6 C	7 D	8 E	9 F	10 G	11 H	12 I	13 J	14	15	16
MANDIBLE	32	31	30	T 29	S 28	R 27	Q 26	P 25	O 24	N 23	M 22	L 21	K 20	19	18	17
12-10-92																
7-6-95																

Figure 9–4 Numeric coding system chart shown with teeth #3, #4, and #5 charted as Porcelain-Fused-To-Non-precious-Metal crowns of a fixed partial denture and teeth #13 and #14 are Porcelain-covered Non-precious metal Crowns

Review Questions

True or False

Directions: Select the letter of the choice that *best* answers the question.

1. Porcelain can only be fused to Non-precious metals. T or F
2. Porcelain-covered Crowns are used on anterior and posterior teeth. T or F
3. A Missing tooth is charted on an anatomic chart with two horizontal lines. T or F
4. The primary code for Porcelain is the letter "H." T or F
5. Pontic is indicated by the secondary code "P." T or F
6. Diagonal lines represent Non-precious metal alloys. T or F
7. Crowns are represented on an anatomic chart by using all three views. T or F
8. Crowns are represented on a numeric coding system chart with the code "C." T or F
9. Porcelain-Fused-To-Metal Crowns are esthetically pleasing. T or F
10. Porcelain must be fused to four or more tooth surfaces to be durable. T or F

Answers

1. **F**, 2. **T**, 3. **F**, 4. **F**, 5. **T**, 6. **F**, 7. **T**, 8. **T**, 9. **T**, 10. **F**

References

Abbate, M. F., Tjan, A., & Fox, W. (1989). Comparison of the marginal fit of various ceramic crown systems. *Journal of Prosthetic Dentistry*, 61, 527–531.

Bader, J. D., Rozier, R. G., McFall, W. T., & Ramsey, D. L. (1991). Effect of crown margins on periodontal conditions in regularly attending patients. *Journal of Prosthetic Dentistry*, 65, 75–79.

Campbell, S. D. (1989). Evalutation of surface roughness and polishing techniques for new ceramic materials. *Journal of Prosthetic Dentistry*, 61, 563–568.

Castellani, D., Clauser, C., & Bernadini, U. (1994). Thermal distortion of different materials in crown construction. *Journal of Prosthetic Dentistry, 72,* 360–366.

Davis, D. R. (1988). Comparison of fit of two types of all-ceramic crowns. *Journal of Prosthetic Dentistry, 59,* 12–16.

Dorland's pocket medical dictionary (28th ed.). (1994). Philadelphia: W. B. Saunders Company.

Felton, D. A., Bayne, S. C., Kanoy, B. E., & White, J. T. (1991). Effect of air abrasives on marginal configurations of porcelain-fused-to-metal alloys: An SEM analysis. *Journal of Prosthetic Dentistry, 65,* 38–43.

Hung, S. H., Hung, K. S., Eick, J. D., & Chappell, R. P. (1990). Marginal Fit of Porcelain-fused-to-metal and two types of ceramic crown. *Journal of Prosthetic Dentistry, 63,* 26–31.

Jendresen, M. D., Allen, E. P., Bayne, S. C., Hansson, T. L., Klooster, J., & Preston, J. D. (1992). Report of the committee on scientific investigation of the American Academy of Restorative Dentistry. *Journal of Prosthetic Dentistry, 68* (1), 137–180.

Miller, L. M. (1992). Porcelain veneer protection plan: Maintenance procedures for all porcelain restorations. *Journal of Esthetic Dentistry,* 2 (3), 63.

Thomas, C. L. (1997). *Taber's cyclopedic medical dictionary.* Philadelphia: F. A. Davis Company.

CHAPTER 10

Nonmetal Restorative Materials: Glass Ionomer, Composite Resin, Porcelain, and Pit and Fissure Sealants

Key Terms

Acrylic Resin
Composite Resin
Composite Resin Veneer
Glass Ionomer
Pit and Fissure Sealants
Porcelain Inlay
Porcelain Jacket Crown
Porcelain Veneer
Silicate
Temporary Crown

PRIMARY CODE	SECONDARY CODE
M = Mesial	-E = Resin (outline blue)
I = Incisal (#6–#11 & #22–#27)	-H = Porcelain
O = Occlusal (#1–#5, #12–#16, #17–#21, & #27–#32)	-Z = Temporary restoration
D = Distal	• = and also
F = Facial (#6–#11 & #22–#27)	• p = Retention Pin
B = Buccal (#1–#5, #12–#16, #17–#21, & #27–#32)	
L = Lingual	
C = Crown	
V = Virgin	

Introduction

Nonmetal restorative materials are used to repair or replace mottled, abraded, eroded, defective, carious, and fractured tooth structures. These tooth-colored materials are used on anterior and posterior tooth surfaces.

In 1871 the first esthetic restorative material was introduced and called **silicate**, which was later followed by acrylic restorative Resins or **acrylic Resin**. **Glass ionomer** restoratives are extremely versatile dental materials and they are used as cavity liners, dentin bonding systems, luting agents, core materials, and Class III and V restorations. These restorative materials can be made radiopaque by adding metal.

Composite Resin restorative materials are used on Class I, III, IV, and V restorations. Due to the presence of quartz, earlier Resins appeared radiolucent on dental radiographs (Figure 10–1). Later development of composite Resin restorative materials with the addition of special fillers produced a restoration that appeared radiopaque on a dental radiograph and these fillers are used today. The photograph in Figure 10–2A

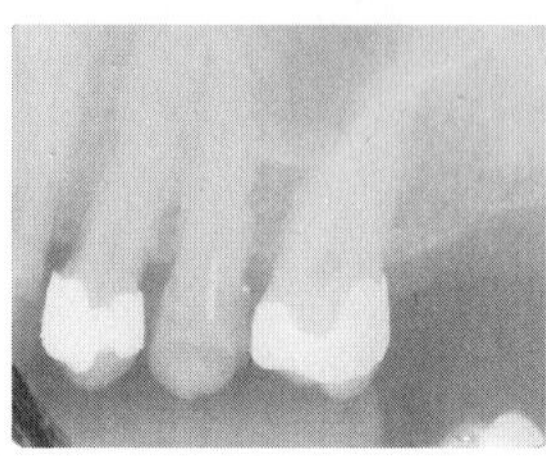

Universal System
#12 #13 #14

Palmer System
|4 |5 |6

ISO/FDI System
24 25 26

Figure 10–1 Periapical radiograph shown with a radiolucent composite Resin restoration with a radiopaque Retention Pin on tooth #13

Universal System
#22 #21 #20 #19 #18

Palmer System
|3 |4 |5 |6 |7

ISO/FDI System
33 34 35 36 37

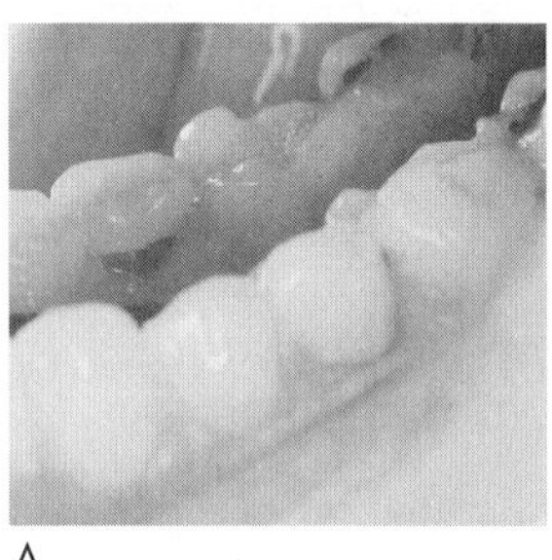

A.

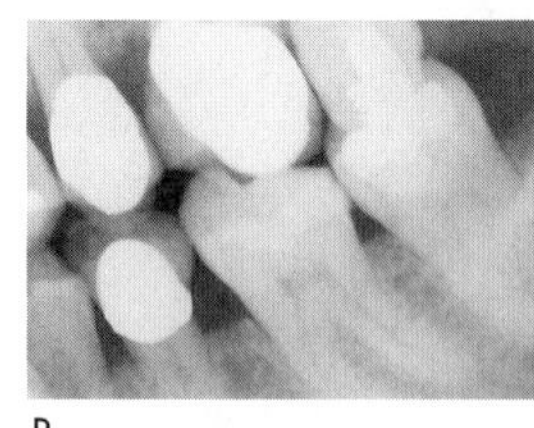

B.

Universal System
#12 #13 #14 #15
#21 #20 #19 #18

Palmer System
|4 |5 |6 |7
|4 |5 |6 |7

ISO/FDI System
24 25 26 27
34 35 36 37

Figure 10–2 (A) Photograph shown with a posterior composite Resin restoration that involves the Distal, Occlusal, and Buccal tooth surfaces on tooth #19 (B) Bitewing radiograph of figure (A) shown with the composite Resin restoration on tooth #19 as a radiopaque image

and the bitewing radiograph in Figure 10–2B show tooth #19 with a composite Resin restoration.

In Figure 10–3A, tooth #7 is shown with a Lingual inclination (linguoversion) and the Distal tooth surface of tooth #8 overlaps the Mesial tooth surface of tooth #7. There is a Class IV Resin restoration involving the Mesial, Incisal, Facial, and Lingual tooth surfaces of tooth #8. The periapical radiograph in Figure 10–3B shows two radiopaque areas on the proximal tooth surfaces of tooth #8.

To distinguish between a radiopaque area caused by the overlap of two teeth and a tooth-colored dental restoration on a dental radiograph, it is necessary to carefully examine the outline where the radiopaque area and the tooth meet. The presence of an undercut indicates a dental restoration. From the evaluation of the dental radiograph alone it is also difficult to establish if either the Facial or Lingual tooth surfaces, or both, have been restored.

The combination of light and chemically activated Resins are used to make **Temporary Crowns**. These Crowns are fabricated in the dental office and transfixed with temporary cement.

Composite Resin veneer is used to restore teeth that have developmental defects, discoloration, or a midline diastema. Veneering is a procedure in which composite Resin is bonded in thin layers to the etched enamel surface of the teeth and reshaped to gain the desired esthetic effect.

Universal System
#6 #7 #8 #9 #10 #11

Palmer System
3| 2| 1| |1 |2 |3

ISO/FDI System
13 12 11 21 22 23

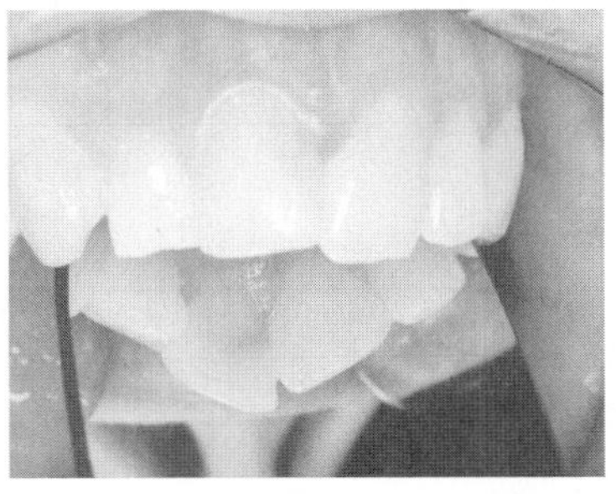

A.

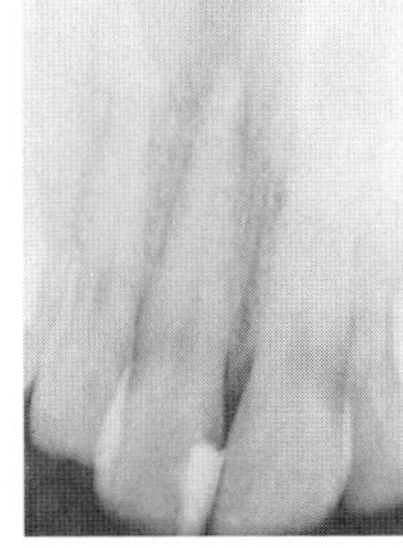

B.

Universal System
#6 #7 #8 #9 #10

Palmer System
3| 2| 1| |1 |2

ISO/FDI System
13 12 11 21 22

Figure 10–3 (A) Photograph shown with an anterior composite Resin restoration that involves the Mesial, Incisal, Facial, and Lingual tooth surfaces on tooth #8 (B) Bitewing radiograph of figure (A) shown with the composite Resin restoration on tooth #8 as a radiopaque image

Charting Glass Ionomer and Composite Resin Restorations on an Anatomic Chart

In Figure 10–2A, tooth #19 has a composite Resin restoration that involves the Distal, Occlusal, and Buccal tooth surfaces and in Figure 10–3A, tooth #8 has a composite Resin restoration that involves the Mesial, Incisal, Facial, and Lingual tooth surfaces. To chart glass ionomer and Resin restorations on an anatomic chart, locate the tooth notation numbers, and with a blue pencil outline the involved areas and use all three views (Figure 10–4).

The restoration on tooth #19 is written as DOB-E and read as a Disto-Occluso-Buccal Resin. The restoration on tooth #8 is written as MIFL-E and read as a Mesio-Inciso-Facio-Lingual Resin.

To chart a Resin veneer restoration, follow the same procedure previously mentioned for charting Resin restorations and follow the rules of dental charting. Figure 10–4 shows a Resin veneer restoration that involves the Facial tooth surface on tooth #24.

To chart a Temporary Resin Crown on an anatomic chart, follow the same procedure for charting Resin restorations except outline all of the tooth sur-

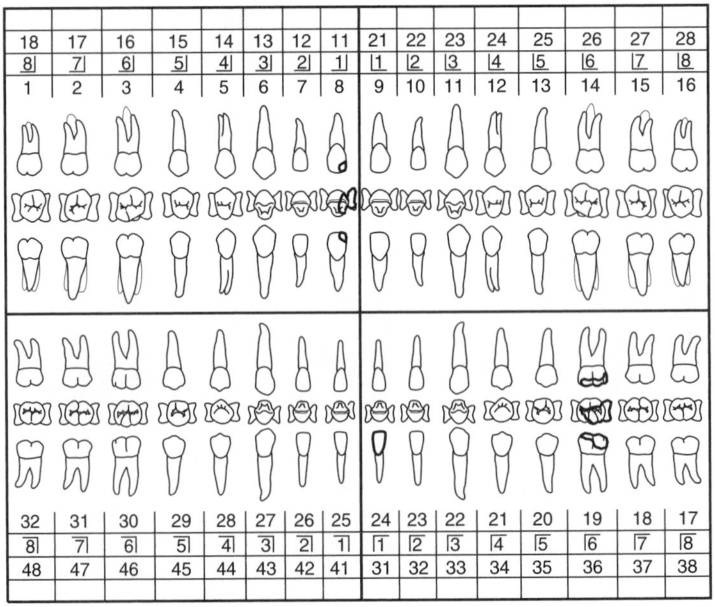

18	17	16	15	14	13	12	11	21	22	23	24	25	26	27	28
8		7		6		5		4		3		2		1			1		2		3		4		5		6		7		8
1	2	3	4	5	6	7	8	9	10	11	12	13	14	15	16

32	31	30	29	28	27	26	25	24	23	22	21	20	19	18	17
8		7		6		5		4		3		2		1			1		2		3		4		5		6		7		8
48	47	46	45	44	43	42	41	31	32	33	34	35	36	37	38

Figure 10–4 Anatomic chart shown with a composite Resin restoration on tooth #8 that involves the Mesial, Incisal, Facial, and Lingual tooth surfaces, a composite Resin restoration on tooth #19 that involves the Distal, Occlusal, and Buccal tooth surfaces, and a Resin veneer restoration on tooth #24 that involves the Facial tooth surface

faces and print the uppercase letter "Z" in the designated box. The Temporary Crown restoration is written with the primary code "C" followed by the secondary codes "EZ" (C-EZ). This is read as Temporary Resin Crown.

Charting Glass Ionomer and Composite Resin Restorations on a Geometric Chart

To chart glass ionomer and composite Resin restorations on a geometric chart, locate the tooth notation numbers, #8 and #19, and with a blue pencil completely outline the involved tooth surfaces. The restoration on tooth #8 involves the Mesial, Incisal, Facial, and Lingual tooth surfaces. When a geometric chart is used, the involved tooth surfaces must be completely outlined whether or not the entire tooth surface actually has a restoration. Tooth #19 has a restoration that involves the Distal, Occlusal, and Buccal tooth surfaces. Because only a small section of the Buccal tooth surface is involved, outline only the first box located on the Buccal view, which indicates one-third of the Buccal tooth surface (Figure 10–5).

To chart a Resin veneer restoration on a geometric chart, follow the same procedure previously mentioned for charting Resin restorations. Figure 10–5

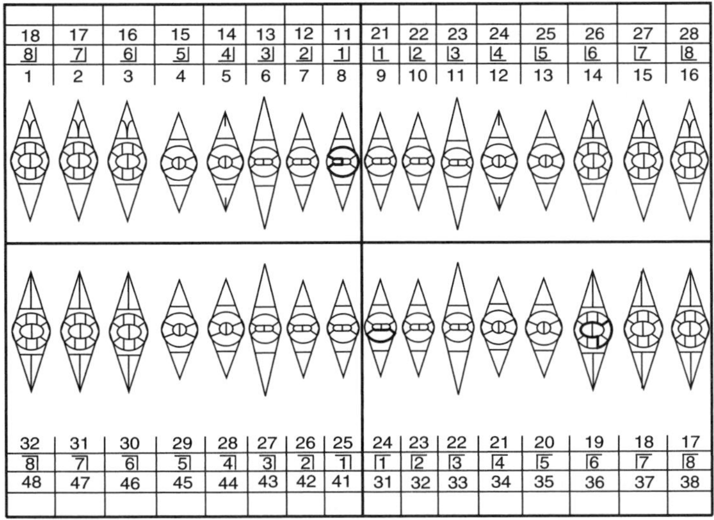

Figure 10–5 Geometric chart shown with a composite Resin restoration on tooth #8 that involves the Mesial, Incisal, Facial, and Lingual tooth surfaces, a composite Resin restoration on tooth #19 that involves the Distal, Occlusal, and Buccal tooth surfaces, and a Resin veneer restoration on tooth #24 that involves the Facial tooth surface

shows a Resin veneer restoration that involves the Facial tooth surface on tooth #24.

To chart a Temporary Resin Crown on a geometric chart, follow the same procedures for charting Resin restorations except outline the entire outer circle and print the uppercase letter "Z" in the designated box. The Temporary Crown restoration is written the same as it was previously described on an anatomic chart.

Charting Glass Ionomer and Composite Resin Restorations on a Numeric Coding System Chart

To show composite Resin restorations are present on teeth #8, #19, and #24 on a numeric coding system chart, use a black pen to enter the date in the specified column. In the rows adjacent to the date entries, locate the tooth notation numbers. With a blue pencil print the letters of the involved tooth surfaces followed by a hyphen (-); then indicate the secondary code for Resin using the uppercase letter "E" (Figure 10–6). The same secondary code is used to indicate glass ionomer restoratives.

Figure 10–6 indicates that on 1-12-95 tooth #8 was restored and shows a MIFL-E, which is read as a Mesio-Inciso-Facio-Lingual Resin; tooth #19 has a DOB-E, which is read as a Disto-Occluso-Buccal Resin; and tooth #24 has an F-E and is read as a Facial Resin restoration.

To chart a Temporary Resin Crown on a numeric coding system chart, enter the date in black ink and use blue pencil to record the appropriate primary and secondary codes above or below the involved tooth notation number. The restoration is written as "C-EZ" and is read as Temporary Resin Crown.

1-12-95								MIFL-E								
MAXILLA	1	2	3	4 A	5 B	6 C	7 D	8 E	9 F	10 G	11 H	12 I	13 J	14	15	16
MANDIBLE	32	31	30	T 29	S 28	R 27	Q 26	P 25	O 24	N 23	M 22	L 21	K 20	19	18	17
1-12-95									F-E					DOB-E		

Figure 10–6 Numeric coding chart that indicates a composite Resin restoration on tooth #8 that involves the Mesial, Incisal, Facial, and Lingual tooth surfaces, a composite Resin restoration on tooth #19 that involves the Distal, Occlusal, and Buccal tooth surfaces, and a Resin veneer restoration on tooth #24 that involves the Facial tooth surface

Porcelain Inlay, Porcelain Veneer, and Porcelain Jacket Crowns

Restorations that are made of Porcelain are constructed outside of the mouth on a working model or die and then they are cemented or bonded into position.

A **Porcelain Inlay** restoration is confined to the tapered cavity preparation and is used for Class III and Class V cavity preparations on anterior and posterior teeth.

A **Porcelain veneer** restoration is bonded with Resin to the etched enamel tooth surfaces. Tooth preparation involves removing some of the Facial and Incisal enamel (Figure 10–7) and some practitioners prefer to continue to remove tooth structure through the contact areas.

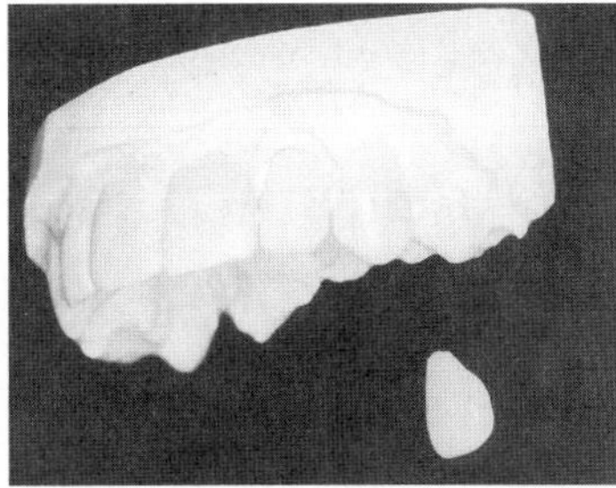

Universal System
#7 #8 #9 #10 #11

Palmer System
2| 1| 1| |2 |3

ISO/FDI System
12 11 21 22 23

Figure 10–7 Plaster model shown with the Facial and Incisal surfaces prepared for the Porcelain veneer restoration on tooth #10

In Figure 10–8A and B Porcelain veneer restorations are shown covering the Incisal and Facial tooth surfaces and each restoration extends through the contact areas on the Mesial and Distal surfaces on teeth #22, #23, #24, #25, #26, and #27. The restorations appear as radiolucent images on the periapical radiograph. Sometimes a thin radiopaque line is visible around the cervical areas of

Universal System
#27 #26 #25 #24 #23 #22

Palmer System
3| 2| 1| |1 |2 |3

ISO/FDI System
43 42 41 31 32 33

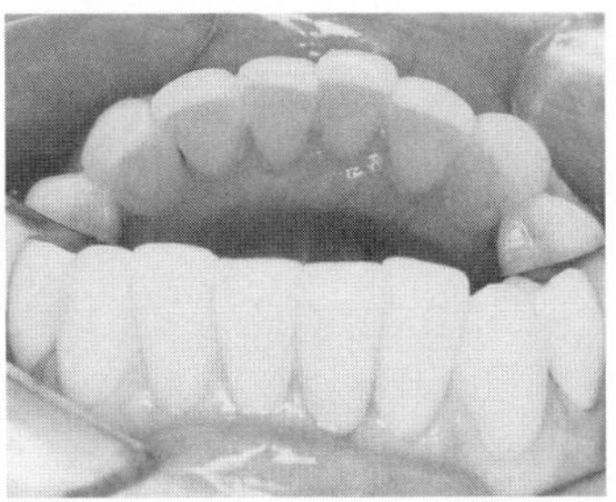

A.

B.

Universal System
#27 #26 #25 #24 #23

Palmer System
3| 2| 1| |1 |2

ISO/FDI System
43 42 41 31 32

Figure 10–8 (A) Photograph shown of Porcelain veneer restorations that involve the Incisal, Facial, and Mesial and Distal tooth surfaces (B) Periapical radiograph showing teeth #22, #23, #24, #25, #26, and #27 appear as radiolucent images (Courtesy Joseph C. Serflek, DDS)

these Resin-bonded veneers that makes them easier to identify. Otherwise, it is often difficult to detect these restorations from radiographs alone.

The **Porcelain jacket Crown** covers the entire coronal portion of the tooth and is used primarily on anterior teeth. In Figure 10–9, the panoramic radiograph shows teeth #6, #7, #8, #9, and #10 with Porcelain jacket Crowns that appear radiolucent. Tooth #8 shows two additional radiopaque areas, the gutta-percha filling within the canal of the root and the Silver Amalgam restoration located on the Lingual tooth surface. The zinc phosphate cement line that surrounds the remaining tooth structure also appears radiopaque.

Charting Porcelain Veneer and Porcelain Jacket Crowns on an Anatomic Chart

To chart the Porcelain veneer restorations in Figure 10–8 on an anatomic chart, locate teeth #22, #23, #24, #25, #26, and #27 and use a blue pencil to outline the involved tooth surfaces on only the Facial and Incisal views and

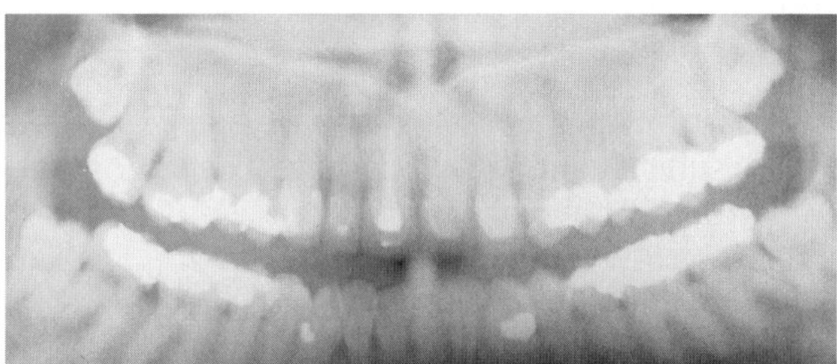

Universal System
#1 #2 #3 #4 #5 #6 #7 #8 #9 #10 #11 #12 #13 #14 #15 #16
#32 #31 #30 #29 #28 #27 #26 #25 #24 #23 #22 #21 #20 #19 #18 #17

Palmer System
8| 7| 6| 5| 4| 3| 2| 1| |1 |2 |3 |4 |5 |6 |7 |8
8| 7| 6| 5| 4| 3| 2| 1| |1 |2 |3 |4 |5 |6 |7 |8

ISO/FDI System
18 17 16 15 14 13 12 11 21 22 23 24 25 26 27 28
48 47 46 45 44 43 42 41 31 32 33 34 35 36 37 38

Figure 10–9 Panoramic radiograph shown with teeth #6, #7, #8, #9, and #10 with Porcelain jacket Crowns that appear as radiolucent images

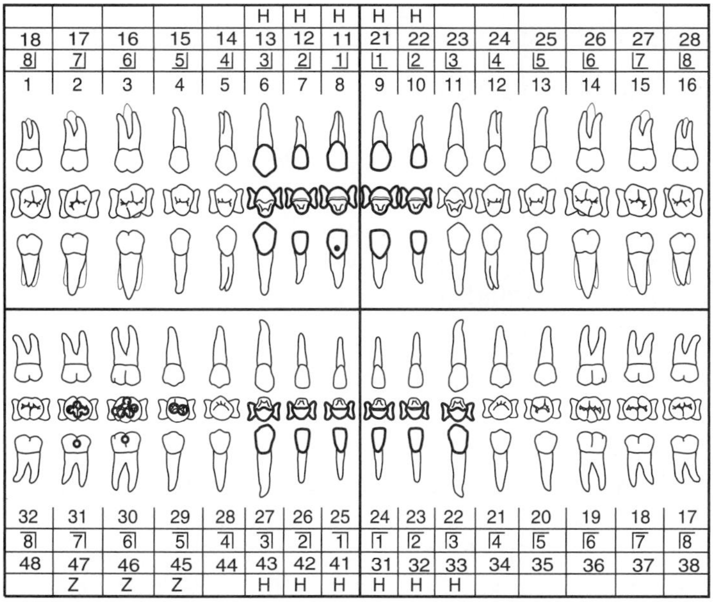

					H	H	H	H	H						
18	17	16	15	14	13	12	11	21	22	23	24	25	26	27	28
8	7	6	5	4	3	2	1	1	2	3	4	5	6	7	8
1	2	3	4	5	6	7	8	9	10	11	12	13	14	15	16
32	31	30	29	28	27	26	25	24	23	22	21	20	19	18	17
8	7	6	5	4	3	2	1	1	2	3	4	5	6	7	8
48	47	46	45	44	43	42	41	31	32	33	34	35	36	37	38
	Z	Z	Z		H	H	H	H	H	H					

Figure 10–10 Anatomic chart with teeth #6, #7, #8, #9, and #10 shown with Porcelain jacket Crowns; teeth #22, #23, #24, #25, #26, and #27 shown with Porcelain veneer restorations; and teeth #29, #30, and #31 shown with pit and fissure sealants

include the Mesial and Distal tooth surfaces. In the box located beneath the tooth notation number, print the secondary code "H" for Porcelain (Figure 10–10).

These restorations are written with the primary codes of the involved tooth surfaces listed first, followed by the secondary code "H." Teeth #22–#27 are written as MIDF-H and are read as Mesio-Inciso-Disto-Facial Porcelain restorations.

In Figure 10–9 teeth #6, #7, #8, #9, and #10 are shown with Porcelain jacket Crowns. To chart these Porcelain jacket Crowns on an anatomic chart, locate the tooth notation numbers and use a blue pencil to outline each of the three surface views and label each box with the secondary code "H" (see Figure 10–10). Tooth #8 also shows a Silver Amalgam restoration on the Lingual tooth surface and endodontic treatment (described in Chapters 5 and 16).

These restorations are written with the primary code "C" separated by a hyphen (-) and followed by the secondary code "H" (C-H). This is read as a Porcelain Crown. Tooth #8 has an additional secondary code "R" for Root Canal and also another restoration that is written as L-S (C-HR•L-S). The restorations present on tooth #8 are read as: Root Canal treatment on a tooth with a Porcelain Crown and also a Silver Amalgam restoration on the Lingual tooth surface.

Charting Porcelain Veneer and Porcelain Jacket Crowns on a Geometric Chart

To chart the six Porcelain veneer restorations in Figure 10–8 on a geometric chart, locate teeth #22 to #27 and use a blue pencil to completely outline the Mesial, Distal, Incisal, and Facial tooth surfaces; then label each diagram with the uppercase letter "H" (Figure 10–11). These Porcelain veneer restorations are written and read as previously indicated on the anatomic chart.

To chart the Porcelain jacket Crowns in Figure 10–9 on a geometric chart, use a blue pencil to completely outline the outside circle located on the stylized diagram and label each box with the secondary code "H" (see Figure 10–11). Tooth #8 must also show a Silver Amalgam restoration on the Lingual surface. The entire Lingual surface diagram must be outlined completely and filled in (described in Chapter 5). The endodontic treatment is drawn the same as it was on an anatomic chart. The restorations are written and read as previously mentioned.

					H	H	H	H	H						
18	17	16	15	14	13	12	11	21	22	23	24	25	26	27	28
8	7	6	5	4	3	2	1	1	2	3	4	5	6	7	8
1	2	3	4	5	6	7	8	9	10	11	12	13	14	15	16

32	31	30	29	28	27	26	25	24	23	22	21	20	19	18	17
8	7	6	5	4	3	2	1	1	2	3	4	5	6	7	8
48	47	46	45	44	43	42	41	31	32	33	34	35	36	37	38
	Z	Z	Z		H	H	H	H	H	H					

Figure 10–11 Geometric chart with teeth #6, #7, #8, #9, and #10 shown with Porcelain jacket Crowns; teeth #22, #23, #24, #25, #26, and #27 shown with Porcelain veneer restorations; and teeth #29, #30, and #31 shown with pit and fissure sealants

Charting Porcelain Veneer and Porcelain Jacket Crowns on a Numeric Coding System Chart

To indicate the Porcelain veneer restorations present in Figure 10–8 on a numeric coding system chart, use a black pen and enter the date in the designated area. In the row of boxes adjacent to the date below teeth #22 to #27, enter the primary codes to designate the involved tooth surfaces followed by the secondary code "H" (Figure 10–12).

The chart indicates that on 2-20-94, restorations were placed on teeth #22 to #27. The Mesio-Inciso-Disto-Facial tooth surfaces were covered with Porcelain restorations. Because of the number of tooth surfaces involved in these restorations, it can be assumed that they are Porcelain veneer restorations.

To show Porcelain jacket Crowns on teeth #6 to #10, enter the primary code "C" followed by the secondary code "H" in the row of boxes adjacent to the date (see Figure 10–12). This chart indicates that on 7-16-95, Porcelain Crowns were placed on teeth #6, #7, #8, #9, and #10. On 2-6-96, Root Canal treatment was completed and a Silver Amalgam restoration was placed on the Lingual surface of the Porcelain Crown.

Pit and Fissure Sealants

Pit and fissure sealants, also known as dental sealants, were designed to protect the fissures, pits, and grooves in the teeth from the effects of bacterial

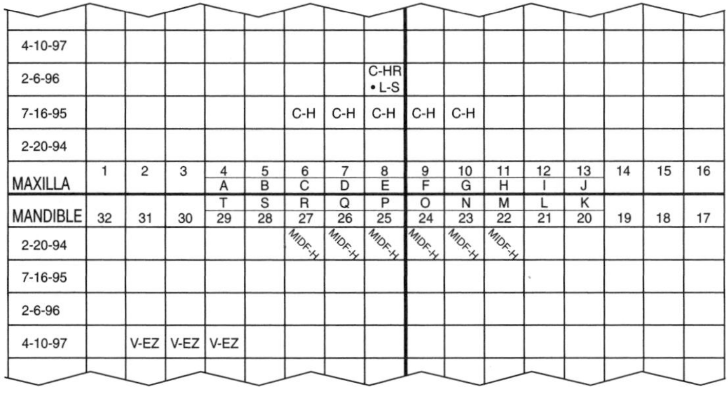

Figure 10–12 Numeric coding system chart with teeth #6, #7, #8, #9, and #10 shown with Porcelain jacket Crowns; teeth #22, #23, #24, #25, #26, and #27 shown with Porcelain veneer restorations; and teeth #29, #30, and #31 shown with pit and fissure sealants

plaque. Occlusal tooth surfaces are the most susceptible to dental caries. It has been determined that the best protection for these surfaces is the placement of dental sealants. Use of fluorides will reduce decay on smooth tooth surfaces. However, fluoride has not been as effective for the prevention of decay on Occlusal tooth surfaces (Figure 10–13A and B).

These dental sealants are easily detected on clinical examination because they appear white. They are shown as radiolucent images that blend together with the existing tooth structures and are extremely difficult to detect from a radiograph alone.

Pit and fissure sealants are retained via the use of mechanical bonding of the sealant material to the enamel surface. To achieve this mechanical bonding, the tooth is conditioned prior to the placement of the sealant material. To complete the conditioning process, the tooth is acid etched, subjected to a 35% to 50% phosphoric acid liquid or gel. The etching creates an irregular surface that allows the sealant material to seep into and mechanically bond to the enamel structure. Sealant failure is usually due to an incomplete or disrupted mechanical bond due to operator technique.

Dental sealants are made from several types of dental material. The most common is bisphenol A glycidyl methacrylate (Bis-GMA). The material is polymerized (set) by either an organic amine or a light source. Materials polymerized by an organic amine are known as self-cured, auto-cured, or chemical-cured dental sealants. This is also referred to as autopolymerizing dental sealants. This type of sealant material is furnished as a two-part system that is mixed immediately prior to placement. The material completes the polymerization automatically. The materials requiring a light source for

Universal System
#31 #30 #29
Palmer System
7┐ 6┐ 5┐
ISO/FDI System
47 46 45

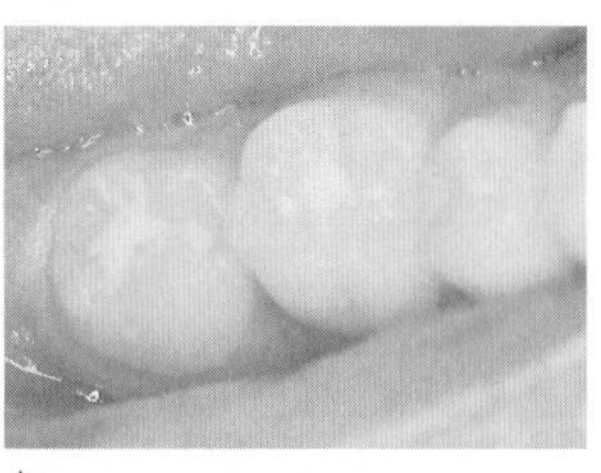

A.

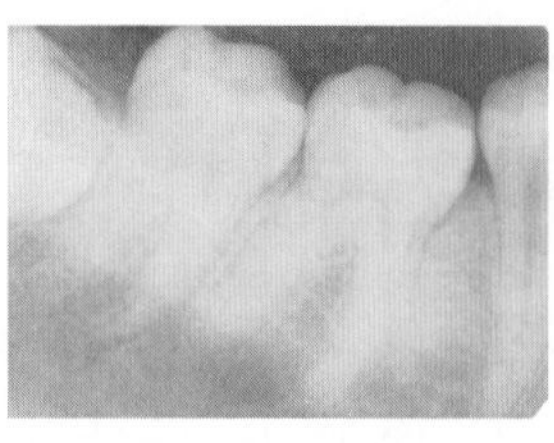

B.

Universal System
#31 #30 #29
Palmer System
7┐ 6┐ 5┐
ISO/FDI System
47 46 45

Figure 10–13 (A) Photograph shown of pit and fissure sealants on the Occlusal tooth surface of tooth #29 and the Occlusal and Buccal tooth surfaces of teeth #30 and #31. (B) Periapical radiograph shown of pit and fissure sealants on teeth #29, #30, and #31

curing are called light-cure or photopolymerizing sealants. The material requires either an ultraviolet or visible light source to complete the polymerization process. Light-cure sealant material requires no mixing, allowing more time for placement. Regardless of the type of material used, studies have shown that the kind of material has no significant difference in the prevention of Occlusal surface caries.

Dental sealants serve as part of a complete preventive program to reduce the incidence of dental caries and are not usually considered to be dental restorations. However, it is important to document their appearance and location so they can be reexamined for any structural deficiencies at maintenance appointments.

Charting Pit and Fissure Sealants on an Anatomic Chart

To show the pit and fissure sealants on teeth #29, #30, and #31 on an anatomic chart, with a blue pencil outline the Occlusal and Buccal surface areas and in the box beneath the tooth designation number, print the secondary code "Z" for Temporary (see Figure 10–10).

The restorations on teeth #29, #30, and #31 are written as "V-EZ" and read as Virgin teeth with Temporary Resin restorations.

Charting Pit and Fissure Sealants on a Geometric Chart

To show the dental sealants on teeth #29, #30, and #31 on the geometric chart, with a blue pencil outline the entire Occlusal surface and only outline the middle section on the Buccal surface view. In the box beneath the tooth designation number, print the secondary code "Z" (see Figure 10–11). The restorations are written and read as previously mentioned on the anatomic chart.

Charting Pit and Fissure Sealants on a Numeric Coding System Chart

To indicate dental sealants on a numeric coding system chart, enter the date in black ink, and in blue ink enter the primary code "V" followed by the secondary codes "EZ" (see Figure 10–12). The dental chart is read as: on 4-10-97 teeth #29, #30, and #31 are Virgin teeth with Temporary Resin restorations placed on them. Some practitioners may prefer to write the word *sealant* with a detailed description of the involved tooth surfaces in the examination progress notes.

Review Questions

Matching

Directions: Place the uppercase letter(s) after the number to match each term with the statement that best defines it.

A Acrylic Resin
B Composite Resin
C Composite Resin veneer
D Glass ionomer
E Pit and fissure sealants
F Porcelain Inlay
G Porcelain jacket Crown
H Porcelain veneer
I Silicate
J Temporary Crown

1. ____ The primary code is "C" and the secondary code is "Z."
2. ____ The first esthetic restorative material introduced in 1871.
3. ____ Ceramic restorations that cover the Facial and Incisal tooth surfaces.
4. ____ This material is used as cavity liners, bonding systems, luting, and core materials.
5. ____ The restorative Resins that followed silicate.
6. ____ The ceramic restoration is confined within a tapered cavity preparation.
7. ____ Material used to restore developmental defects and discolored teeth.
8. ____ This restoration covers all of the surfaces of the teeth.
9. ____ The general name for tooth-colored materials.
10. ____ Used to prevent dental decay on occlusal tooth surfaces.

Answers

1. **J,** 2. **I,** 3. **H,** 4. **D,** 5. **A,** 6. **F,** 7. **C,** 8. **G,** 9. **B,** 10. **E**

References

American National Standards Institute/American Dental Association, Council on Dental Materials and Equipment. (1985) *Dental glass ionomer cements* (ANSI/ADA Spec. No.66). Chicago: Author.

Arcoria, C. J., Gonzalez, J. P., & Vitasek, B. A. (1992). Effects of ultrasonic instrumentation on microleakage in composite restorations with glass ionomer liners. *Journal of Oral Rehabilitation*, 19, 21–29.

Brownbill, J. W. & Setcos, J. C. (1990). Treatment selections for fissured grooves of permanent molar teeth. ASDC *Journal of Dentistry for Children*, 54(4), 274–278, July–August.

Burke, F. J. T. & McCaughey, A. D. (1995). The four generations of dentin bonding. *American Journal of Dentistry*, 8, 88.

Cohen, L. D. (1990). Pit and fissure sealants: An underutilized preventive technology. *International Journal of Technology Assessment in Health Care*, (6)3, 378–391.

Corbin, S. B. & Kohn, W. G. (1994). The benefits and risks of dental amalgam:current findings reviewed. *Journal of the American Dental Association*, 125, 381–388.

Curtis, P. M., von Fraunhofer, A., & Farman, A. G. (1990). The radiographic density of composite restorative resins. *Oral Surgery, Oral Medicine, and Oral Pathology*, 70.

DeCraene, G. P., Martins, L. C., Dermaut, L. R., & Surmount, P. A. (1989). A clinical evaluation of a light-cured fissure sealant (helioscal). *Journal of Dentistry for Children*, 56(2), 97–102, March–April.

Dietschi, D. & Holy, J. (1990). A clinical trial of four light-curing posterior composite resins: Two-year report. *Quintessence International*, 21, 965.

Dorland's pocket medical dictionary (28th ed.). (1994). Philadelphia: W. B. Saunders Company.

Douvitsas, G. (1991). Effect of cavity design on gap formation in class II composite resin restorations. *Journal of Prosthetic Dentistry*, 65, 475–479.

Eldiway, M., Powers, J. M., & George, L. A. (1993). Mechanical properties of direct and post-cured composities. *American Journal of Dentistry*, 6, 222.

Ferracane, J. L., & Condon, J. R. (1990). Rate of elution of leachable components from composite. *Dental Materials*, 6, 282–287.

Fissore, B. J., Nicholls, I., & Yuodelis, R. A. (1991). Load fatigue of teeth restored by a dentin bonding agent and a posterior composite resin. *Journal of Prosthetic Dentistry*, 65, 80–85.

Forsten, L. (1991). Fluoride release and uptake by glass ionomers. *Scandinavian Journal of Dental Research*, 99, 241–245.

Garber, D. A. (1989). Direct composite veneers versus etched porcelain laminate veneers. *Dental Clinics of North America*, 33, 301–304.

Gray, H. S. (1963). The Porcelain Jacket Crown. *New Zealand Dental Journal*, 59, 283.

Harasani, M. R., Isidor, F., & Kaaber, S. (1991). Marginal fit of porcelain and indirect composite laminate veneers under in vitro conditions. *Scandinavian Journal of Dental Research*, 99, 262–268.

Jendresen, M. D., Allen, E. P., Bayne, S. C., Hansson, T. L., Klooster, J., & Preston, J. D. (1992). Report of the committee on scientific investigation of the american academy of restorative dentistry. *Journal of Prosthetic Dentistry*, 68(1), 137–180.

Johnson, G. H., Bales, D. J., Gordon, G. E., & Powell, L. V. (1992). Clinical performance of posterior composite resin restorations. *Quintessence International*, 23, 705.

Johnson, G. H., Gordon, G. E., & Bales, D. J. (1988). Postoperative sensitivity associated with posterior composite and amalgam restorations. *Operative Dentistry*, 13(2), 66.

Matis, B. A., Carlson, T., Cochran, M., & Phillips, R. W. (1991). How finishing effects glass ionomers. Results of a five year evaluation. *Journal of the American Dental Association*, 122, 43–46.

Milleding, P., Ortengren, V., & Karlsson, S. (1995). Ceramic inlay systems: Some clinical aspects. *Journal of Oral Rehabilitation*, 22, 571.

Miller, L. M. (1992). Porcelain veneer protection plan: Maintenance procedures for all porcelain restorations. *Journal of Esthetic Dentistry*, 2(3), 63.

Mjor, I. A., Jokstad, A., & Qvist, V. (1990). Longevity of posterior restorations. *International Dental Journal*, 40, 11–17.

Oilo, G. (1992). Biodegradation of dental composites/glassionomer cements. *Advances in Dental Research*, 6, 50–54.

Suzuki, H., Taira, M., Wakasa, K., & Yamaki, M. (1991). Refractive-index-adjustable fillers for visible-light-cured dental resin composites: Preparation of TiO_2-SiO_2 glass powder by the sol-gel process. *Journal of Dental Research*, 70, 883–888.

Svanberg, M., Mjor, I. A., & Orstavik, D. (1990). Mutans streptococci in plaque from margins of amalgam, composite and glass-ionomer restorations. *Journal of Dental Research*, 69, 861–864.

Thomas, C. L. (1997). *Taber's cyclopedic medical dictionary*. Philadelphia: F. A. Davis Company.

Torstenson, B. (1988). *Contraction gaps around dental composite resin restorations*. (Thesis). Stockholm.

Van Zeghbroeck, L. M., Feilzer, A. J., & Davidson, C. L. (1989). Spontaneous failure of glass ionomer cements. *Journal of Dental Research*, 68, 613.

Willems, G., Noack, M. J., Inokoshi, S., et al. (1991). Radiopacity of composites compared with human enamel and dentine. *J Dent*, 19, 362–365.

Winkler, M. M., Greener, E. H., & Lautenschlager, E. P. (1991). Non-linear in vitro wear of posterior composites with time. *Dental Materials*, 7(4), 258–262.

Wright, G. Z., Friedman, C. S., Plotzke, O., & Feasby, W. H. (1988). A comparison between autopolymerizing and visible-light activated sealants. *Clinical Preventive Dentistry*, 10(1), 14–17, Jan–Feb.

CHAPTER 11

Fixed Prosthesis

Key Terms

- Abutment
- Bilateral Bridge
- Blade
- Cantilever Bridge
- Dental Implants
- Dental Prosthesis
- Endosseous Implant
- Fixed Partial Denture
- Maryland Bridge
- Osseointegration
- Pontic
- Root Form
- Subperiosteal
- Transosseous Implant

PRIMARY CODE	SECONDARY CODE
C = Crown	-H = Porcelain
X = Missing	-N = Non-precious (blue cross-hatch)
	-P = Pontic
	-Pi = Pontic Implant (blue symbol)
	-Q = Three-Quarter
	-R = Root Canal (blue vertical line)
	-T = Denture

Introduction

The replacement of a Missing tooth or several teeth with an artificial substitute is referred to as **dental prosthesis.** There are two types of artificial replacements for Missing teeth: fixed prosthesis, which is discussed in this chapter, and removable prosthesis (discussed in Chapter 12). A **fixed partial denture,** formerly referred to as dental bridge, provides the replacement of one or more Missing teeth either by being secured and supported to existing natural teeth or to structures implanted within the body tissues.

The natural teeth used to support the fixed partial denture are referred to as **abutment** teeth. The abutments are attached to the artificial replacement tooth that replaces the Missing tooth called the **Pontic**. There are three types of fixed partial dentures that utilize natural tooth abutments. The **bilateral bridge** consists of one or more abutment teeth attached to the sides of one or more replacement teeth (Figure 11–1A and B and Plate 3). The **cantilever bridge** involves an artificial tooth connected to one or more abutment teeth on the same end (Figure 11–2A and B). In Figure 11–2B, the Pontic is shown only attached to one side, the Mesial surface, of the abutment tooth. A **Maryland bridge** is a cast metal Pontic attached to bilateral retainers that are Resin-bonded to the etched enamel surfaces of the abutment teeth (Figure 11–3A and B).

Universal System
#2 #3 #5 #6 #7 #8

Palmer System
7| 6| 4| 3| 2| 1|

ISO/FDI System
17 16 14 13 12 11

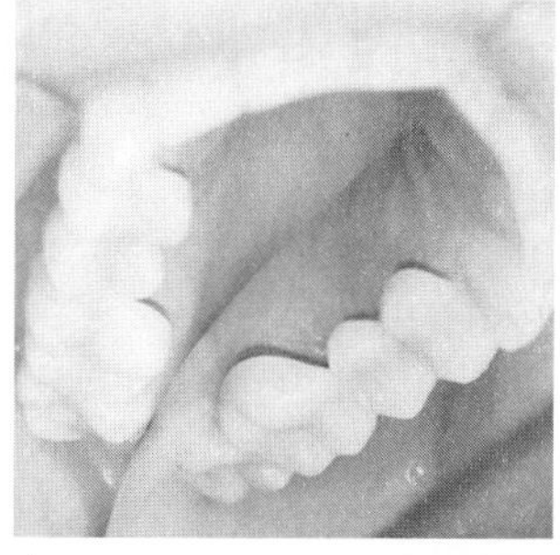

A.

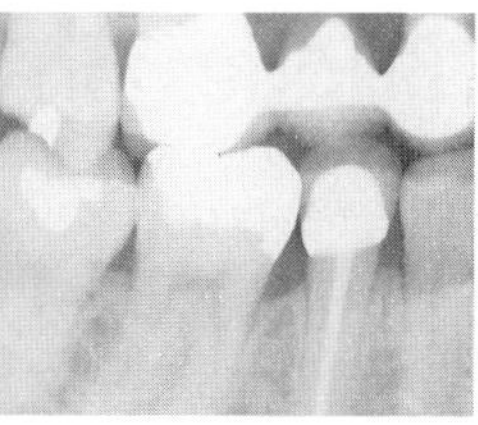

B.

Universal System
#2 #3 #5
#31 #30 #29 #28

Palmer System
7| 6| 4|
7| 6| 5| 4|

ISO/FDI System
17 16 14
47 46 45 44

Figure 11–1 (A) Photograph shown with a Porcelain-Fused-To-Metal fixed partial denture (B) Bitewing radiograph showing bilateral abutment teeth on teeth #3 and #5 and tooth #4 is shown Missing and replaced with a Pontic; the bilateral bridge appears as a radiopaque image

Universal System
#3 #4 #5 #6 #8

Palmer System
6| 5| 4| 3| 1|

ISO/FDI System
16 15 14 13 11

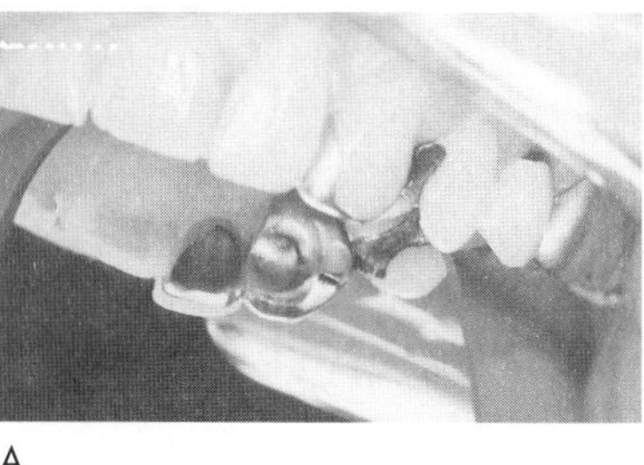

A.

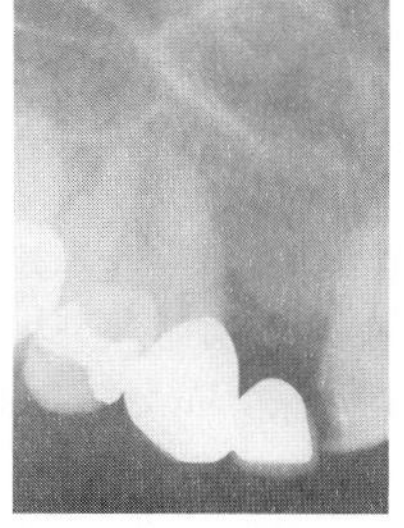

B.

Universal System
#4 #5 #6 #8

Palmer System
5| 4| 3| 1|

ISO/FDI System
15 14 13 11

Figure 11–2 (A) Photograph shows a cantilever bridge with the abutment tooth #6 shown with a Three-Quarter Gold Crown (B) Periapical radiograph showing tooth #7 is Missing and replaced with a Porcelain-Fused-To-Gold Pontic; the cantilever bridge appears as a radiopaque image

Universal System
#6 #7 #8 #10 #11 #12

Palmer System
3| 2| 1| |2 |3 |4

ISO/FDI System
13 12 11 22 23 24

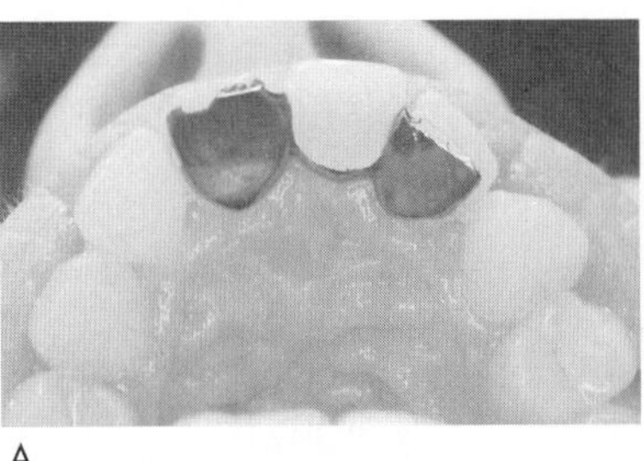

A.

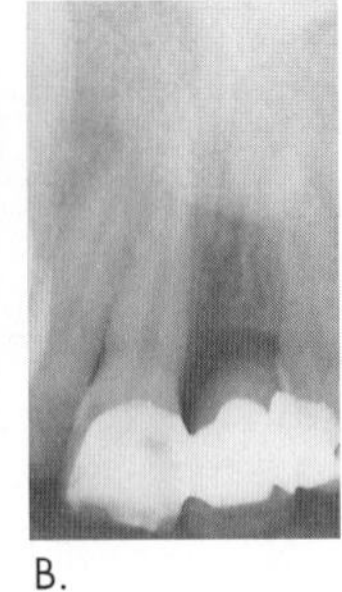

B.

Universal System
#7 #8 #10

Palmer System
2| 1| |2

ISO/FDI System
12 11 22

Figure 11–3 (A) Photograph showing a Maryland bridge with Resin-bonded retainers on teeth #8 and #10 (B) Periapical radiograph showing tooth #9 is Missing and replaced with a Porcelain-Fused-To-Metal Pontic

Charting Bilateral, Cantilever, and Maryland Bridges on an Anatomic Chart

To chart the bilateral bridge shown in Figure 11–1A and B on an anatomic chart, locate tooth #4 and with a blue pencil cross out all three views to indicate the tooth is Missing. On teeth #3, #4, and #5 outline all three views and completely cross-hatch all of the areas to indicate full cast Crowns made of Non-precious metal. In the box located above the tooth notation numbers, with a blue pencil print the uppercase letter "H" to indicate the Crowns are Porcelain covered (described in Chapter 9). Draw three horizontal lines from each view that extend away from both sides of the Pontic, tooth #4, to the abutment teeth #3 and #5 to indicate a fixed partial denture (Figure 11–4).

The fixed partial denture is written as: teeth #3 and #5 will show the primary code "C" for Crown followed by a hyphen (-), then followed by the secondary codes "N" for Non-precious metal, and "H" for Porcelain covered (C-NH). Tooth #4 is written with the primary code "X" to indicate Missing followed by the secondary code "P" for Pontic, then "N" for Non-precious metal and "H" to indicate Porcelain covered (X-PNH). These restorations are read as: tooth abutments #3 and #5 have Porcelain-covered Non-precious metal Crowns and tooth #4 is Missing and replaced with a Porcelain-covered Non-precious metal Pontic.

Figure 11–2A and B shows that tooth #6 is a cantilever bridge abutment with a Three-Quarter Gold Crown and tooth #7 is a Porcelain-covered Gold Pontic. To indicate this on an anatomic chart, locate tooth #6 and with a

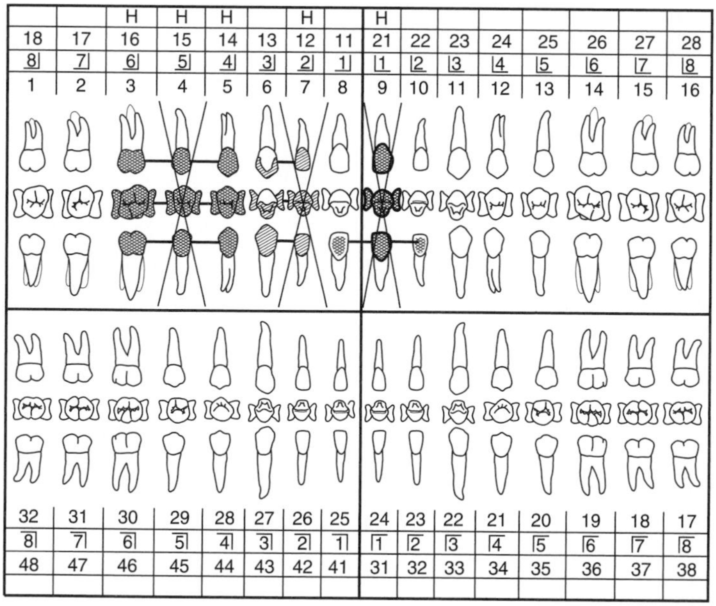

		H	H	H		H		H							
18	17	16	15	14	13	12	11	21	22	23	24	25	26	27	28
8⌋	7⌋	6⌋	5⌋	4⌋	3⌋	2⌋	1⌋	⌊1	⌊2	⌊3	⌊4	⌊5	⌊6	⌊7	⌊8
1	2	3	4	5	6	7	8	9	10	11	12	13	14	15	16
32	31	30	29	28	27	26	25	24	23	22	21	20	19	18	17
8⌉	7⌉	6⌉	5⌉	4⌉	3⌉	2⌉	1⌉	⌈1	⌈2	⌈3	⌈4	⌈5	⌈6	⌈7	⌈8
48	47	46	45	44	43	42	41	31	32	33	34	35	36	37	38

Figure 11–4 Anatomic chart shown with a bilateral bridge that involves teeth #3, #4, and #5, a cantilever bridge on teeth #6 and #7, and a Maryland bridge replacing tooth #9

blue pencil completely outline the Lingual view, partially outline the Incisal view, then fill in the areas with diagonal lines (described in Chapter 8). Cross out tooth #7 and outline all of the views, completely fill in the areas with diagonal lines, then place the letter "H" in the box located above the tooth notation number (see Figure 11–4).

The cantilever bridge restorations are written as: tooth #6, C-QG, and tooth #7, X-PGH. These are read as: tooth #6 has a Three-Quarter Gold Crown and tooth #7 is Missing and replaced with a Porcelain-covered Gold Pontic.

In Figure 11–3A and B, tooth #9 is replaced with a Maryland bridge. To indicate a Porcelain-Fused-To-Non-precious metal Pontic on tooth #9 on an anatomic chart, use a blue pencil and cross out the tooth. Outline all of the views and completely cross-hatch the areas, then label the tooth with the secondary code "H." To indicate teeth #8 and #9 are attached to the Pontic with Resin-bonded retainers, cross-hatch the areas just slightly within the perimeter of the Lingual tooth surfaces (see Figure 11–4).

On an anatomic chart, a Maryland bridge is written as: tooth #9, X-PNH and teeth #8 and #10, L-N. This is read as: tooth #9 is Missing and replaced with a Porcelain-covered Non-precious metal Pontic, and teeth #8 and #10 have Non-precious metal bonded to the Lingual tooth surfaces.

Charting Bilateral, Cantilever, and Maryland Bridges on a Geometric Chart

To show the bilateral bridge in Figure 11–1 charted on a geometric chart, locate the tooth notation numbers, and with a blue pencil cross out the diagram on tooth #4, then outline the outside circle and completely cross-hatch the area inside. In the box located above, print the secondary code "H." On teeth #3 and #5, outline and completely cross-hatch the diagrams and draw a single short horizontal line that extends off each side of tooth # 4 to the other diagrams. Label the boxes with the same secondary code that was previously recorded for tooth #4 (Figure 11–5). The restorations on teeth #3, #4, and #5 are written and read the same way as they were for the anatomic chart.

To draw the cantilever bridge in Figure 11–2 on a geometric chart, use a blue pencil to mark tooth #7 as Missing and outline the diagram, then completely fill in the area with diagonal lines. Label the diagram with the letter "H." On tooth #6, outline all views except the Facial view and fill in the area with diagonal lines, then print an uppercase "H" in the designated box located at the top of the diagram. Draw a single horizontal line that extends from the Mesial surface of tooth #6 to the Distal surface of tooth #7 (see Figure 11–5). These restorations are written and read as previously mentioned.

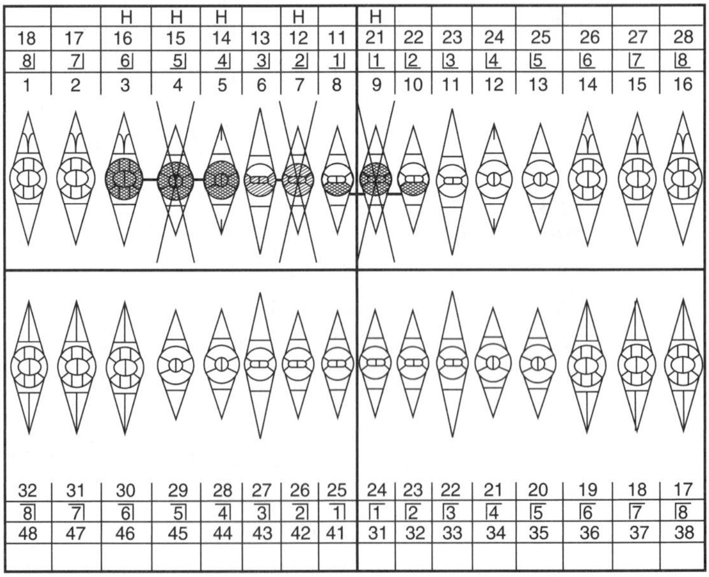

Figure 11–5 Geometric chart shown with a bilateral bridge that involves teeth #3, #4, and #5, a cantilever bridge on teeth #6 and #7, and a Maryland bridge replacing tooth #9

		H	H	H		H		H							
18	17	16	15	14	13	12	11	21	22	23	24	25	26	27	28
8⌋	7⌋	6⌋	5⌋	4⌋	3⌋	2⌋	1⌋	⌊1	⌊2	⌊3	⌊4	⌊5	⌊6	⌊7	⌊8
1	2	3	4	5	6	7	8	9	10	11	12	13	14	15	16
32	31	30	29	28	27	26	25	24	23	22	21	20	19	18	17
8⌉	7⌉	6⌉	5⌉	4⌉	3⌉	2⌉	1⌉	⌈1	⌈2	⌈3	⌈4	⌈5	⌈6	⌈7	⌈8
48	47	46	45	44	43	42	41	31	32	33	34	35	36	37	38

To chart the Maryland bridge in Figure 11–3 on a geometric chart, use a blue pencil to draw and label the restoration on tooth #9 in the same manner as tooth #4 was charted. Outline and cross-hatch the entire Lingual surface views of teeth #8 and #10, then draw short horizontal lines from these restorations to tooth #9 (see Figure 11–5). The primary and secondary codes previously specified for these restorations remain the same.

Charting Bilateral, Cantilever, and Maryland Bridges on a Numeric Coding System Chart

Figure 11–6 represents a numeric coding system chart indicating a bilateral bridge that involves teeth #3, #4, and #5.

Use a black pen to enter the date in the designated column and with a blue pencil in the row of boxes adjacent to the date above teeth #3 and #5, print the primary code "C" followed by a hyphen (-), then the secondary codes "N" and "H" (C-NH). In the box above tooth #4, print the primary code "X" followed by the secondary codes "PNH" (X-PNH). On the vertical grid line between teeth #3 and #4 and teeth #4 and #5, place a short horizontal line to indicate that the restorations are attached to each other.

The chart is read as: on 1-12-94, a three-unit fixed partial denture was placed and teeth #3 and #5 are abutments with Porcelain-covered Non-precious metal Crowns, and tooth #4 is Missing and replaced with a Porcelain-covered Non-precious metal Pontic.

3-5-96								L-N	X-PNH	L-N						
7-12-95						C-QG	X-PGH									
1-12-94			C-NH	X-PNH	C-NH											
MAXILLA	1	2	3	4 A	5 B	6 C	7 D	8 E	9 F	10 G	11 H	12 I	13 J	14	15	16
MANDIBLE	32	31	30	T 29	S 28	R 27	Q 26	P 25	O 24	N 23	M 22	L 21	K 20	19	18	17
1-12-94																
7-12-95																
3-5-96																

Figure 11–6 Numeric coding system chart indicating a bilateral bridge that involves teeth #3, #4, and #5, a cantilever bridge on teeth #6 and #7, and a Maryland bridge replacing tooth #9

To document the cantilever bridge in Figure 11–2, enter the date, then above tooth #6 enter the primary code "C" followed by the secondary codes "QG" (C-QG). To indicate tooth #7 is Missing, enter the primary code "X" followed by the secondary codes "PGH" (X-PGH), then place a short line on the grid line between the two teeth involved (see Figure 11–6). The chart indicates that on 7-12-95, a cantilever bridge was placed and tooth #6 has a Three-Quarter Gold Crown attached to tooth #7 that was replaced with a Porcelain-covered Gold Pontic.

To indicate a Maryland bridge is present and involves teeth #8, #9, and #10, locate the row of boxes adjacent to the date above tooth #9, then enter the same primary and secondary codes used for tooth #4. Above teeth #8 and #10, print the primary code "L" for Lingual surface followed by the secondary code "N" (L-N), then connect the two as previously described. The chart indicates that on 3-5-96, a Maryland bridge was inserted to replace tooth #9, which is Missing and has a Porcelain-covered Non-precious metal Pontic secured to the Lingual tooth surfaces of tooth #8 and #10 with Non-precious metal (see Figure 11–6).

Dental Implants

The three types of **dental implants** most commonly used today include the **root form** (screw-type or cylinder), **blade** (plate), and the **subperiosteal**. The first two Pontic Implants are placed directly into the alveolar bone tissue (**endosseous implants**). The third type of Pontic Implant sits on top of the alveolar bone and is held in place with the periosteum, as well as mechanical retention. A fourth type of Pontic Implant, called the staple, is rarely used today. It is a **transosseous implant** previously used in the anterior mandible, penetrating both superior and inferior cortical plates.

The desired physiologic mechanism of a successful endosseous implant is through **osseointegration** (fusion) with the bone tissue. The latest research involved the use of differing bone densities throughout the mouth to influence the characteristics of the Pontic Implant (i.e., surface area, thread design, surface coatings). The optimal properties of the Pontic Implant are matched to the quality of the surrounding bone tissue.

In Plates 4 and 5, four screw-type root form Pontic Implants are shown placed in the anterior mandible and they are connected with a bar. These endosseous Pontic Implants serve as anchors for a removable overdenture,

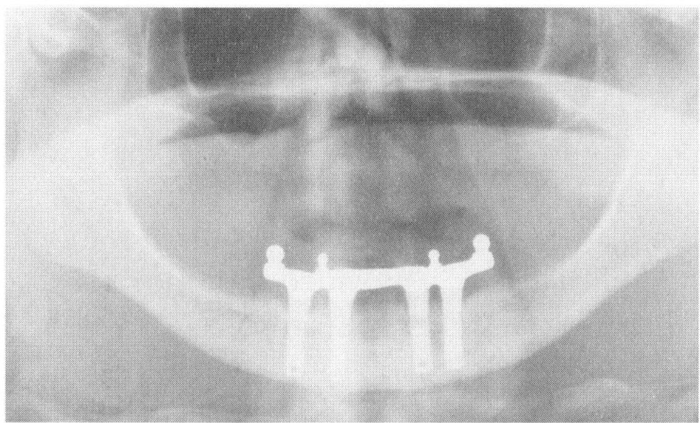

Figure 11–7 Panoramic radiograph showing the endosseous implant with four screw-type root form implants that appear radiopaque (Courtesy Paul A. Johnson, DDS)

which is attached with O-rings for retention. The overdenture is partially supported by the connecting bar and also the soft tissue of the posterior mandible. The ridges on the screw-type Pontic Implants are easily identified on the panoramic radiograph and they appear as radiopaque images (Figure 11–7).

Figure 11–8A and B show a subperiosteal implant with Dr. Carl Misch's nine-post design. The removable lower overdenture is retained with O-rings and is thoroughly implanted and supported with no contact on the soft tissue. The panoramic radiograph shows the subperiosteal implant in Figure 11–8A as a radiopaque image (Figure 11–8C).

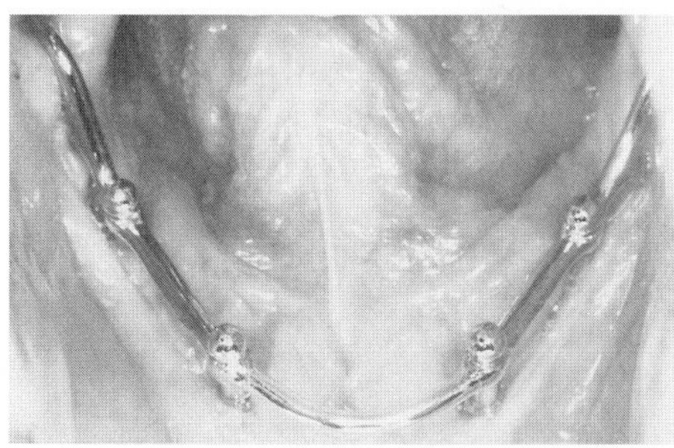

A.

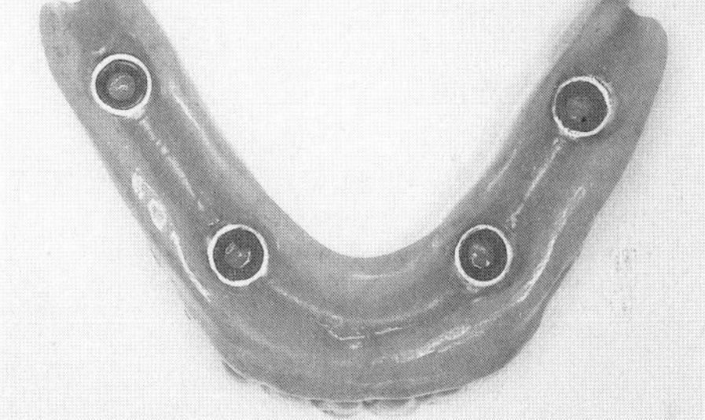

B.

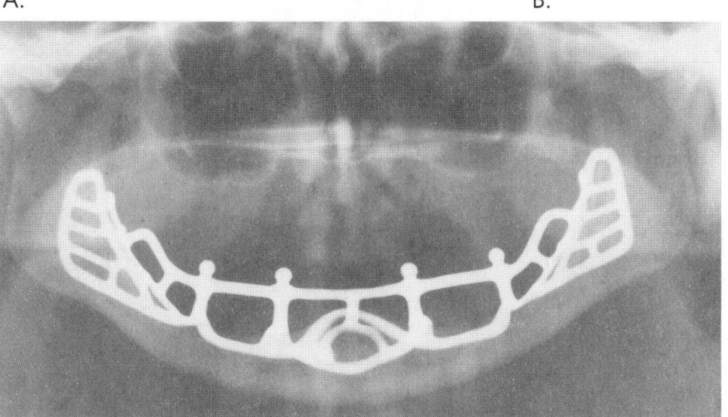

C.

Figure 11–8 (A) Photograph showing mandibular subperiosteal implant (B) Photograph shown of an overdenture for the subperiosteal implant in figure (A) (C) Panoramic radiograph showing the subperiosteal implant in figure (A) with the nine-post design that appears radiopaque (Courtesy Paul A. Johnson, DDS)

The panoramic radiograph in Figure 11–9A shows two types of endosseous implants, screw-type root form and blade. There are ten screw-type root form Pontic Implants placed in the maxilla. Bilaterally, sinus augmentation procedures with bone grafting were required. Two blade Pontic Implants were placed in the posterior mandible. Porcelain-Fused-To-Metal fixed partial denture restorations connect the Pontic Implants and are non-removable by the patient. Allowance for mandibular flexure is provided with the use of an interlock attachment between the two lower bridges (Figure 11–9B).

Charting Dental Implants on an Anatomic Chart

To chart endosseous implants on an anatomic chart, use a blue pencil and cross out all three views for each Missing tooth. On the Facial surface

Universal System
#27 #22

Palmer System
3⌉ ⌈3

ISO/FDI System
43 33

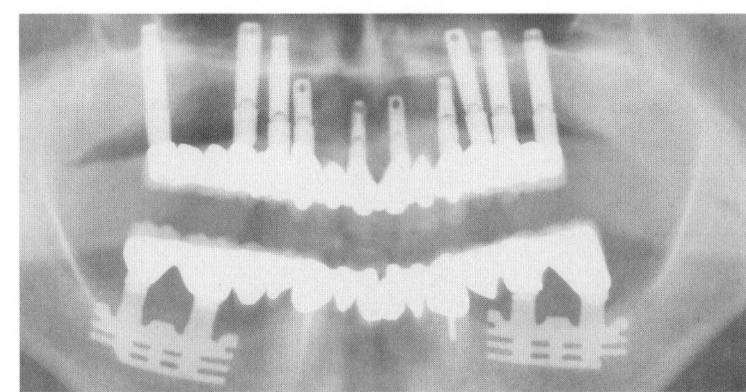

A.

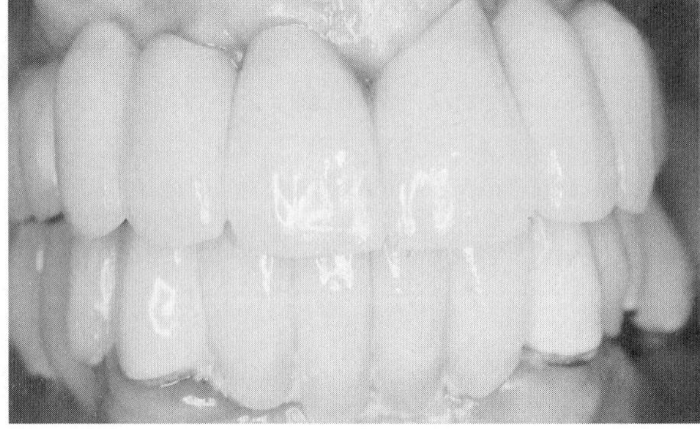

B.

Figure 11–9 (A) Panoramic radiograph shown with ten screw-type root form Pontic Implants on the maxillary arch and two posterior blade Pontic Implants connected to abutment teeth #22 and #27 with full mouth Porcelain-Fused-To-Metal fixed partial dentures on the maxillary and mandibular arches (B) Photograph shown of full mouth Porcelain-Fused-To-Metal restorations attached to the endosseous implants in figure (A) (Courtesy Paul A. Johnson, DDS)

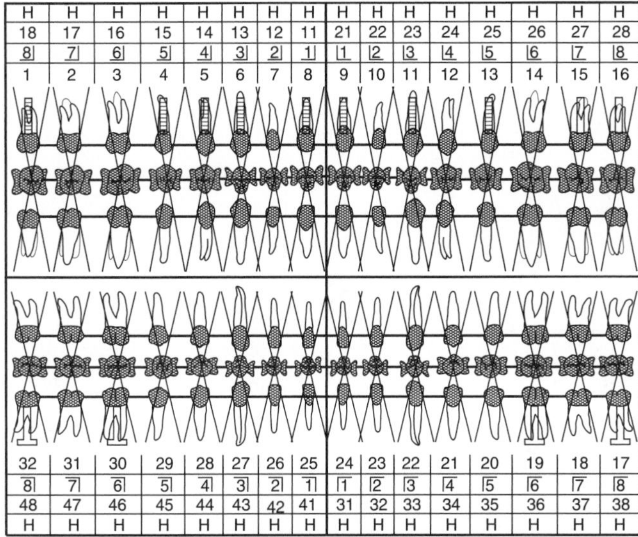

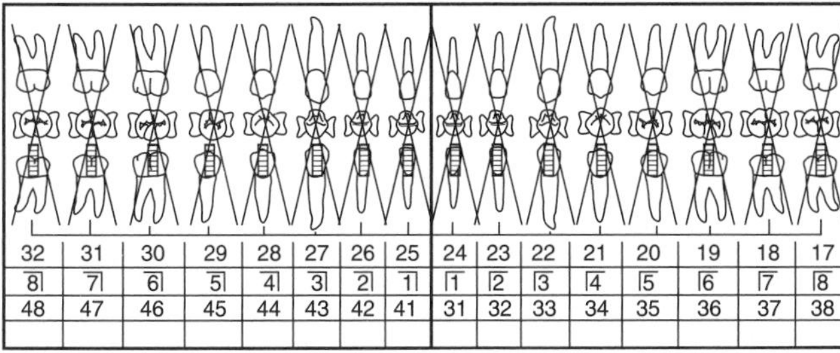

Figure 11–10 (A) Anatomic chart showing the maxillary and mandibular arches replaced with Porcelain-Fused-To-Non-precious-Metal Pontics attached to endosseous implants (B) Anatomic chart shown with teeth #17 to #32 replaced with an overdenture attached to a subperiosteal implant

views, draw a vertical rectangle on the root diagrams. To indicate a screw-type root form Pontic Implant, fill in the rectangle with short horizontal lines and to indicate a cylinder root form leave the rectangle blank. To show a blade Pontic Implant, draw the same diagram that was used to indicate a cylinder Pontic Implant, then at the base of the vertical rectangle draw a small horizontal rectangle that appears as "⊥." Chart each tooth diagram with cross-hatched lines to indicate the Porcelain-Fused-To-Non-precious metal Crowns and label the designated box with the letter "H" (described in Chapter 9). Draw three horizontal lines that extend from each tooth diagram to the adjacent tooth diagrams to indicate a fixed partial denture. The screw-type root form and blade Pontic Implants shown in Figure 11–9 are shown charted in Figure 11–10. Teeth #15 and #16 are shown charted as cylinder Pontic Implants.

To chart a subperiosteal implant, follow the same procedure mentioned previously for an endosseous implant with the exception that the rectangle is drawn from the CEJ to the top of the Crown on the tooth diagram. The subperiosteal implant in Figure 11–8 is shown charted in Figure 11–10B. Some practitioners may prefer to document the number and type of Pontic Implants in the examination progress notes.

Charting Dental Implants on a Geometric Chart

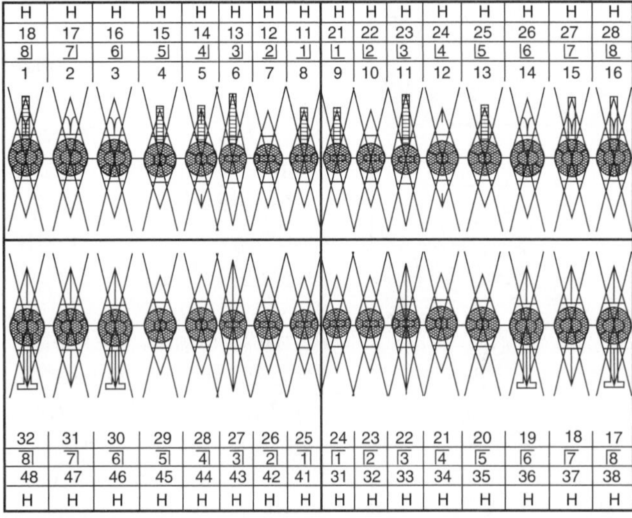

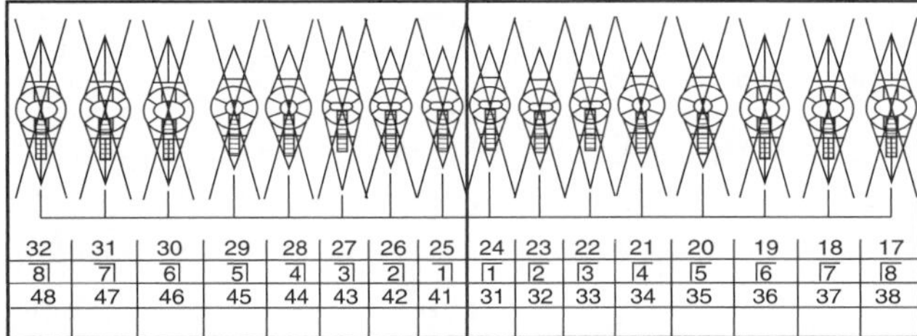

Figure 11–11 (A) Geometric chart showing the maxillary and mandibular arches replaced with Porcelain-Fused-To-Non-precious-Metal Pontics attached to endosseous implants (B) Geometric chart shown with teeth #17 to #32 replaced with an overdenture attached to a subperiosteal implant

To indicate the endosseous implants on a geometric chart, follow the same procedures that were previously mentioned for an anatomic chart; then to indicate a fixed partial denture, draw a single short horizontal line between each tooth diagram (Figure 11–11A).

To chart a subperiosteal implant on a geometric chart, follow the same procedures that were previously mentioned with the exception that the rectangle be drawn from the edge of the inner circle and extend to the middle third of the root. The subperiosteal implant shown in Figure 11–8 is charted in Figure 11–11B.

Charting Dental Implants on a Numeric Coding System Chart

To indicate the endosseous Pontic Implants present in Plate 4 and Figure 11–7 on a numeric coding system chart, use a black pen to enter the date in the designated column. Use a blue pencil to place the letter "X" in the box located above and below the tooth notation numbers followed by a hyphen (-), then the secondary codes "PiNH" (X-PiNH). For teeth #22 and #27, print the primary code "C" followed by the secondary codes "NHR" (Figure 11–12A). In the row of boxes above and below, draw two horizontal lines with the word "endosseous implant" printed in between them.

The chart in Figure 11–12A is read as: on 4-3-97 teeth #1–#21, #23–#26, and #28–#32 are Missing and replaced with endosseous Pontic Implants attached to Porcelain-covered Non-precious metal restorations. Teeth #22 and #27 have Root Canal treatment and are Porcelain-covered Non-precious metal Crowns that are attached to the endosseous Pontic Implants.

To indicate the subperiosteal implants and the Denture on teeth #17 to #32, use a blue pencil to print the primary code "X" followed by the secondary code for Denture "T" (X–T), then in the row of boxes located below draw two horizontal lines and print the words "subperiosteal implant" in between them (Figure 11–12B). The chart is read as: on 11-1-95 teeth #17–#32 are Missing and replaced with a Denture attached to a subperiosteal implant.

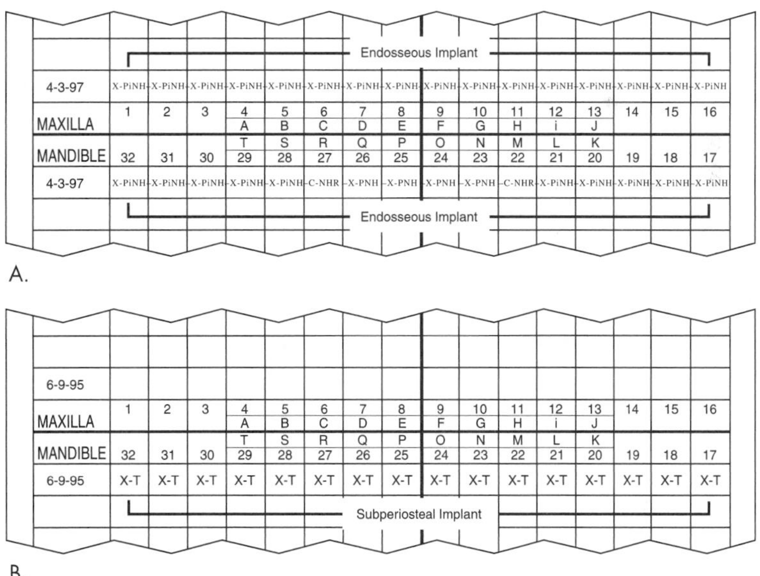

Figure 11–12 (A) Numeric coding system chart showing the maxillary and mandibular arches replaced with Porcelain-Fused-To-Non-precious-Metal Pontics attached to endosseous implants (B) Numeric coding system chart shown with teeth #17 to #32 replaced with an overdenture attached to a subperiosteal implant

Review Questions

Matching

Directions: Place the uppercase letter(s) after the number to match each term with the statement that best defines it.

A Abutment
B Bilateral bridge
C Cantilever bridge
D Pontic implant
E Dental prosthesis
F Fixed partial denture
G Maryland bridge
H Pontic

1. ___ The Crown is secured by a structure inserted into the bone tissue.
2. ___ The artificial replacement of a tooth.
3. ___ The replacement of a Missing tooth with an artificial tooth.
4. ___ The tooth used to support a fixed partial denture.
5. ___ This tooth is charted with the primary code "X."
6. ___ This restoration consists of an artificial tooth supported by a single tooth.
7. ___ This structure is supported by two resin-bonded retainers.
8. ___ Fixed prosthesis.
9. ___ An artificial tooth with a supporting tooth located on each end.
10. ___ The restoration has a structure that is only charted on the Lingual surface view.

Answers

1. **D,** 2. **E,** 3. **H,** 4. **A,** 5. **H,** 6. **C,** 7. **G,** 8. **F,** 9. **B,** 10. **G**

References

Albrektsson, T., & Sennerby, L. (1990). Direct bone anchorage of oral implants: Clinical and experimental considerations of the concept of osseointegration. *International Journal of Prosthodontics*, 3, 30–41.

Andersson, J. E. & Svartz, K. (1988). CT-scanning in the preoperative planning of osseointegrated implants in the maxilla. *International Journal of Oral Maxillofacial Surgery*, 17, 33–35.

Bader, J. D., Rozier, R. G., McFall, W. T., & Ramsey, D. L. (1991). Effect of crown margins on periodontal conditions in regularly attending patients. *Journal of Prosthetic Dentistry*, 65, 75–79.

Balkin, B. E. (1988). Implant dentistry: Historical overview with current perspective. *Journal of Dental Education*, 52, 684–685.

Campbell, S. D. (1989). Evalutation of surface roughness and polishing techniques for new ceramic materials. *Journal of Prosthetic Dentistry*, 61, 563–568.

Castellani, D., Clauser, C., & Bernadini, U. (1994). Thermal distortion of different materials in crown construction. *Journal of Prosthetic Dentistry*, 72, 360–366.

Clark, D. E., Danforth, R. A., Barnes, R. W., & Burtch, M. L. (1990). Radiation absorbed from dental implant radiography: A comparison of linear tomography. *Journal of Oral Implantology* 16(3), 156–164.

Davis, D. R. (1988). Comparison of fit of two types of all-ceramic crowns. *Journal of Prosthetic Dentistry*, 59, 12–6.

Donley, T. G. & Gillette, W. B. (1991). Titanium endosseous implant-soft tissue interface: A literature review. *Journal of Periodontology*, 62, 153.

Dorland's pocket medical dictionary, (28th ed.) Philadelphia: W. B. Saunders Company.

Frielich, M. A., Niekrash, C. E., Katz, R. V., & Simonsen, R. J. (1992). Periodontal effects of fixed partial denture retainer margins: Configuration and location. *Journal of Prosthetic Dentistry*, 67, 184–190.

Hamada, M. O. (1989). Implantology: Radiographic resources. *Journal of California Dental Association*, 17, 20–31.

Harris, B. W. (1990). A new technique for the subperiosteal implant. *Journal of the American Dental Association*, 121, 422.

Hensten-Pettersen, A., & N. Jacobsen (1991). Perceived Side Effects of Biomaterials in Prosthetic Dentistry. *Journal of Prosthetic Dentistry*, 65, 138–144.

Hung, S. H., Hung, K. S., Eick, J. D., & Chappell, R. P. (1990). Marginal fit of porcelain-fused-to-metal and two types of ceramic crown. *Journal of Prosthetic Dentistry*, 63, 26–31.

Jendresen, M. D., Allen, E. P., Bayne, S. C., Hansson, T. L., Klooster, J., & Preston, J. D., (1992). Report of the committee on scientific investigation of the american academy of restorative dentistry. *The Journal of Prosthetic Dentistry*, 68(1), 137–180.

Johansson, C., Hansson, H. A., & Albrektsson, T. (1989). A qualitative, interfacial study between bone and tantalum, niobium, or commercially pure titanium. *Biomaterials*, 4, 27–280.

Lemons, J. E. (1990). Dental Implant Biomaterials. *Journal of the American Dental Association*, 121, 716.

Lyman, D. & Boucher, L. J. (1990). Radiographic examination of edentulous mouths. *Journal of Prosthetic Dentistry*, 64, 180–182.

Meffert, R. (1995). Implantology and the dental hygienist's role. *Journal of Practical Hygiene*, 4, 11–13.

Meijer, H. J. A., Steen, W. H. A., & Bosman, F. (1992). Standardized radiographs of the alveolar crest around implants in the mandible. *Journal of Prosthetic Dentistry*, 68, 318.

Schnitman, P. A. (1993). Implant dentistry: Where are we now? *Journal of the American Dental Association*, 124, 39.

Schulman, L. & Koch, G. (1988). Three-year survival results: Blade implant vs. Cantilever clinical trial. *Journal of Dental Research*, 347.

Small, I. A. (1990). The fixed mandibular implant: Its use in reconstructive prosthetics. *Journal of the American Dental Association*, 121, 369.

Smith, R. A., Berger, R., & Dodson, T. B. (1992). Risk factors associated with dental implants in healthy and medically compromised patients. *International Journal of Oral Maxillofacial Implants*, 7, 367,3.

Thomas, C. L. (1997). *Taber's Cyclopedic Medical Dictionary*. Philadelphia: F. A. Davis Company.

Tjellstrom, A., Jacobsson, M., & Albrektsson, T. (1988). Removal torque of osseointegrated craniofacial implants. *International Journal of Oral Maxillofacial Implants*, 3, 287–289.

Wolff, L. F., Pihlstrom, B. L. Bakdash, M. B. et al. (1988). Current implant usage. *Journal of Dental Education*, 52, 692–695.

Zarb, G. A. & Schmitt, A. (1991). Osseointegration and the edentulous predicament: The 10-year old toronto study. *British Dental Journal*, 170, 439.

CHAPTER 12

Removable Prosthesis

Key Terms

Artificial Replacement
Clasp
Complete Denture
Denture Teeth
Gaskets
Kennedy Classification System
Overdenture
Removable Partial Denture
Rest
Treatment Partial

PRIMARY CODE	SECONDARY CODE
M = Mesial	-T = Denture
I = Incisal (#6–#11 and #22–#27)	-R = Root Canal
O = Occlusal (#1–#5, #12–#16, #17–#21, and #27–#32)	• = and also
D = Distal	• p = Retention Post
F = Facial (#6–#11 and #22–#27)	-Z = Temporary Restoration
B = Buccal (#1–#5, #12–#16, #17–#21, and #27–#32)	= is the symbol that is placed between adjacent teeth on the numeric coding system chart to indicate the teeth are connected and replaced with a Denture (partial or complete).
L = Lingual	⊤ (maxillary) or ⊥ (mandibular) = the symbol that is placed at the root tips of adjacent teeth on anatomic and geometric charts to indicate that the teeth are connected and replaced with a Denture (partial or complete).
X = Missing	

Introduction

The **artificial replacement** of a missing body part is referred to as prosthesis. The removable dental prosthesis that is used to replace missing teeth and their surrounding structures is called a **removable partial denture**. This type of Denture system is supported by the remaining natural teeth.

Removable partial dentures can be utilized for certain partially edentulous conditions and the **Kennedy Classification System** classifies these edentulous situations into the following categories:

- Class I: Bilateral edentulous area with only the anterior teeth remaining
- Class II: Unilateral edentulous area with the anterior teeth present and the remainder of the teeth on the right or left
- Class III: Unilateral edentulous area with surrounding teeth that cannot assume the support of the prosthesis
- Class IV: Anterior edentulous area with the remaining teeth located bilaterally

Universal System
#4 #5 #6 #7 #8 #9 #10 #11 #12 #13

Palmer System
5| 4| 3| 2| 1| |1 |2 |3 |4 |5

ISO/FDI System
15 14 13 12 11 21 22 23 24 25

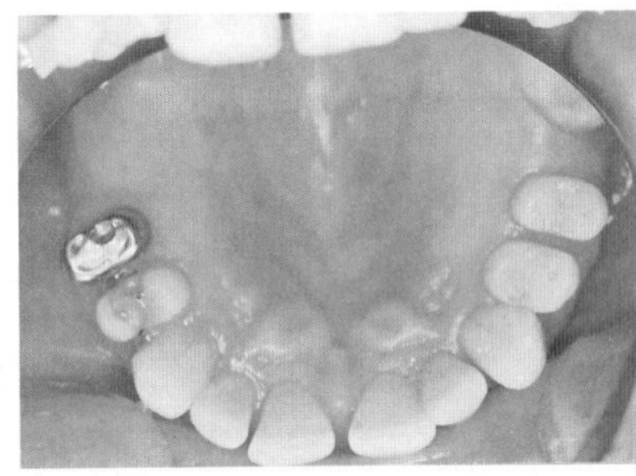

A.

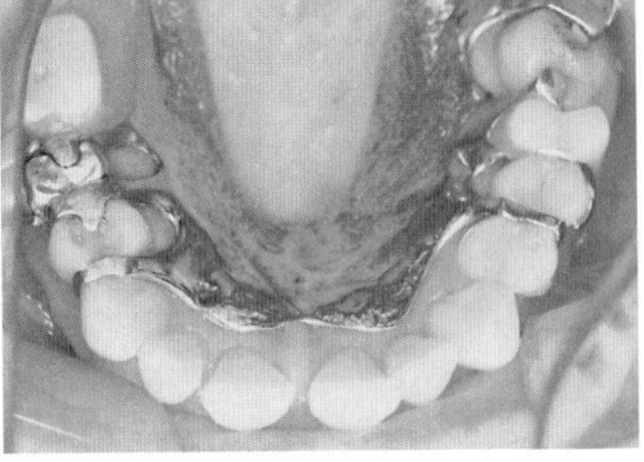

B.

Universal System
#4 #5 #6 #7 #8 #9 #10 #11 #12 #13

Palmer System
5| 4| 3| 2| 1| |1 |2 |3 |4 |5

ISO/FDI System
14 13 12 11 21 22 23 24 25

Figure 12–1 (A) Photograph shown with teeth #1, #2, #3, and #14 Missing (B) Photograph shown of figure (A) with a removable partial denture

- Class V: Anterior and posterior edentulous area with anterior teeth that cannot assume the support of the prosthesis
- Class VI: Edentulous area where the abutment teeth are capable of supporting the prosthesis

Cast cobalt-chromium and nickel-chromium alloys are used to fabricate the framework for partial dentures. Figure 12–1A shows teeth #1, #2, #3, and #14 as Missing and Figure 12–1B shows the teeth replaced with a removable partial denture.

The components on the partial denture include the **clasp**, **rest**, and **denture teeth**. The clasp is made of metal alloy and surrounds and secures the Denture to the existing natural teeth. The rest, which is an extension of the clasp, stabilizes and prevents movement of the partial denture and fits onto the remaining tooth structures. The Gold Crown on tooth #4 is shown with the receptacle area for the clasp to fit into. The denture teeth are made from Porcelain or modified acrylic materials and are set into the Denture base.

Another type of removable partial denture that uses rubber **gaskets** instead of metal clasps to surround and support the remaining natural teeth is shown in Figure 12–2 and Plate 8.

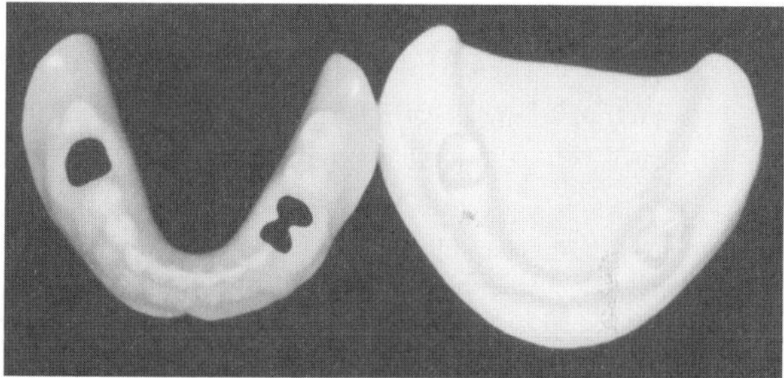

Figure 12–2 Photograph shown with a removable partial denture with rubber gaskets

A **treatment partial** is made from acrylic and is used to temporarily replace one or more Missing teeth. This is not supposed to be used as the permanent replacement but used until the area can be restored with a fixed partial denture. Figure 12–3 shows three different types of treatment partials.

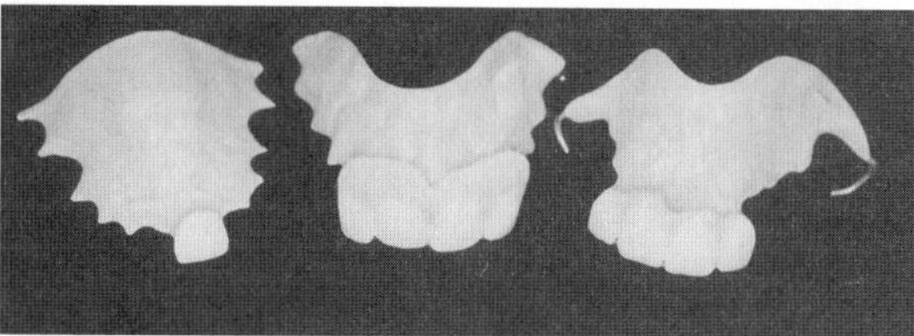

Figure 12–3 Photograph shown with three different treatment partials (Courtesy Olsen Dental)

Charting Removable Partial Dentures on an Anatomic Chart

To indicate that teeth #1, #2, #3, and #14 (see Figure 12–1B) are replaced with a removable partial denture, use a blue pencil to mark the teeth Missing (described in Chapter 4). Then located at the Root Tip of each Missing tooth, draw a horizontal line over the Root Tips and then attach this to a short vertical line that extends off the Root Tip of each tooth (Figure 12–4).

This is written as: the primary code "X" followed by a hyphen (-) then the secondary code "T" "X-T." This is read as: teeth #1, #2, #3, and #14 are Missing and replaced with a Denture.

The photograph in Figure 12–2 shown of the partial denture with rubber gaskets is shown charted in Figure 12–4.

To indicate the presence of a treatment partial, follow the same procedures above except draw the brackets that connect to the roots in red pencil. In Figure 12–4, the chart shows that the central and lateral incisors are replaced with a treatment partial. This is written as "X-TZ." This is read as: teeth #7, #8, #9, and #10 are Missing and replaced with a Temporary Denture.

Figure 12–4 Anatomic chart shown with removable partial dentures on the maxillary and mandibular arches and a treatment partial on the maxillary arch replacing teeth #7, #8, #9, and #10

18	17	16	15	14	13	12	11	21	22	23	24	25	26	27	28
8	7	6	5	4	3	2	1	1	2	3	4	5	6	7	8
1	2	3	4	5	6	7	8	9	10	11	12	13	14	15	16

32	31	30	29	28	27	26	25	24	23	22	21	20	19	18	17
8	7	6	5	4	3	2	1	1	2	3	4	5	6	7	8
48	47	46	45	44	43	42	41	31	32	33	34	35	36	37	38

Charting Removable Partial Dentures on a Geometric Chart

To show the removable partial dentures in Figure 12–1B and Figure 12–2 and Plate 8 on a geometric chart, follow the same procedure that was previously mentioned for charting on an anatomic chart (Figure 12–5).

The treatment partial shown in Figure 12–3 is shown charted as was previously mentioned.

Charting Removable Partial Dentures on a Numeric Coding System Chart

To indicate teeth #1, #2, #3, and #14 (see Figure 12–1B) are replaced with a removable partial denture on a numeric coding system chart, use a black pen to enter the date in the appropriate column. With a blue pencil, print the primary code "X" followed by the secondary code "T" in the row of boxes adjacent to the date. To indicate one or more teeth are connected together, locate the vertical line between each tooth and draw two short horizontal lines through it (Figure 12–6).

18	17	16	15	14	13	12	11	21	22	23	24	25	26	27	28
8	7	6	5	4	3	2	1	1	2	3	4	5	6	7	8
1	2	3	4	5	6	7	8	9	10	11	12	13	14	15	16

32	31	30	29	28	27	26	25	24	23	22	21	20	19	18	17
8	7	6	5	4	3	2	1	1	2	3	4	5	6	7	8
48	47	46	45	44	43	42	41	31	32	33	34	35	36	37	38

Figure 12–5 Geometric chart shown with removable partial Dentures on the maxillary and mandibular arches and a treatment partial on the maxillary arch replacing teeth #7, #8, #9, and #10

8-20-93	X-T	X-T	X-T				X-T	X-T	X-T	X-T				X-T		
MAXILLA	1	2	3	4 A	5 B	6 C	7 D	8 E	9 F	10 G	11 H	12 I	13 J	14	15	16
MANDIBLE	32	31	30	T 29	S 28	R 27	Q 26	P 25	O 24	N 23	M 22	L 21	K 20	19	18	17
8-20-93	X-T	X-T		X-T	X-T	X-T	X-T	X-T	X-T	X-T	X-T			X-T	X-T	X-T

Figure 12–6 Numeric coding system chart shown with removable partial Dentures on the maxillary and mandibular arches and a treatment partial on the maxillary arch replacing teeth #7, #8, #9, and #10

The teeth on this chart are written and read as they were previously mentioned. The partial denture shown in Figure 12–2 and Plate 8 and the treatment partial in Figure 12–3 are shown charted here.

Complete Dentures

The dental prosthesis that replaces all of the teeth either in the maxillary, mandibular, or both arches, is referred to as a **complete denture**. The Denture is constructed of a base made of acrylic resins or plastics and the teeth are made of plastic resins or Porcelain.

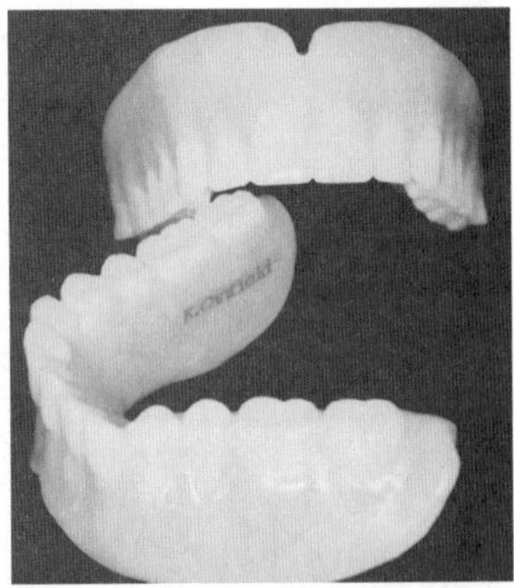

Figure 12–7 Photograph shown of complete dentures (Courtesy Olsen Dental)

Figure 12–7 is a photograph that shows an upper and lower Denture. It is common practice today for dental laboratories to incorporate a label with the name of the Denture owner directly into the Denture base material for identification purposes.

Charting Complete Dentures on an Anatomic Chart

To indicate the maxillary and mandibular teeth are Missing and replaced with dentures, follow the same procedure used to chart removable partial dentures. Mark all of the teeth Missing and connect all the teeth present on the Denture with a horizontal line attached to each tooth with a vertical line (Figure 12–8).

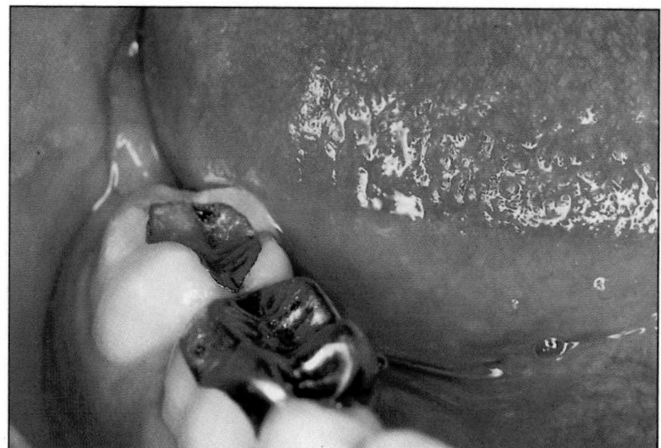

Plate 1 Gold Inlay and Gold Onlay restorations

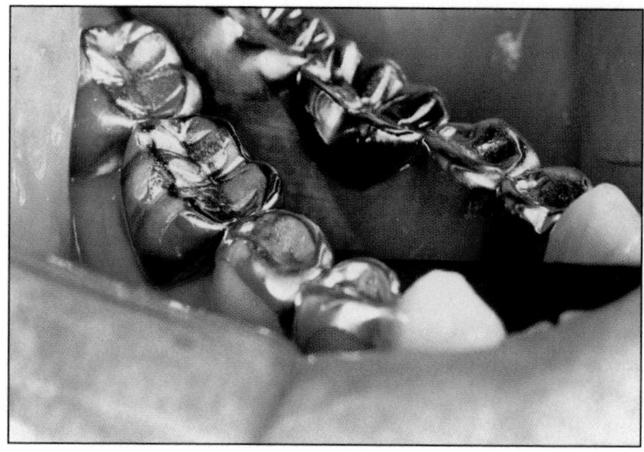

Plate 2 Gold Onlay restorations, Non-precious Crown, and Gold Crown restorations

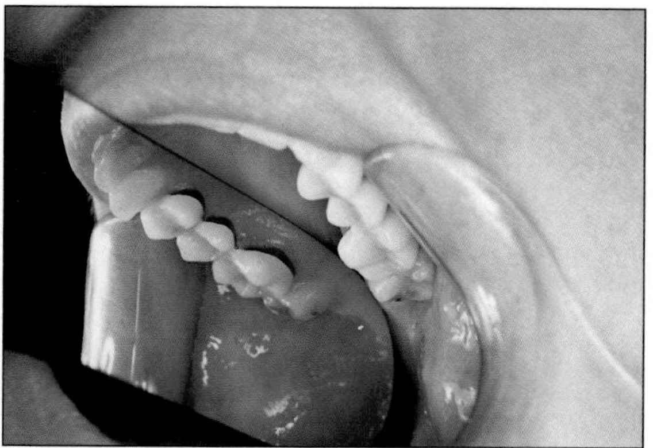

Plate 3 Fixed partial denture with Porcelain-Fused-To-Metal Crowns

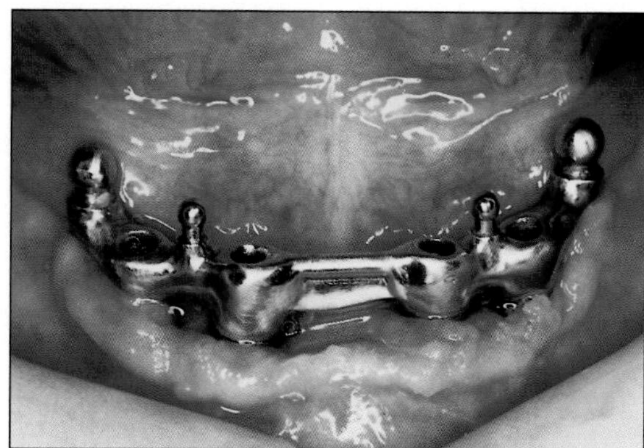

Plate 4 Endosseous implant (Courtesy Paul A. Johnson, DDS)

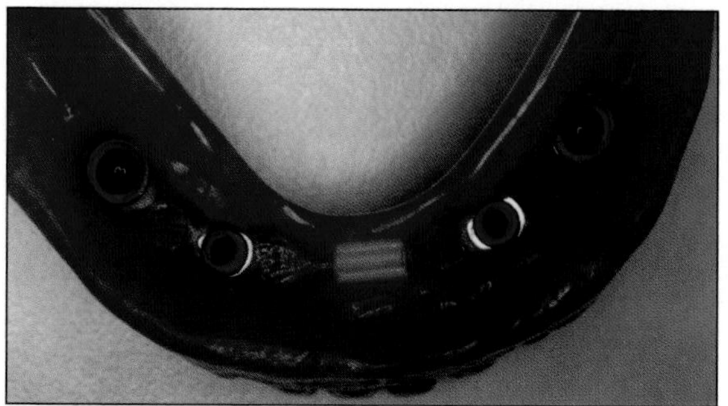

Plate 5 Overdenture for the endosseous implant (Courtesy Paul A. Johnson, DDS)

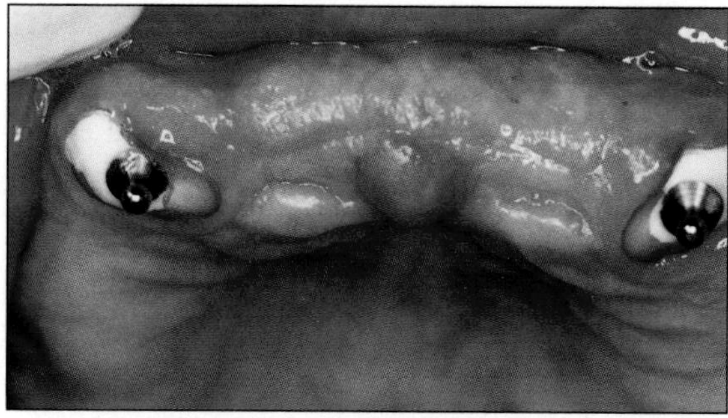

Plate 6 Retention roots with prefabricated posts and overdenture attachment apparatus (Courtesy Paul A. Johnson, DDS)

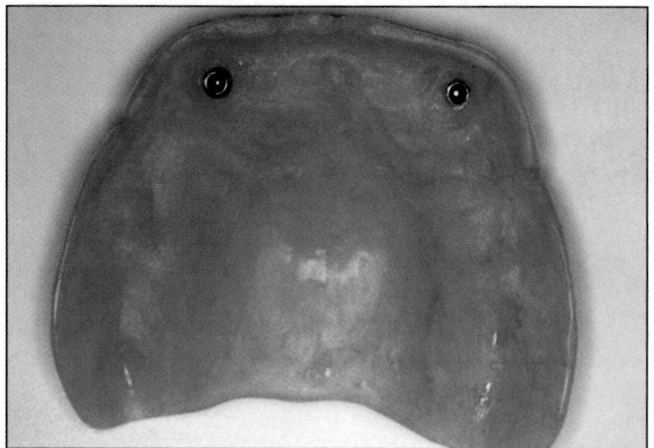

Plate 7 Complete maxillary overdenture (Courtesy Paul A. Johnson, DDS)

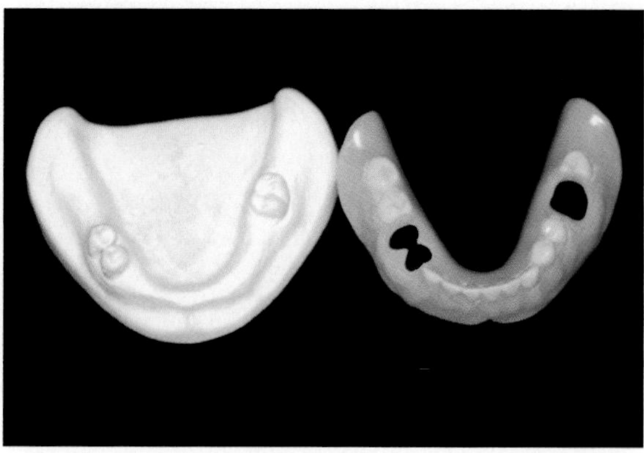

Plate 8 Removable partial denture with rubber gaskets

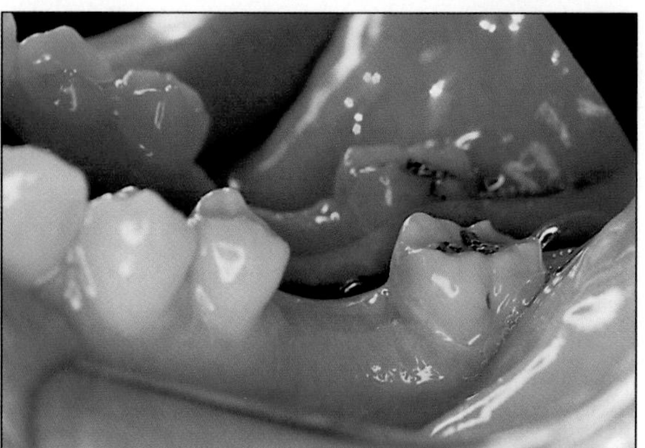

Plate 9 Dental caries

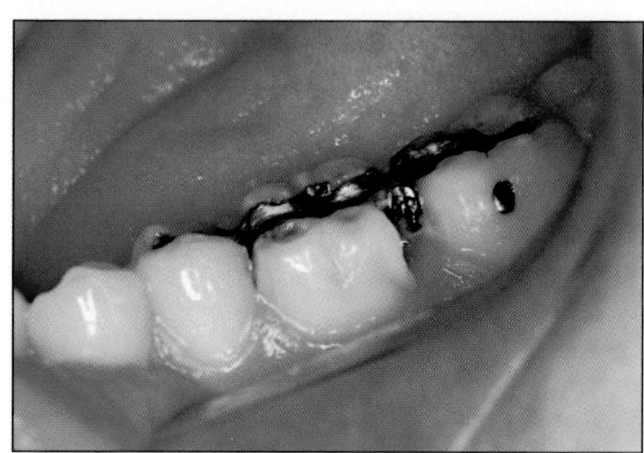

Plate 10 Recurrent caries

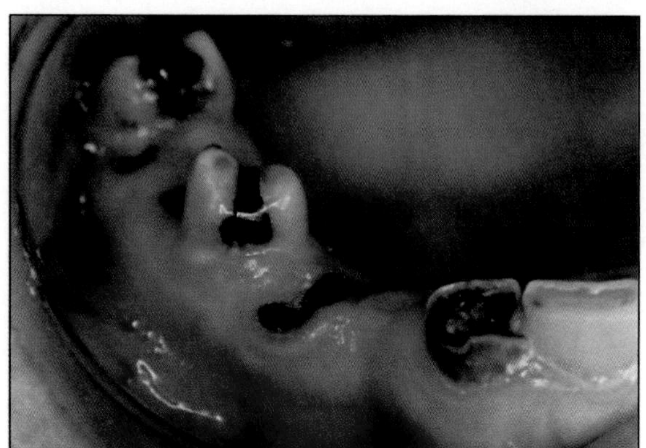

Plate 11 Rampant caries

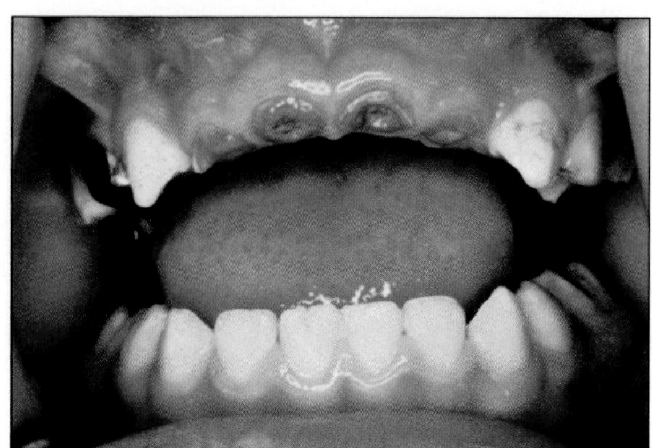

Plate 12 Baby bottle tooth decay

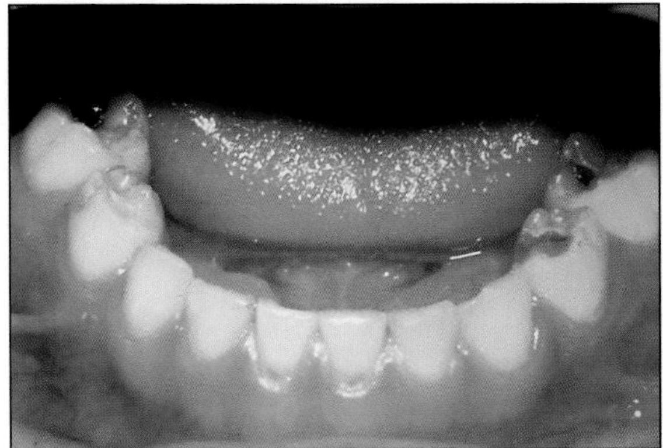

Plate 13 Chronic medication-related caries

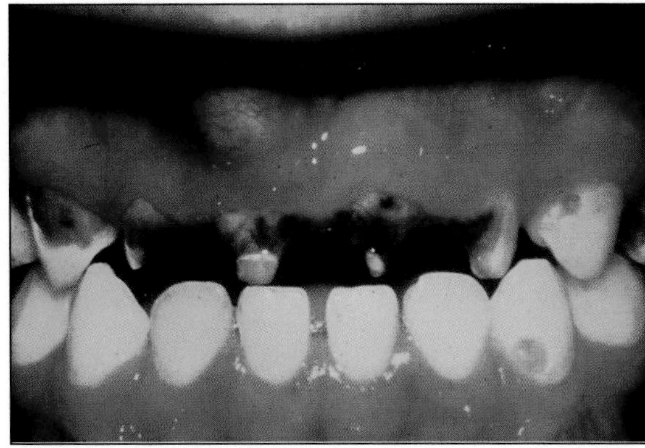

Plate 14 Pacifier caries

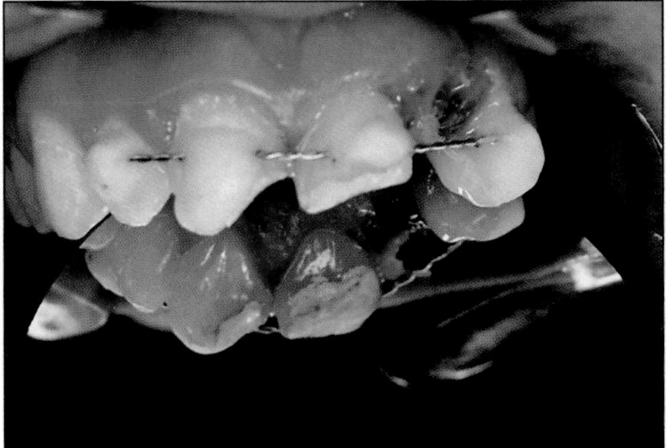

Plate 15 Fractured crowns and the teeth are stabilized with a splint

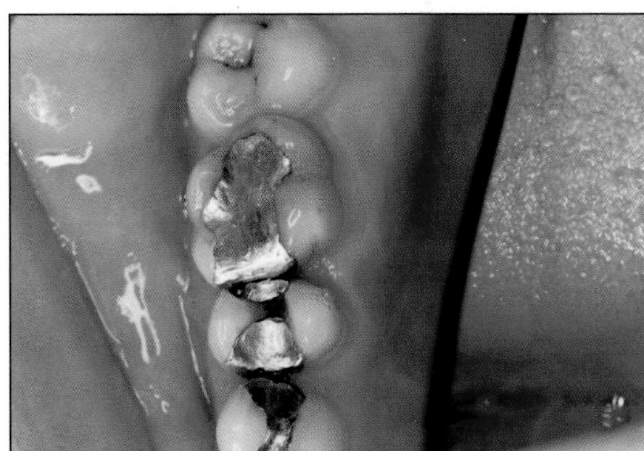

Plate 16 Fractured restoration

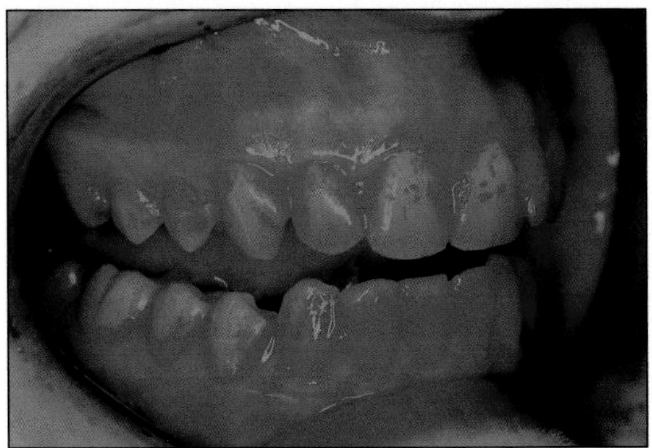

Plate 17 Disclosed bacterial plaque and pellicle with erythrosin disclosing agent

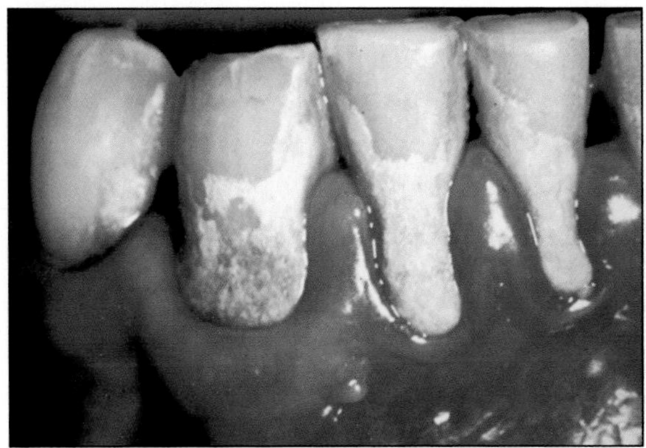

Plate 18 Generalized calculus

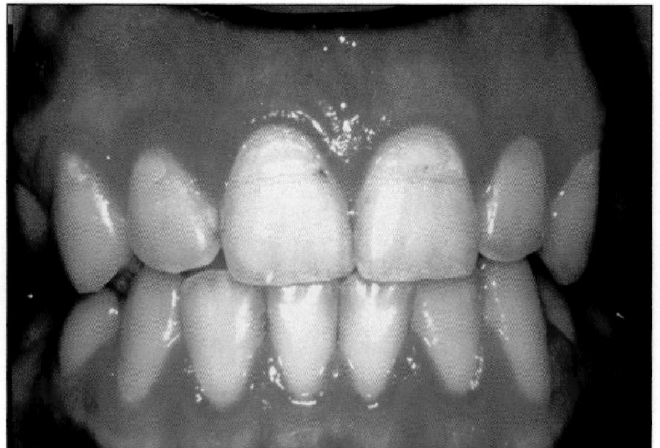

Plate 19 Marginal gingivitis

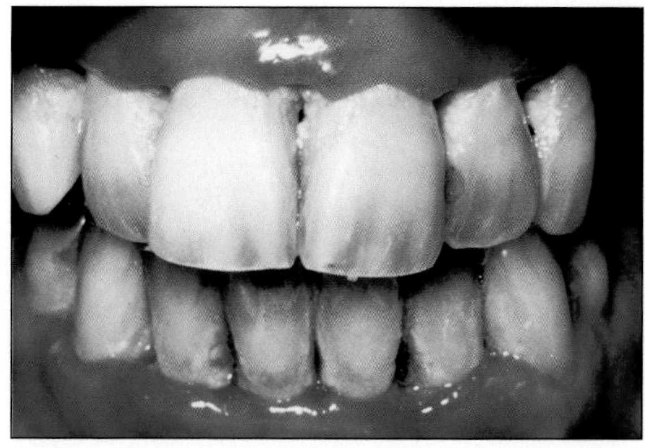

Plate 20 Necrotizing ulcerative gingivitis (NUG)

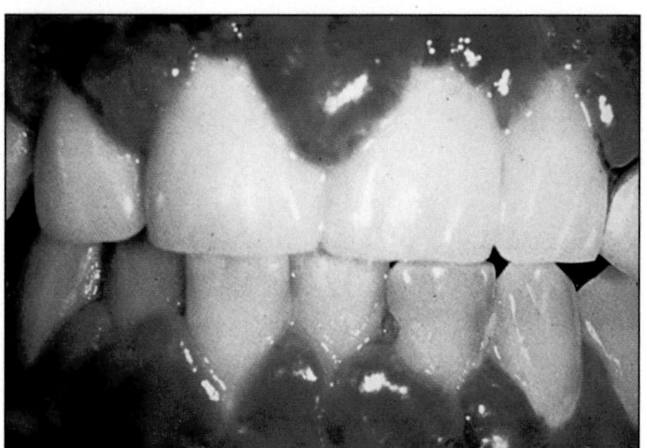

Plate 21 Hormone-induced gingivitis due to pregnancy

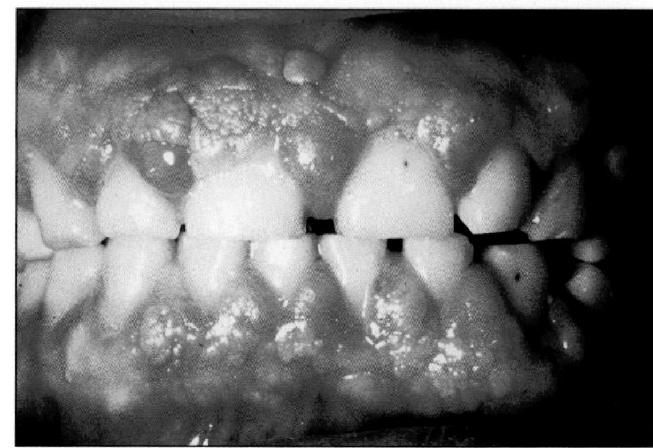

Plate 22 Drug influenced gingivitis (phenytoin)

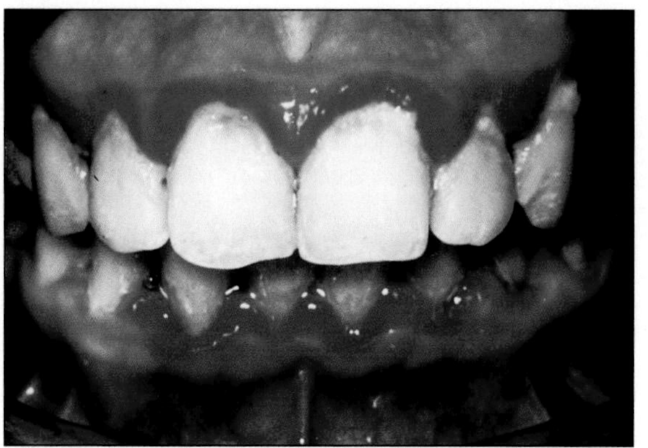

Plate 23 Linear gingival erythema (LGE) (previously called HIV-gingivitis)

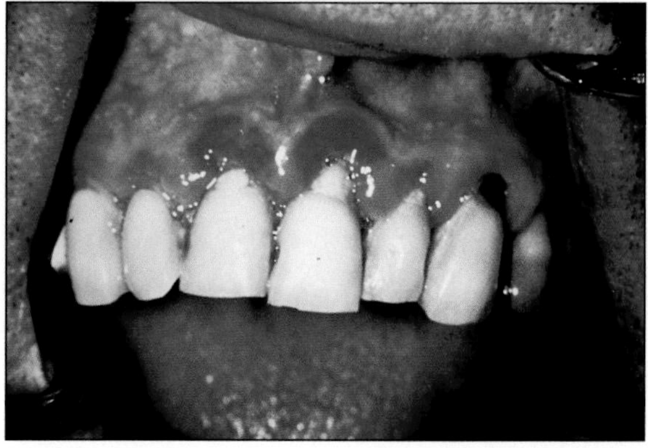

Plate 24 Periodontitis

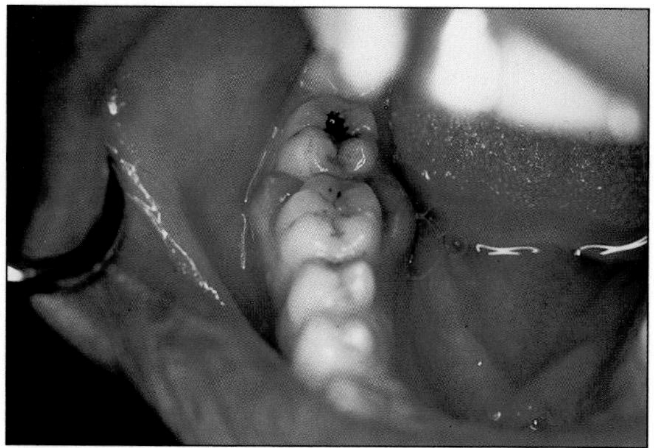

Plate 25 Food impaction (Courtesy Ronald E. Gier, DMD, MSD)

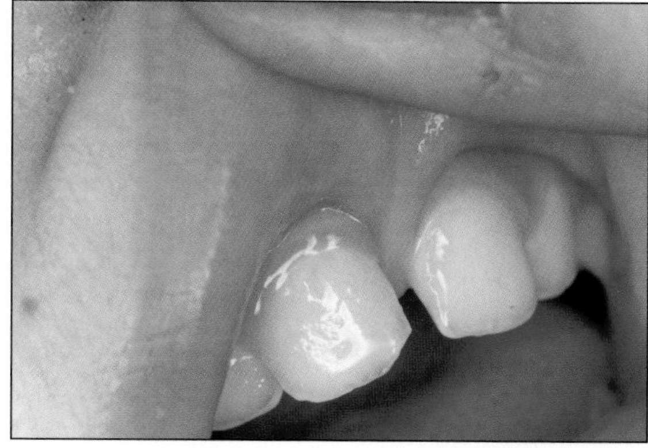

Plate 26 Diastema and pathologic frenum attachment

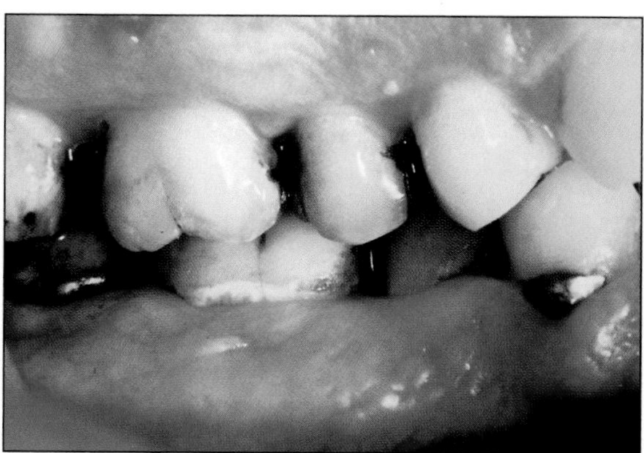

Plate 27 Demineralization on the cervical third of tooth #30

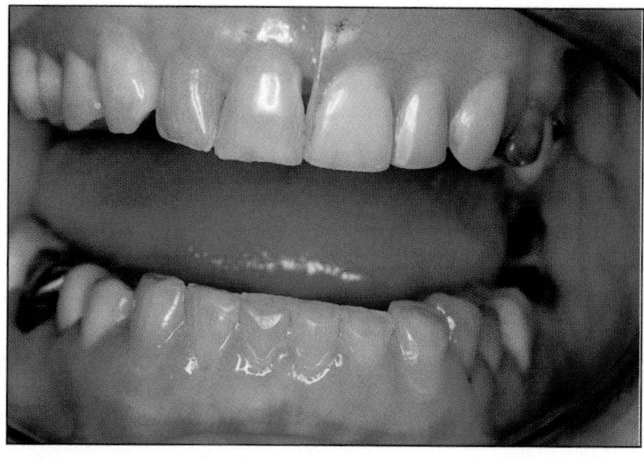

Plate 28 Attrition and wear facets

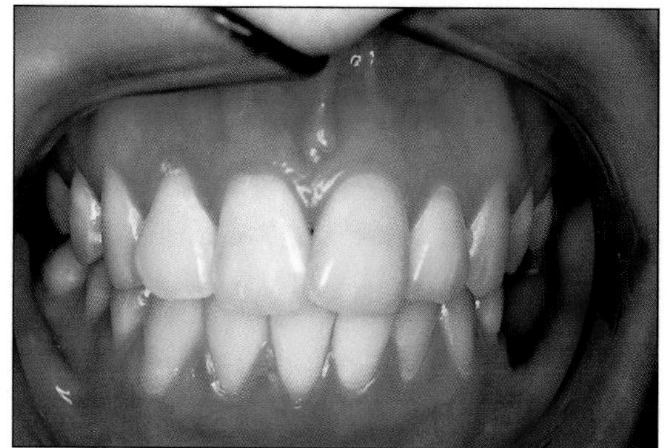

Plate 29 Erosion

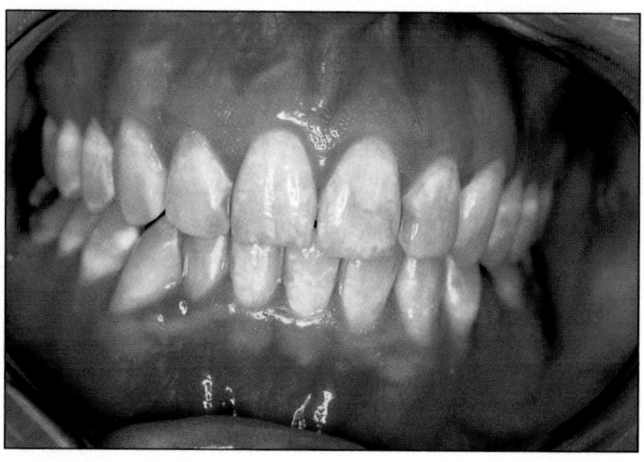

Plate 30 Fluorosis

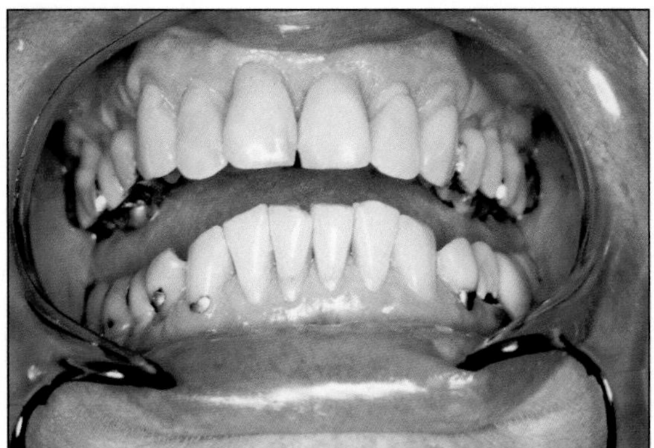

Plate 31 Abrasion

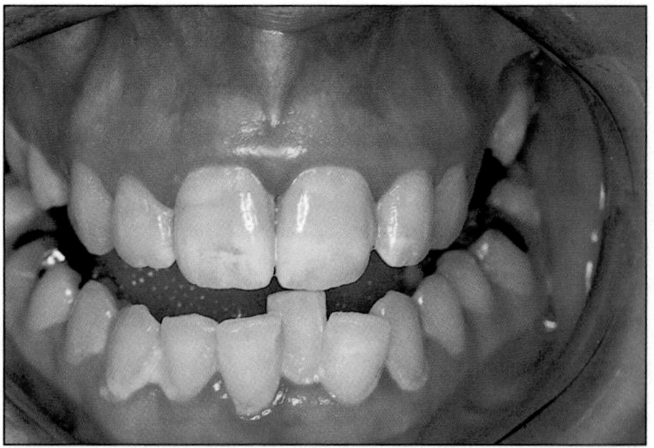

Plate 32 Endogenous intrinsic stain due to tetracycline antibiotics

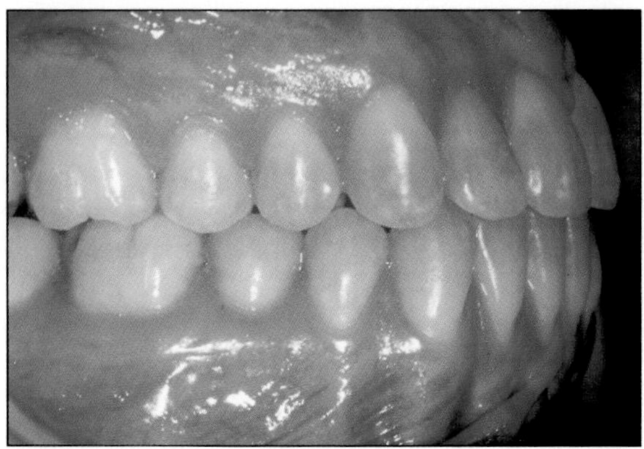

Plate 33 Normal "ideal" occlusion

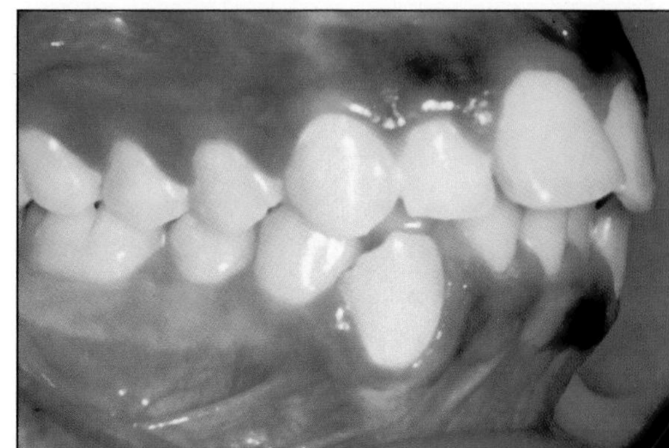

Plate 34 Class I malocclusion

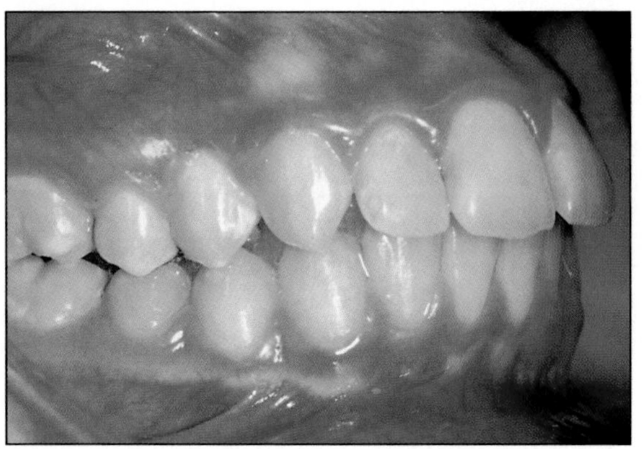

Plate 35 Class II, Division 1 with a 2 mm discrepancy

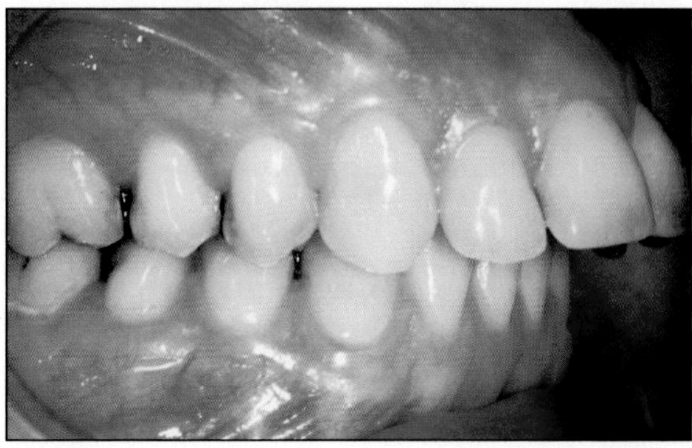

Plate 36 Class II, Division 2 with a > 2 mm discrepancy

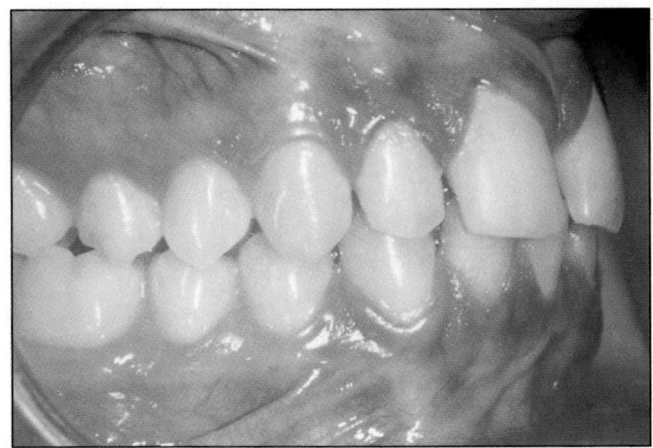

Plate 37 Class III malocclusion—molars

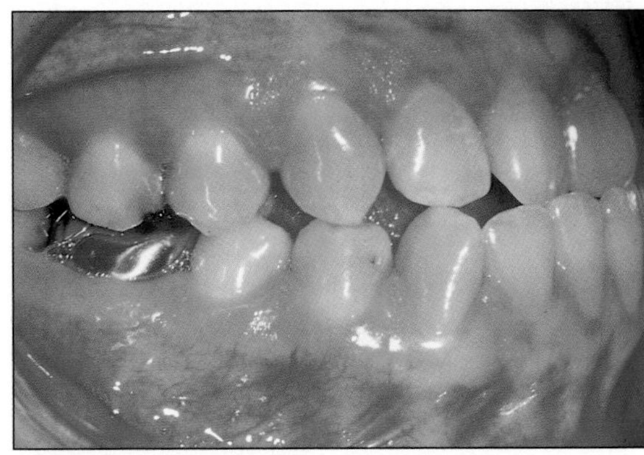

Plate 38 Class III malocclusion with underjet

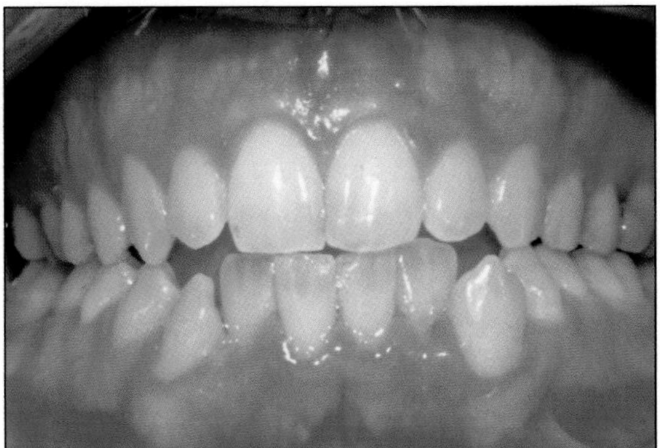

Plate 39 End-to-end bite

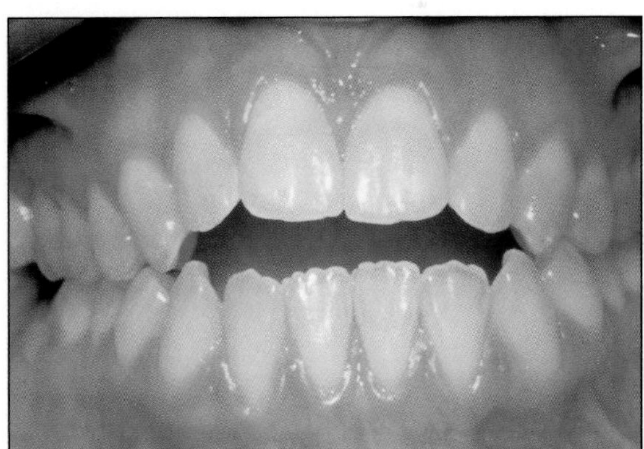

Plate 40 Openbite

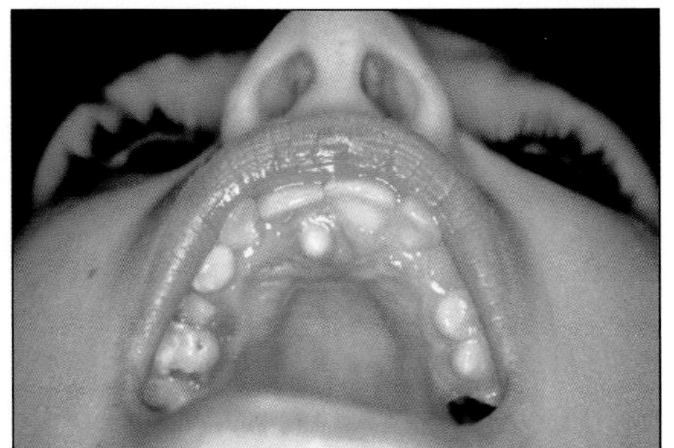

Plate 41 Mesiodens

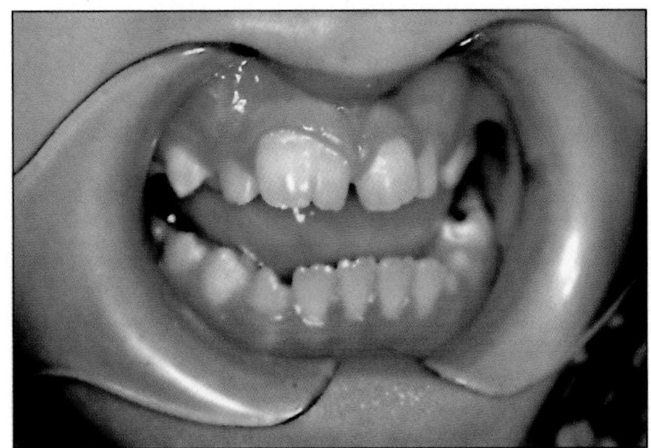

Plate 42 Gemination

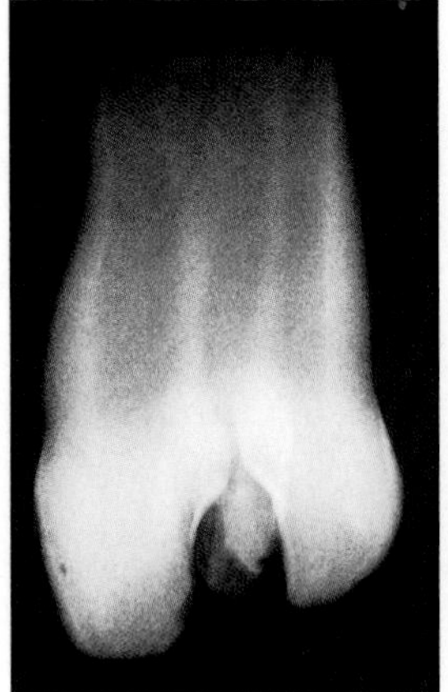

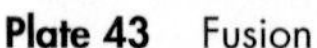

Plate 43 Fusion

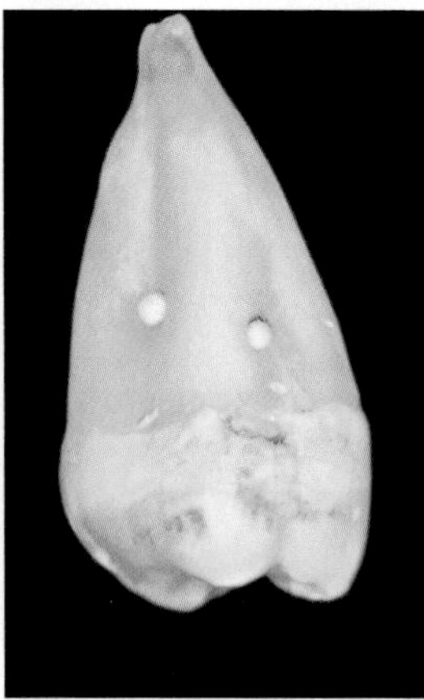

Plate 44 Enamel pearls

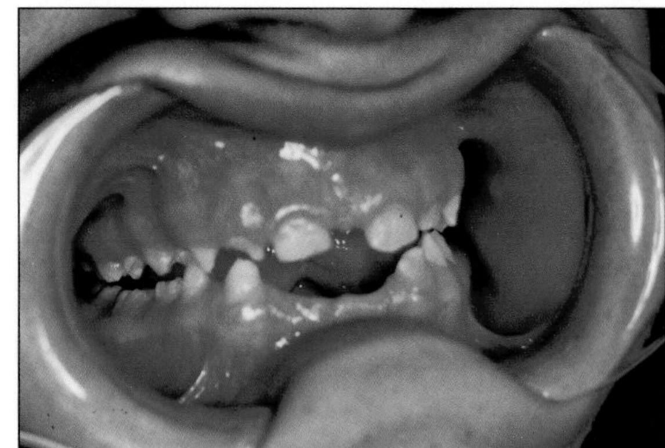

Plate 45 Amelogenesis imperfecta (Courtesy Ronald E. Gier, DMD, MSD)

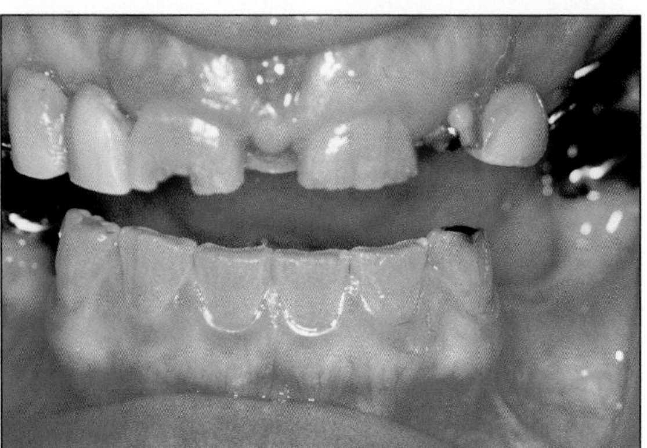

Plate 46 Dentinogenesis imperfecta (Courtesy Ronald E. Gier, DMD, MSD)

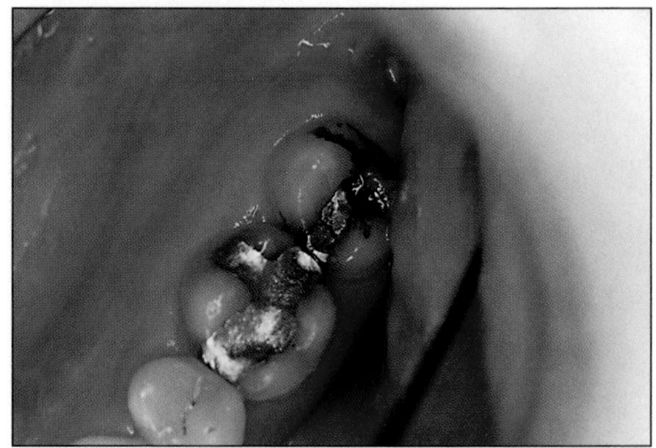

Plate 47 Fractured restoration

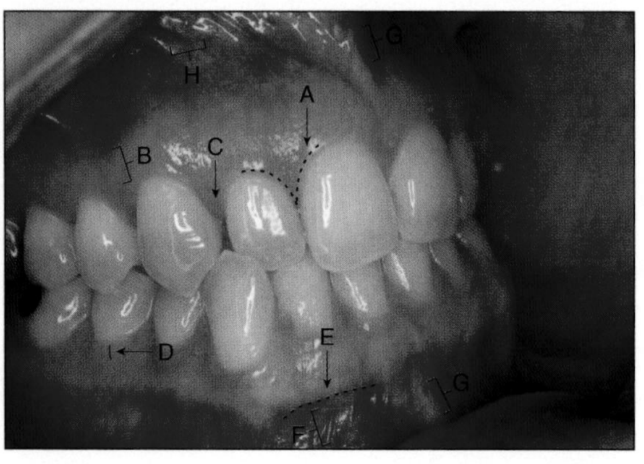

Plate 48 Healthy gingiva and associated structures: (A) Free gingival groove (B) Attached gingiva (C) Interdental papilla (D) Free gingiva (E) Mucogingival junction (F) Alveolar mucosa (G) Labial frenum (H) Buccal frenum

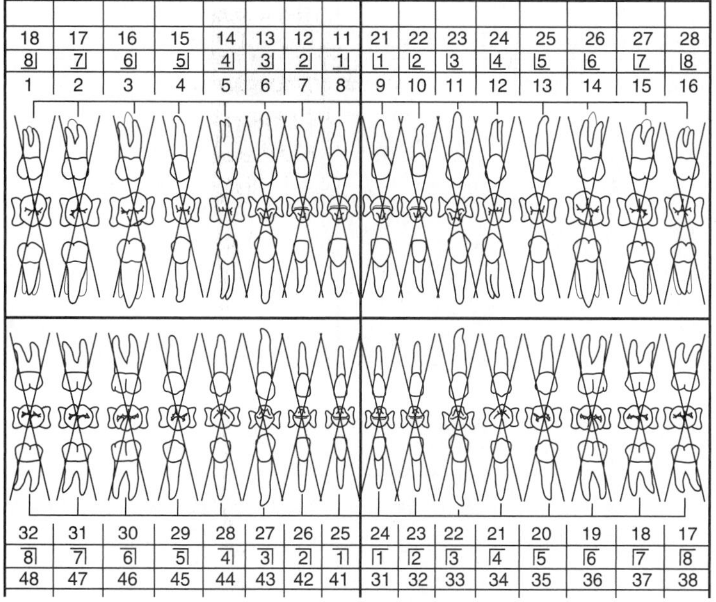

Figure 12–8 Anatomic chart shown with complete dentures on the maxillary and mandibular arches

The primary and secondary codes are the same as they are for documenting a removable partial denture.

Charting Complete Dentures on a Geometric Chart

To chart complete dentures on a geometric chart, follow the same procedures that are used for indicating removable partial dentures on an anatomic chart. Figure 12–9 shows complete upper and lower dentures charted. These are written and read as previously described.

Charting Complete Dentures on a Numeric Coding System Chart

To indicate complete dentures on a numeric coding system chart, follow the same procedure for charting removable prosthesis. Figure 12–10 indicates complete upper and lower Dentures. This chart is read and written following the same procedures that were previously described.

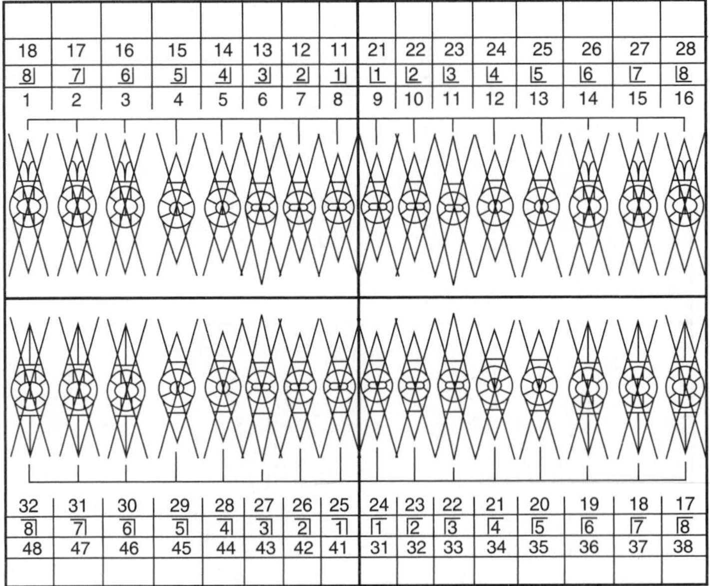

Figure 12–9 Geometric chart shown with complete dentures on the maxillary and mandibular arches

1-12-96	X-T	X-T	X-T	X-T	X-T	X-T	X-T	X-T	X-T	X-T	X-T	X-T	X-T	X-T	X-T	X-T
MAXILLA	1	2	3	4	5	6	7	8	9	10	11	12	13	14	15	16
				A	B	C	D	E	F	G	H	I	J			
				T	S	R	Q	P	O	N	M	L	K			
MANDIBLE	32	31	30	29	28	27	26	25	24	23	22	21	20	19	18	17
1-12-96	X-T	X-T	X-T	X-T	X-T	X-T	X-T	X-T	X-T	X-T	X-T	X-T	X-T	X-T	X-T	X-T

Figure 12–10 Numeric coding system chart shown with complete dentures on the maxillary and mandibular arches

Complete Overdenture

An **overdenture**, also known as coping or overlay Denture, is a complete Denture supported by retained teeth that have had their crowns reduced and treated endodontically or by dental implants (described in Chapter 11). The residual roots following endodontic treatment are restored with custom cast posts fabricated with special attachments that are cemented into place. The Denture has metal-encapsulated O-rings that insert onto the attachment apparatus.

Universal System
#6 #11
#27 #22

Palmer System
3⌋ ⌊3
3⌉ ⌈3

ISO/FDI System
13 23
43 33

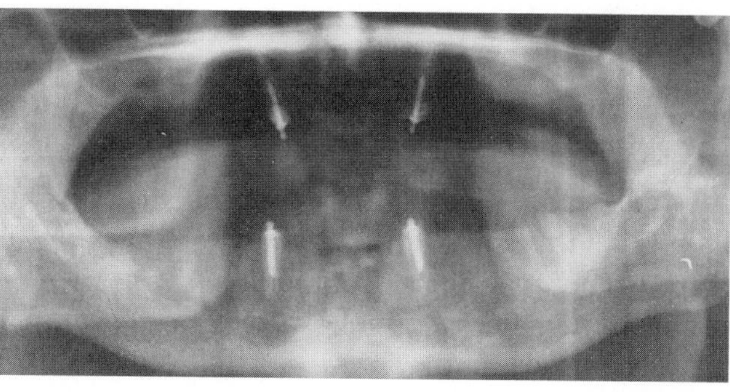

Figure 12–11 Panoramic radiograph shown of teeth #6, #11, #22, and #27 as retained roots that have Root Canal treatment with cast Retention Posts and attachment apparatus for complete overdentures (Courtesy Paul A. Johnson, DDS)

The panoramic radiograph in Figure 12–11 shows teeth #6, #11, #22, and #27 with endodontically treated roots, prefabricated cast posts, and the overdenture attachment apparatus. These restorations appear as radiopaque images.

Plate 6 shows the reduced crowns on teeth #6 and #11 with the metal copings and Plate 7 shows the complete maxillary overdenture with metal encapsulated O-rings.

Charting a Complete Overdenture on an Anatomic Chart

To indicate two retained roots and an overdenture in Figure 12–11, Plate 6, and Plate 7 on an anatomic chart, follow the same procedures for charting a complete Denture except on teeth #6 and #11 only cross out the crowns on the three surface views. Indicate each Root Canal and custom Retention Post with a single line that is expanded near the cervical third of the root (described in Chapter 16). To show that the teeth are replaced with a Denture, draw a single horizontal line with short vertical lines that are connected to the roots of each tooth diagram (Figure12–12).

Charting a Complete Overdenture on a Geometric Chart

To chart an overdenture on a geometric chart, follow the same procedures that were previously mentioned when using an anatomic chart (Figure 12–13).

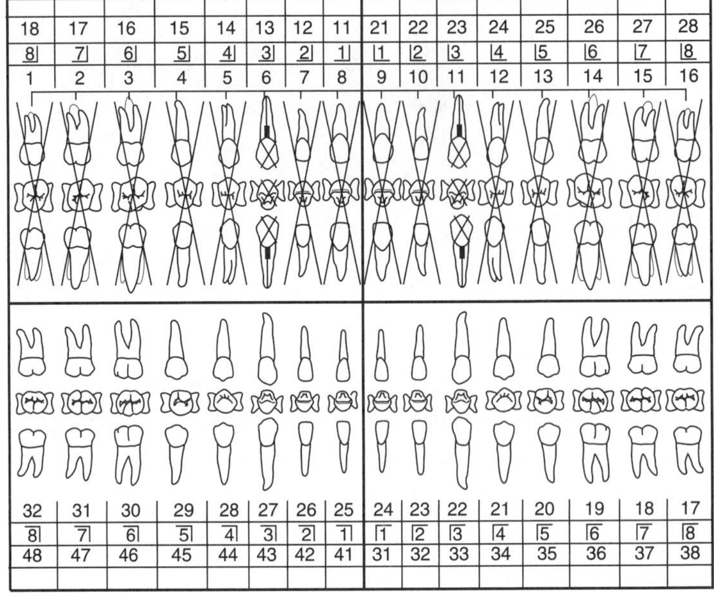

Figure 12–12 Anatomic chart shown with teeth #1–#5, #7–#10, and #12–#16 Missing. Teeth #6 and #11 crowns are Missing and the retained roots have Root Canals with cast Retention Posts and fabricated attachment apparatus for a complete maxillary overdenture

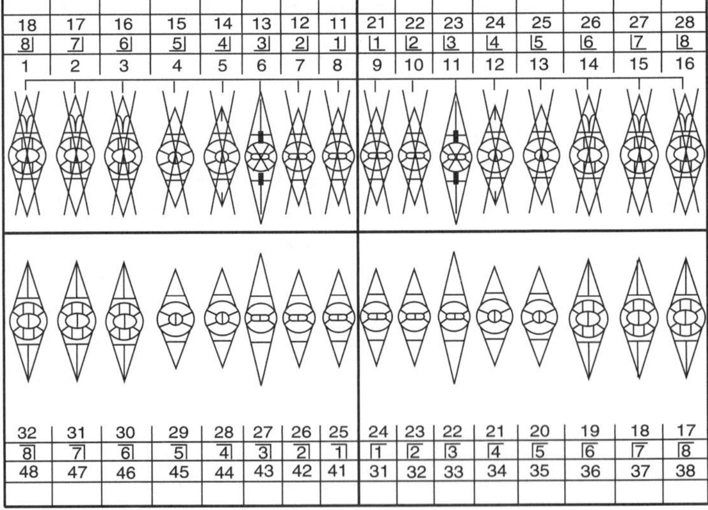

Figure 12–13 Geometric chart shown with teeth #1–#5, #7–#10, and #12–#16 Missing. Teeth #6 and #11 crowns are Missing and the retained roots have Root Canals with cast Retention Posts and fabricated attachment apparatus for a complete maxillary overdenture

Charting a Complete Overdenture on a Numeric Coding System Chart

To indicate an overdenture on a numeric coding system chart, use a black pen to enter the date in the designated column. In the row of boxes adjacent to the date column, use a blue pencil to place the primary code "X" followed by the secondary code "T" (X-T) in each of the boxes except for teeth #6 and #11. To show that teeth #6 and #11 crowns are Missing, have retained roots with Root Canal treatment with Retention Posts, and support an overdenture, print the primary codes "MIDFLX" and the secondary code "R," then the symbol "•" followed by "•p" and "• T"(MIDFLX-R • •p • T) (Figure 12–14).

The chart is written as: teeth #1–#5, #7–#10, #12–#16, "X-T" are Missing and replaced with a Denture. For teeth #6 and #11: "MIDFLX-R • •p • T," the Mesio-Inciso-Disto-Facio-Lingual tooth surfaces are Missing. The root is present and restored with a Root Canal and also a Retention Post and also covered with a Denture.

11-1-95	X-T	X-T	X-T	X-T	X-T	MIDFLX-R •p•T	X-T	X-T	X-T	X-T	MIDFLX-R •p•T	X-T	X-T	X-T	X-T	X-T
MAXILLA	1	2	3	4 A	5 B	6 C	7 D	8 E	9 F	10 G	11 H	12 I	13 J	14	15	16
MANDIBLE	32	31	30	T 29	S 28	R 27	Q 26	P 25	O 24	N 23	M 22	L 21	K 20	19	18	17
11-1-95																

Figure 12–14 Numeric coding system chart shown with teeth #1–#5, #7–#10, and #12–#16 Missing. Teeth #6 and #11 crowns are Missing and the retained roots have Root Canals with cast Retention Posts and fabricated attachment apparatus for a complete maxillary overdenture

Review Questions

Matching

Directions: Place the uppercase letter(s) after the number to match each term with the statement that *best* defines it.

A Clasp
B Complete denture
C Denture teeth
D Kennedy Classification System
E Overdenture
F Removable partial denture
G Prosthesis
H Rest
I Treatment partial

1. ____ The system for classifying edentulous situations.
2. ____ An artificial replacement.
3. ____ A replacement for an entire arch of Missing teeth.
4. ____ They are made of Porcelain or acrylic.
5. ____ A support that is located on the Denture clasp.
6. ____ Is identified by the secondary code as "Z."
7. ____ A removable prosthesis that fits on the tops of remaining roots.
8. ____ Is made of acrylic teeth and cast nickel-chromium alloys.
9. ____ This surrounds the existing natural tooth.
10. ____ Charted as "X-T."

Answers

1. **D,** 2. **G,** 3. **B,** 4. **C,** 5. **H,** 6. **I,** 7. **E,** 8. **F,** 9. **A,** 10. **B** and **F**

References

Blackman, R., Gaghi, N., & Tran, C. (1991). Dimensional changes in casting titanium removable partial denture frameworks. *Journal of Prosthetic Dentistry*, 65, 309–315.

Chan, E. C., Iugovaz, I., Siboo, R., Bilyk, M., Barolet, R., Amsel, R., Wooley, C., & Klitorinos, A. (1991). Comparison of two popular methods for removal and killing of bacteria from dentures. *Journal/Canadian Dental Association*, 57, 937.

Dorland's pocket medical dictionary (28th ed.). (1994). Philadelphia: W. B. Saunders Company.

Ettinger, R. L., & Jakobsen, J. (1990). Caries: A problem in an overdenture population. *Community Dentistry and Oral Epidemiology*, 18, 42.

Gomes, B. C., & Renner, R. P. (1990). Periodontal considerations of the removable partial overdenture. *Dental Clinics of North America*, 34, 653.

Hensten-Pettersen, A., & Jacobsen, N. (1991). Perceived side effects of biomaterials in prosthetic dentistry. *Journal of Prosthetic Dentistry*, 65, 138–144.

Jendresen, M. D., Allen, E. P., Bayne, S. C., Hansson, T. L., Klooster, J., & Preston, J. D. (1992). Report of the committee on scientific investigation of the American Academy of Restorative Dentistry. *Journal of Prosthetic Dentistry*, 68 (1), 137–180.

Keltjens, H. M. A. M., Schaeken, M. J. M., van der Hoeven, J. S., & Hendriks, J. C. M. (1990). Caries control in overdenture patients: 18-month evaluation on fluoride and chlorhexidine therapies. *Caries Research*, 24, 371.

Lyman, S., & Boucher, L. J. (1990). Radiographic examination of edentulous mouths. *Journal of Prosthetic Dentistry*, 64, 180–182.

Marinello, C. P., Scharer, P., & Meyenberg, K. (1991). Resin-bonded etched castings with extracoronal attachments for removable partial dentures. *Journal of Prosthetic Dentistry*, 66, 52–55.

McDermott, I. G., & Samant, A. (1990). An overview of removable partial overdentures. *Compendium*, 11, 106.

Norman, A. L. (1964). Frictional resistance and dental prosthetics. *Journal of Prosthetic Dentistry*, 14, 45.

Seals, R. R., Williams, E. O., & Jones, J. D. (1992). Panoramic radiographs: Necessary for edentulous patients? *Journal of the American Dental Association*, 123.

Taylor, T. D., & Morton, T. H. (1991). Ulcerative lesions of the palate associated with removable partial denture castings. *Journal of Prosthetic Dentistry*, 66, 213.

Thomas, C. L. (1997). *Taber's cyclopedic medical dictionary*. Philadelphia: F. A. Davis Company.

Wallace, P. W., Graser, G. N., Myers, M. L., & Proskin, H. M. (1991). Dimensional accuracy of denture resin cured by microwave energy. *Journal of Prosthetic Dentistry*, 66: 403–409.

CHAPTER 13

Conditions and Lesions of Hard Dental Tissues

Key Terms

- Arrested Caries
- Classification of Cavities
- Dental Caries
- Early Childhood Caries
- Incipient Carious Lesion
- Interproximal Carious Lesion
- Occlusal Carious Lesion
- Radiation Caries
- Rampant Caries
- Recurrent Caries
- Root Surface Caries
- Slow Caries Activity

PRIMARY CODE	SECONDARY CODE
M = Mesial	-C = Carious (clinical/radiographic) (solid red)
I = Incisal (#6–#11 and #22–#27)	-C^{W} = Carious Watch (incipient) (red outline)
O = Occlusal (#1–#5, #12–#16, #17–#21, and #27–#32)	-C^{R} = Carious Recurrent (red outline restoration)
D = Distal	-Z = Carious (CAPMI4 for missing or unidentified)
F = Facial (#6–#11 and #22–#27)	-S = Silver Amalgam (solid blue)
B = Buccal (#1–#5, #12–#16, #17–#21, and #27–#32)	• = and also
L = Lingual	
X = Missing	

Introduction

Dental caries has been defined as a disease of the hard structures of the teeth. This is usually seen as a demineralization or degradation of the enamel and underlying tooth structures. Development of dental caries requires a susceptible tooth surface, presence of bacterial plaque, and a source of sucrose. The developmental phases of dental caries are:

- Phase I: Formation of the primary lesion
  - Demineralization of the subsurface of the enamel. Acid produced by bacterial plaque begins to dissolve minerals in the enamel.
  - Visualization. The area of demineralization is not yet visible clinically. A very thin layer of enamel is still present on the tooth surface.
  - Clinical evidence. A white spot appears on the enamel surface. No break in the enamel surface is present. The color of the lesion may change from white to brown from exposure to food, tobacco, and beverages.
  - Remineralization potential. The demineralized areas can absorb low concentrations of fluoride if applied frequently during this phase.
- Phase II: Progression of the primary lesion
  - Enamel breakdown. The demineralized area of enamel becomes visible clinically and an irregular surface is noted with an explorer (Plate 27).
  - Caries progression. The carious lesion will follow the direction of the enamel rods.
  - Dentin involvement and progression. Once the caries reaches the dentinoenamel junction (DEJ), the lesion will continue to spread by following the dentinal tubules.

G.V. Black's Standard Classification of Cavities

Dr. G.V. Black developed the method for classifying dental caries. His classification was based on the location and appearance of the Carious lesion. It must be noted that Dr. Black's **Classification of Cavities** does not include root caries or recurrent caries (Figure 13–1).

Classification	Location	Assessment method
Class I Cavities in pits or fissures a. Occlusal surfaces of premolars and molars b. Facial and lingual surfaces of molars c. Lingual surfaces of maxillary incisors	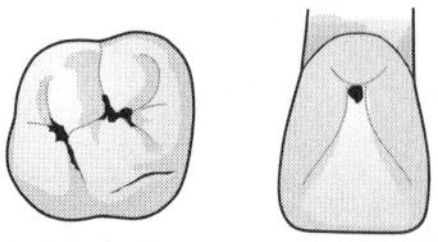	Visualization Exploration
Class II Cavities in proximal surfaces of premolars and molars	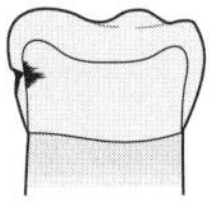	Dental radiographs Visualization Exploration
Class III Cavities in proximal surfaces of incisors and canines that do not involve the incisal angle	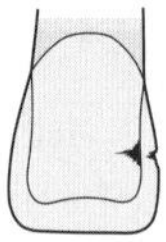	Dental radiographs Visualization Transillumination Exploration
Class IV Cavities in proximal surfaces of incisors and canines that involve the incisal angle	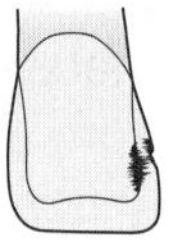	Visualization Transillumination
Class V Cavities in the Cervical 1/3 of facial or lingual surfaces (not pit or fissure)	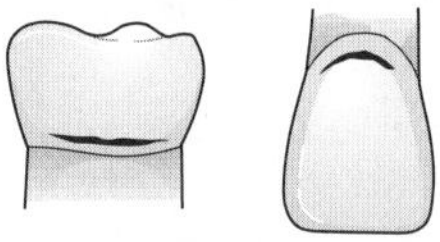	Visualization Exploration
Class VI Cavities on incisal edges of anterior teeth and cusp tips of posterior teeth	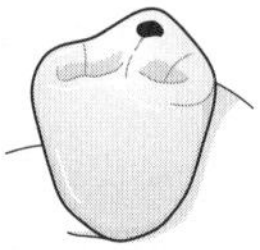	Visualization

Figure 13–1 G. V. Black's Standard Classification of Cavities

Types of Carious Lesions

The **incipient carious lesion** is characterized as an early lesion occurring on an enamel surface for the first time. These lesions are also referred to as primary caries, or initial caries. An Occlusal incipient Carious lesion is not usually detected on a dental radiograph until the dentin becomes involved.

Through exploration, the Distal pits on the Occlusal surfaces on teeth #20 and #28 have been assessed as having incipient Carious lesions. These caries are not seen on the bitewing radiographs and will be considered as areas to watch (Figures 13–2 and 13–3A and B).

Universal System
#2 #3 #4
#31 #30 #29

Palmer System
7| 6| 5|
7| 6| 5|

ISO/FDI System
17 16 15
47 46 45

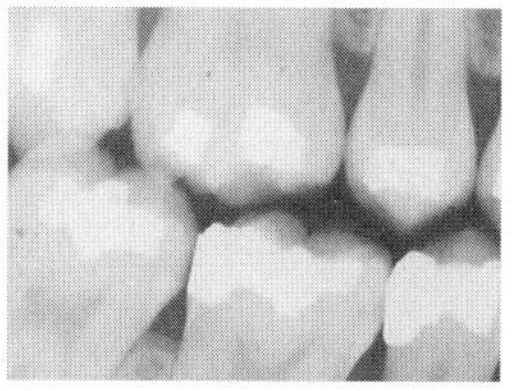

A.

B.

Figure 13–2 (A) Bitewing radiograph showing interproximal Carious lesions involving the Mesial surface of teeth #30 and #31 (B) Bitewing radiograph shown with the previous Carious lesions repaired with Silver Amalgam restorations

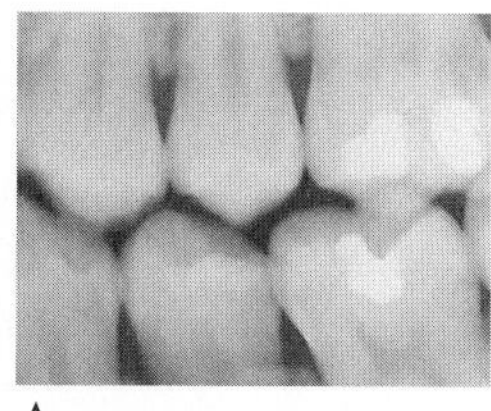

A.

B.

Universal System
#12 #13 #14
#21 #20 #19

Palmer System
|4 |5 |6
|4 |5 |6

ISO/FDI System
24 25 26
34 35 36

Figure 13–3 (A) Bitewing radiograph showing interproximal Carious lesions on the Distal surface of tooth #14 and on the Mesial and Distal surfaces of tooth #19; an incipient Carious lesion shown present on the Occlusal surface and an interproximal Carious lesion shown present on the Distal surface of tooth #20 (B) Bitewing radiograph shown with the previous Carious lesions repaired with Silver Amalgam restorations

The **interproximal Carious lesion** usually occurs just below the contact area and is best detected from bitewing radiographs. This type of lesion shows the classic "V" shape with the smallest part of the "V" pointing toward the dentinoenamel junction (DEJ) (see Figures 13–2 and 13–3).

Occlusal Carious lesions occur in the pits and fissures of the premolars and molars. These lesions can be detected with an explorer. Once the lesion moves into the dentin, a radiograph becomes more useful for assessment (Figure 13–4).

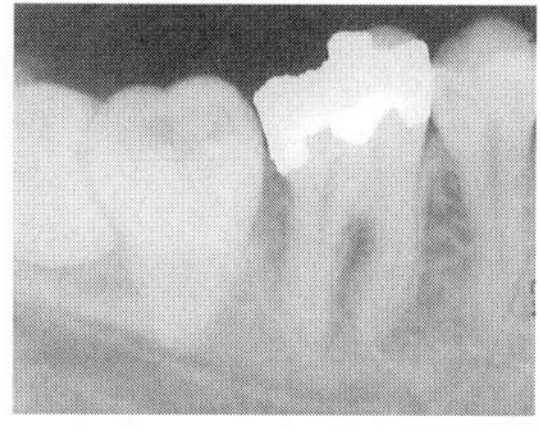

Universal System
#32 #31 #30 #29

Palmer System
8| 7| 6| 5|

ISO/FDI System
48 47 46 45

Figure 13–4 Periapical radiograph shown with Occlusal Carious lesions on tooth #29 and #31 and recurrent caries on tooth #30

Root surface caries or cemental caries are described as lesions involving the cementum and dentin tooth structures that become exposed from abrasion, attrition, erosion, and gingival recession. The Facial surfaces of the roots are most frequently affected by caries.

The destructive process of root caries begins near the cementoenamel junction (CEJ), which produces cavitation of the cementum and does not usually invade the enamel. Figure 13–5 shows the progression of root surface caries.

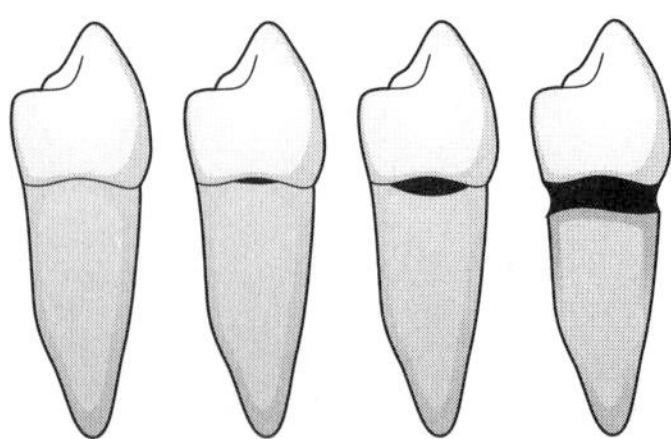

Figure 13–5 Progression of root surface caries

Carious lesions of the cementum appear discolored and have a soft and leathery texture when explored. Lesions are frequently found in older patients or those suffering from a debilitating disease. The application of fluorides can help arrest the involved root surfaces.

Recurrent caries may be observed next to, or under, existing dental restorations often caused by incorrectly designed cavity preparations, improperly placed restorations, or poor oral hygiene with subsequent bacterial invasion. Although there may be other contributing factors, these situations can lead to loss of integrity of the margins of the restorations and allow for the invasion of oral *Streptococcus*, *Lactobacillus*, *Actinomyces*, and other microorganisms to initiate and cause the progression of the caries process (Figures 13–6 and 13–7 and Plates 9 and 10).

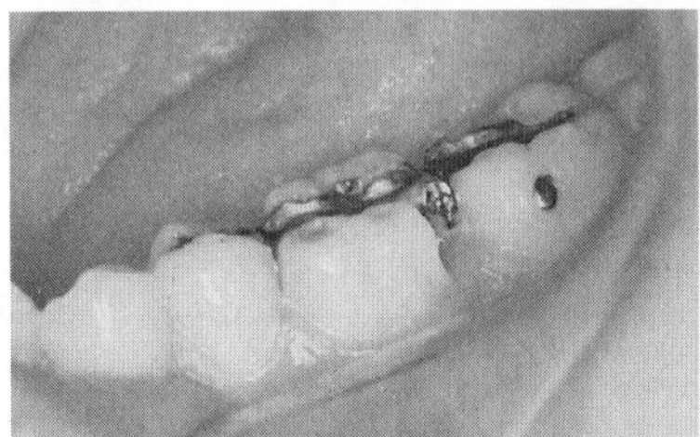

Universal System
#21 #20 #19 #18

Palmer System
⌈4 ⌈5 ⌈6 ⌈7

ISO/FDI System
34 35 36 37

Figure 13–6 Photograph of the mandibular left molar and premolar region that shows recurrent caries on the Mesial surface of tooth #18, the Mesial and Distal surfaces of tooth #19, and the Distal surface of tooth number #20

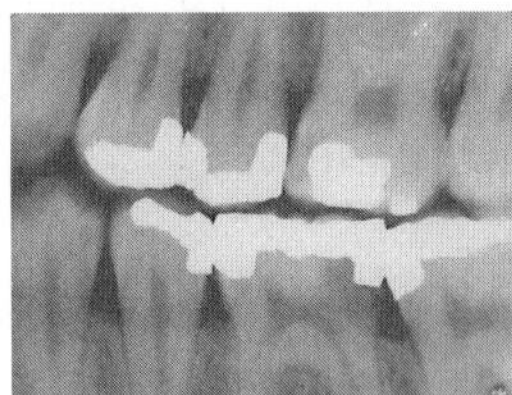

Universal System
#11 #12 #13 #14 #15
#21 #20 #19 #18

Palmer System
⌊3 ⌊4 ⌊5 ⌊6 ⌊7
⌈4 ⌈5 ⌈6 ⌈7

ISO/FDI System
23 24 25 26 27
34 35 36 37

Figure 13–7 Bitewing radiograph that shows recurrent caries on the Mesial surface of tooth #18, the Mesial and Distal surfaces of tooth #19, and the Distal surface of tooth #20; an interproximal Carious lesion shown on the Mesial surface of tooth #14

Advanced Carious lesions that produce extensive damage to the interproximal, Occlusal, and smooth tooth surfaces are referred to as **rampant caries** (Figure 13–8 and Plate 11). This condition is more prevalent in children but can also occur in adults. Factors that intensify the progression of caries are poor oral hygiene, dietary habits, and financial constraints. In rampant Carious lesions, the enamel tooth surfaces may be covered with diffuse patches of white chalky enamel, showing an attack over a broad front.

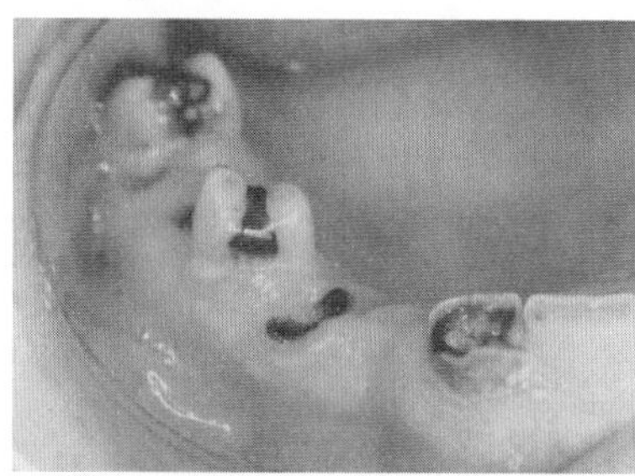

Universal System
#31 #30 #29 #28 #26 #25

Palmer System
7┐ 6┐ 5┐ 4┐ 2┐ 1┐

ISO/FDI System
47 46 45 44 42 41

Figure 13–8 Photograph showing rampant caries

The dentin tooth structure will have a soft texture when explored due to the rapid dissolution and removal of the mineral salts. Because the tooth structure is lost at such a rapid rate, it has little opportunity to be discolored by coffee, berry juices, or other foods.

In direct contrast to rampant caries is **slow caries activity**. The enamel and dentin of a Carious lesion that progresses slowly will appear discolored, dark brown, or black, due to repeated subjection to foods that stain (e.g., coffee or berries). Enamel and dentin tooth structures that are discolored should not be identified as Carious by color alone. Exploration of the enamel and dentin tooth structures and radiographic assessment are necessary to determine if caries activity is progressing, slowed, or arrested. The term that refers to a Carious lesion that no longer shows progression and has become stable is **arrested caries**.

Radiation therapy to the head and neck may cause xerostomia, a condition that produces decreased salivary flow due to the partial or total loss of salivary gland function. This condition, if left untreated, can result in severe and rampant destruction of the teeth often referred to as **radiation caries**. The Carious lesions appear as dark brown or black stains with no visible demineralization of the enamel, cervical decay sometimes encircling the entire tooth, or caries that begins on the Incisal surface or cusp of the tooth. This type of caries progresses rapidly.

Early childhood caries is a group of rampant caries that is found in very young children. Other names for this condition are nursing caries, nursing bottle mouth, baby bottle tooth decay, and prolonged nursing habit. The etiology of these rampant types of caries brought about the name change to encompass all of the forms. The early childhood caries occur in young children who are given a nursing bottle of milk, juice, or other sucrose sweetened drinks, or allowed at-will breastfeeding for prolonged periods.

The following list describes the various types of early childhood caries, and the etiology and clinical manifestations associated with them:

- Baby bottle tooth decay. The etiology is a child is put to bed with a bottle containing milk, juice, or other sucrose sweetened liquid. Maxillary anterior teeth have severe decay (Plate 12).
- Breastfeeding caries. Caries due to prolonged breastfeeding, or allowing child to breastfeed on demand throughout the night. Caries are generalized.
- Chronic medication-related caries. The child is required to ingest drugs for a medical condition. These medications are placed in a sucrose-based suspension. Caries are generalized on anterior teeth but can be seen on posterior teeth as well (Figure 13–9 and Plate 13).
- Pacifier caries. Prolonged use of a pacifier dipped in honey or other sweet liquid. Caries are generalized and severe (Plate 14).
- Caries secondary to developmental defects. This form of caries can be due to a defect in the development of the teeth or other anatomic systems. Caries are present where the defects exist.

Charting Incipient and Interproximal Carious Lesions on an Anatomic Chart

In Figures 13–2A and 13–3A, the Distal pits located on the Occlusal surfaces of teeth #20 and #29 do not show the incipient Carious lesions that were detected during exploration. These two incipient Carious lesions need to be recorded as areas to watch for further progression of the decay.

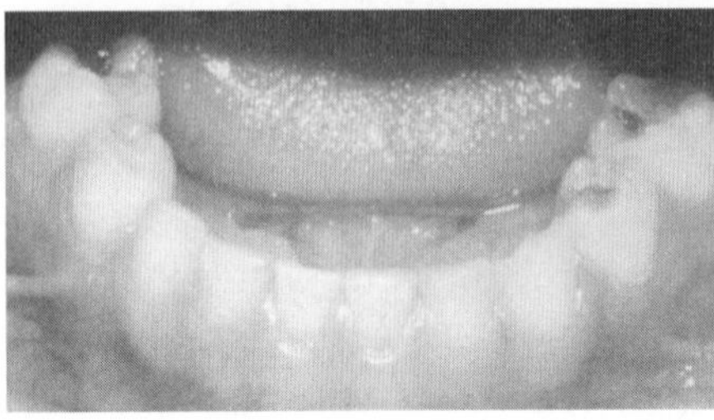

Universal System
T S R Q P O N M L K

Palmer System
E| D| C| B| A| |A |B |C |D |E

ISO/FDI System
85 84 83 82 81 71 72 73 74 75

Figure 13–9 Chronic medication-related caries

To chart these incipient caries on an anatomic chart, locate the tooth notation numbers and with a red pencil draw a circle around the area that designates the Distal pits on the Occlusal tooth surfaces of teeth #20 and #29. The outlined area represents an area that needs to be watched (Figure 13–10).

Figures 13–2A and 13–3A show interproximal Carious lesions on teeth #14, #19, #20, #30, and #31. To indicate interproximal caries that are advanced on an anatomic chart, use a red pencil to draw a circle and fill it in on the designated area of the involved tooth surface (see Figure 13–10). When only one tooth surface is involved, it is only necessary to chart the condition on one view.

Charting Incipient and Interproximal Carious Lesions on a Geometric Chart

To chart incipient Carious lesions on the Occlusal tooth surfaces of teeth #20 and #29 using a geometric chart, outline the entire tooth surface that represents the involved area with a red pencil. The Occlusal tooth surfaces on teeth #20 and #29 indicate that the Distal pits have incipient Carious lesions (Figure 13–11).

18	17	16	15	14	13	12	11	21	22	23	24	25	26	27	28
8	7	6	5	4	3	2	1	1	2	3	4	5	6	7	8
1	2	3	4	5	6	7	8	9	10	11	12	13	14	15	16

32	31	30	29	28	27	26	25	24	23	22	21	20	19	18	17
8	7	6	5	4	3	2	1	1	2	3	4	5	6	7	8
48	47	46	45	44	43	42	41	31	32	33	34	35	36	37	38

Figure 13–10 Anatomic dental chart shown with incipient Carious lesions charted on teeth #20 and #29 and interproximal Carious lesions charted on teeth #14, #19, #20, #30, and #31

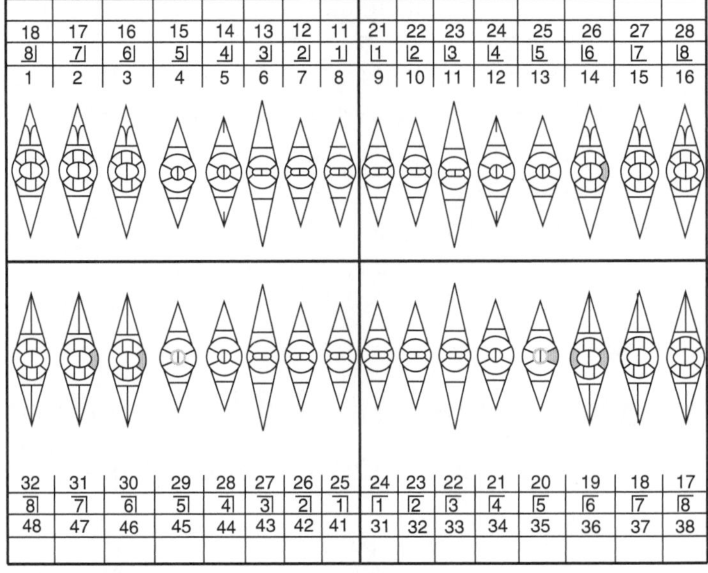

Figure 13–11 Geometric chart shown with incipient Carious lesions charted on teeth #20 and #29 and interproximal Carious lesions charted on teeth #14, #19, #20, #30, and #31

To indicate interproximal caries, use a red pencil and on the Mesial and/or Distal tooth surfaces outline the entire area and fill it in completely. Figure 13–3 shows advanced interproximal caries on teeth #14, #19, #20, #30, and #31.

Charting Incipient and Interproximal Carious Lesions on a Numeric Coding System Chart

To indicate incipient Carious lesions on a numeric coding system chart, with a black pen enter the date above and below the words "Maxilla" and "Mandible" in the column marked "Date." Locate the tooth notation numbers #20 and #29 and in the box below using a red pencil, print the uppercase letter "O" followed by a hyphen (-) and then the uppercase letter (C) with a superscript "W," O-C^{W}. This reads as Occlusal Carious Watch (Figure 13–12).

To describe interproximal Carious lesions on a numeric coding system chart, use a red pencil and indicate the separate interproximal surfaces "M" and "D" by using the symbol (•) between them, followed by a hyphen (-) then the uppercase letter "C." In Figure 13–12 tooth #19 is shown with the letters "M-C • D-C" that is read as Mesial and also Distal Carious lesions.

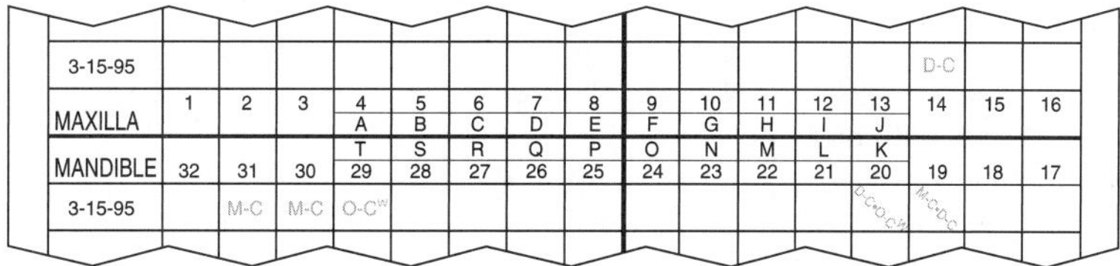

Figure 13–12 Numeric coding system chart with incipient Carious lesions described on teeth #20 and #29 and interproximal Carious lesions depicted on teeth #14, #19, #20, #30, and #31

Charting Advanced and Recurrent Carious Lesions on an Anatomic Chart

Figure 13–4 shows teeth #29 and #31 with advanced dental decay on the Occlusal tooth surfaces, and recurrent caries that involve the Occlusal and Buccal tooth surfaces of tooth #30. Figures 13–6 and 13–7 show recurrent caries on the Mesial surface of tooth #18, the Mesial and Distal surfaces of tooth #19, and the Distal surface of tooth #20.

To chart the advanced caries on an anatomic chart, locate the tooth notation numbers and with a red pencil outline the areas involved and fill them in completely. The Occlusal tooth surfaces of teeth #29 and #31 indicate large Carious lesions (Figure 13–13).

Tooth #30 has a MODB-S restoration with recurrent caries on the Occlusal and Buccal tooth surfaces. To indicate recurrent decay on the anatomic chart, with a red pencil outline the Occlusal and Buccal areas of the restoration to indicate the location of the recurrent caries (see Figure 13–13). Figures 13–6 and 13–7 show recurrent caries on teeth #18, #19, and #20, and the recurrent caries are shown charted around the existing restorations in Figure 13–13.

Charting Advanced and Recurrent Carious Lesions on a Geometric Chart

To chart the advanced caries on a geometric chart, locate the tooth notation numbers and with a red pencil outline the entire Occlusal area on each tooth diagram involved and fill them in completely. The Occlusal tooth surfaces of teeth #29 and #31 indicate large Carious lesions (Figures 13–14).

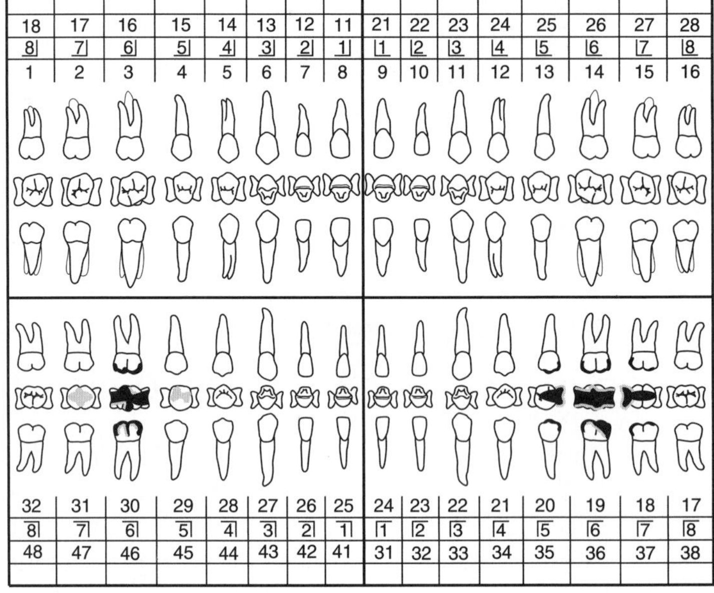

Figure 13–13 Anatomic dental chart shown with recurrent Carious lesions charted on teeth #18, #19, #20, and #30, and advanced Carious lesions charted on teeth #29 and #31

Figure 13–14 Geometric chart shown with recurrent Carious lesions charted on teeth #18, #19, #20, and #30, and advanced Carious lesions charted on teeth #29 and #31

To indicate recurrent decay on the geometric chart, with a red pencil outline the Occlusal and Buccal areas of the restoration to indicate the location of the recurrent caries (see Figure 13–14). Figures 13–6 and 13–7 show recurrent caries on teeth #18, #19, #20, and #30, and the recurrent caries are shown charted around the existing restorations in Figure 13–14.

Charting Advanced and Recurrent Carious Lesions on a Numeric Coding System Chart

Figure 13–4 shows teeth #29 and #31 with advanced dental decay on the Occlusal tooth surfaces, and recurrent caries that involve the Occlusal and Buccal tooth surfaces of teeth #18, #19, #20, and #30. Figures 13–6 and 13–7 show recurrent caries on the Mesial surface of tooth #18, the Mesial and Distal surfaces of tooth #19, and the Distal surface of tooth #20.

To indicate advanced decay on the numeric coding system chart, follow the same procedure as for depicting interproximal Carious lesions and use uppercase letters M, D, I, O, F, B, or L followed by a hyphen and the uppercase letter "C" (Figure 13–15).

To indicate recurrent decay on a numeric coding system chart, print the date in black ink and in red pencil enter the involved tooth surfaces followed by a hyphen and an uppercase letter "C" with a superscript "R" (C^R). In Figure 13–15, restorations were placed on teeth #18, #19, and #20 on 7-26-97. On 7-30-98 Carious Recurrent lesions were detected on the same teeth.

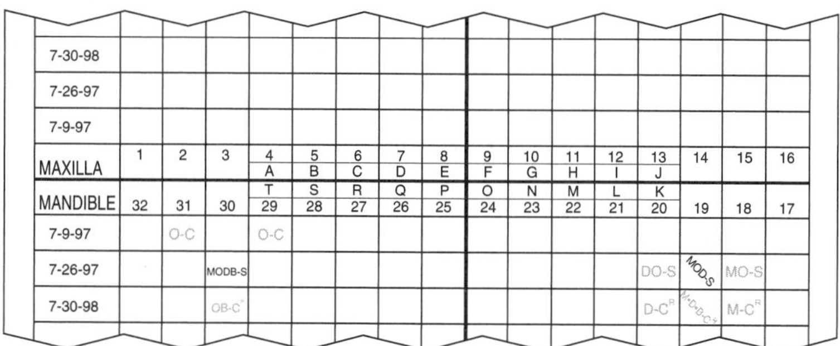

Figure 13–15 Numeric coding system chart with recurrent Carious lesions described on teeth #18, #19, #20, and #30, and advanced Carious lesions charted on teeth #29 and #31

Charting Rampant, Radiation, and Early Childhood Caries on Anatomic, Geometric, and Numeric Coding System Charts

Rampant, radiation, and early childhood caries are all forms of advanced Carious lesions that usually affect large numbers of teeth. To chart these lesions on the three different types of dental charts, follow the same procedures as indicated for charting advanced Carious lesions. Locate the section on the dental chart designated as clinical examination or progress notes and document the specific condition that has produced the pattern of dental caries.

Review Questions

Matching

Directions: Place the uppercase letter(s) after the number to match each term with the statement that *best* defines it.

A Arrested caries
B Early childhood caries
C Incipient Carious lesions
D Interproximal Carious lesion
E Radiation caries
F Rampant caries

1. ____ A disease involving the hard structures of the teeth.
2. ____ A Carious lesion usually not apparent on a dental radiograph.
3. ____ Carious lesions occurring around the margins of a dental restoration.
4. ____ Extensive caries occurring throughout the mouth.
5. ____ A Carious lesion that no longer progresses.
6. ____ A Carious lesion that involves the chewing surface of the tooth.
7. ____ A form of nursing caries.
8. ____ This caries is associated with attrition, erosion, and gingival recession.

G Recurrent caries
H Root surface caries
I Occlusal Carious lesion
J Dental caries

9. ____ Severe Carious lesions due to xerostomia.
10. ____ A Carious lesion apparent on a dental radiograph and involves either the Mesial or Distal tooth surfaces.

Answers

1. **J,** 2. **C,** 3. **G,** 4. **F,** 5. **A,** 6. **I,** 7. **B,** 8. **H,** 9. **E,** 10. **D**

References

Berkey, C. S., Douglass, C. W., Valachovic, R. W., & Chauncey, H. H. (1988). Longitudinal radiographic analysis of carious lesion progression. *Community Dentistry and Oral Epidemiology*, 16, 83–90.

Dorland's pocket medical dictionary (28th ed.). (1994). Philadelphia: W. B. Saunders Company.

Farman, A. G. (1990). Prediction of efficacy of bitewing radiographs for caries detection. *Oral Surgery, Oral Medicine, and Oral Pathology*, 69 (4), 506–513.

Gornbein, J. A. (1990). Prediction of efficacy of bitewing radiographs for caries detection. *Oral Surgery, Oral Medicine, and Oral Pathology*, 69.

Kidd, E. A. M., & Pitts, N. B. (1990). A reappraisal of the value of the bitwe-ing radiograph in the diagnosis of posterior approximal caries. *British Dental Journal*, 169, 195–200.

Kronmiller, J. E., Nirschl, R. F., & Zullo, T. G. (1988). Patient's age at the initial detection of interproximal caries. *Journal of Dentistry for Children*, 55, 105–109.

Matteson, S. R., Phillips, C., Kantor, M. L., & Leinedecker, T. (1989). The effect of lesion size, restorative material, and film speed on the detection of recurrent caries. *Oral Surgery, Oral Medicine, and Oral Pathology*, 68.

Sidi, A. D., & Naylor, M. N. (1988). A comparison of bitewing radiography and interdental transillumination as adjuncts to the clinical identification of approximal caries in posterior teeth. *British Dental Journal*, 164, 15–18.

Thomas, C. L. (1997). *Taber's cyclopedic medical dictionary*. Philadelphia: F. A. Davis Company.

White, S. C., Gratt, B. M., & Bauer, J. G. (1988). A clinical comparison of xeroradiography film radiography for the detection of proximal caries. *Oral Surgery, Oral Medicine, and Oral Pathology*, 65.

White, S. C., Kaffe, I., & Gornbein, J. A. (1990). A prediction of efficacy of bitewing radiographs for caries detection. *Oral Surgery, Oral Medicine, and Oral Pathology*, 69.

CHAPTER 14

Traumatic Injury of the Tooth

Key Terms

Classification of Fractures
Concussion
Dislocation
Extraction
Fracture
International Classification of Diseases
Luxation
Splint
Tooth Avulsion
Traumatic Injury

PRIMARY CODE	SECONDARY CODE
M = Mesial	FX = Fracture (red zigzag line)
I = Incisal (#6–#11 and #22–#27)	RT = Root Tip (solid red Root Tip)
O = Occlusal (#1–#5, #12–#16, #17–#21, and #27–#32)	• = and also
D = Distal	To Be Extracted = | | Red vertical lines
F = Facial (#6–#11 and #22–#27)	
B = Buccal (#1–#5, #12–#16, #17–#21, and #27–#32)	
L = Lingual	
C = Crown	
X = Missing	

Introduction

Restorative procedures and **traumatic injury** to the head and face can cause tooth **Fracture** and bone and soft tissue injuries.

The World Health Organization has developed the **Classification of Fractures** of the teeth and the following is an excerpt from the **International Classification of Diseases**:

- 873.60 Fracture of only the enamel (Fissures, chips, and cracks.)
- 873.61 Fracture of the Crown without affecting the pulp
- 873.62 Fracture of the Crown with involvement of the pulp
- 873.63 Fracture of only the root of the tooth
- 873.64 Fracture of a Crown and root with/without the involvement of the pulp
- 873.65 Fracture of the root of the tooth
- 873.66 Luxation, concussion, and subluxation of the tooth
- 873.67 Extrusion and intrusion of the tooth
- 873.68 Avulsion of the tooth

Figure 14–1 is an illustration of a maxillary central incisor, which shows the various types of Fractures.

Fractures that involve the Crown of a tooth can range from minimal to severe. A minimal Fracture either produces an infraction in the enamel, or a small area of tooth is Missing and does not involve the dentin. A severe and more complex Fracture of the tooth shows signs of bleeding and a relatively large section of the enamel and dentin is Missing (Figure 14–2).

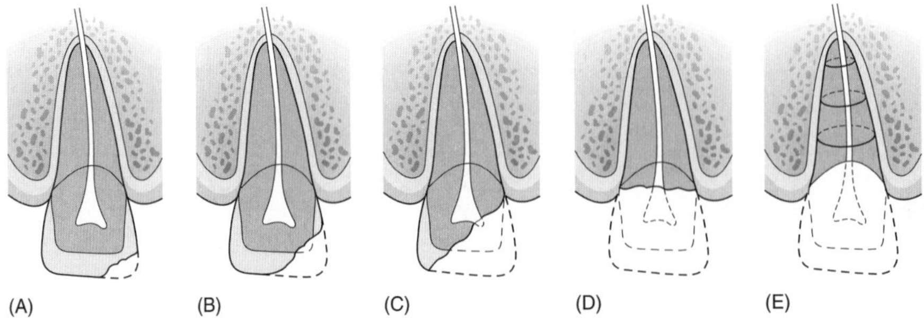

Figure 14–1 Types of tooth Fractures: (A) Fracture of the enamel (B) Fracture of the Crown without the involvement of the pulp (C) Fracture of the Crown with the involvement of the pulp (D) Fracture of the Crown and root with involvement of the pulp (E) Fractures of the root

Fractures of the root can sometimes be difficult to detect on a radiograph and most often occur in the middle third of the root. Figure 14–3 is a periapical radiograph that shows tooth #10 with a Root Tip fragment present following a traumatic injury. When a Root Fracture of a tooth occurs and the prognosis is poor, an **extraction** is indicated.

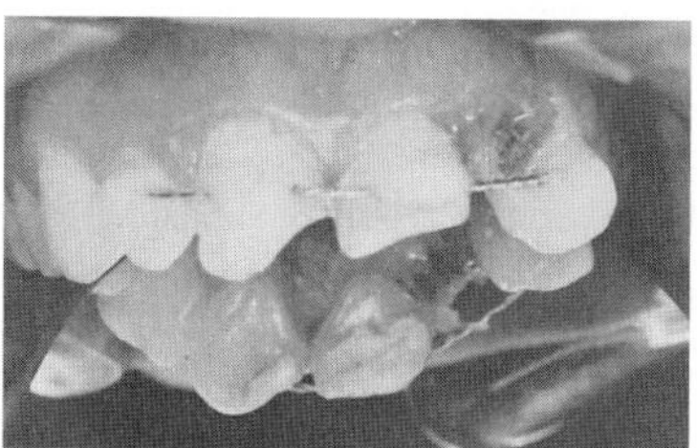

Universal System
#6 #7 #8 # 9 #11
Palmer System
3| 2| 1| |1 |3
ISO/FDI System
13 12 11 21 23

Figure 14–2 Anterior photograph showing Crown Fractures involving teeth #8 and #9

The term **concussion** is used to describe a traumatic injury that has affected the supporting structures of the tooth but does not produce abnormal displacement or mobility. The appearance of a dental concussion on a radiograph shows widening of the periodontal ligament space.

Traumatic injury can cause **luxation**, which results in damage to the supporting structures of the teeth. The clinical manifestations of a **dislocated** tooth are the tooth is displaced and shows a high degree of mobility. Figure 14–4 is an anterior radiograph, which shows a widened periodontal ligament space at the root apices.

The clinical features of an intruded tooth show the Crown depressed below the line of occlusion; the radiographic examination shows partial or total destruction of the periodontal ligament space and obliteration of the apical

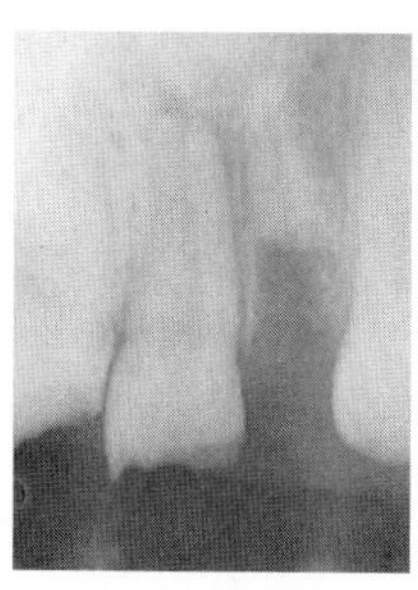

Universal System
#8 #9 #11
Palmer System
1| |1 |3
ISO/FDI System
11 21 23

Figure 14–3 Anterior periapical radiograph showing Root Tip fragment of tooth #10 (Courtesy J. S. Goetz, D.D.S. and Robert C. Urquhart, D.D.S.)

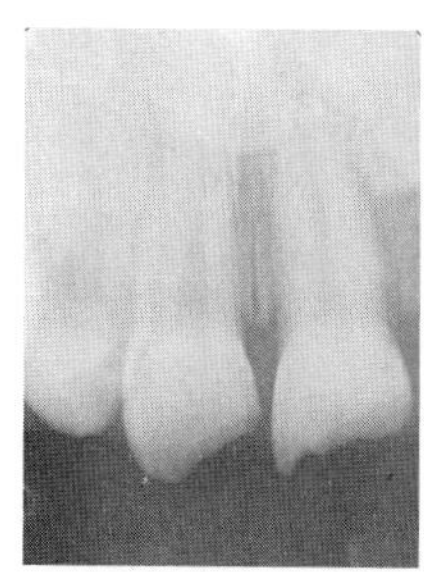

Universal System
#7 #8 #9
Palmer System
2| 1| |1
ISO/FDI System
12 11 21

Figure 14–4 Anterior periapical radiograph showing luxated teeth #8 and #9 (Courtesy J. S. Goetz, D.D.S and Robert C. Urquhart, D.D.S.)

lamina dura. An extruded tooth shows widening of the periodontal space and the Crown extends below the line of occlusion.

When a tooth is completely displaced from the alveolar bony socket and is Missing it is referred to as **tooth avulsion**. Depending on the extent of injury to the tooth and alveolus, an avulsed tooth can be reimplanted and stabilized with a **splint**. A splint is composed of wire that is attached to the tooth with acrylic. Figure 14–2 shows teeth #7, #8, #9, and #11 splinted together.

Charting Crown and Root Fractures on an Anatomic Chart

Figure 14–2 and Plate 15 show teeth #8, #9, and #11 with Fractured Crowns. To chart a Crown Fracture on teeth #8, #9, and #11, locate the tooth designation numbers and with a red pencil draw a zigzag line over the involved tooth surfaces, which indicate the Fractured areas (Figure 14–5). In the box located above the tooth notation numbers, with a red pencil print the uppercase letters "FX," which indicates Fracture.

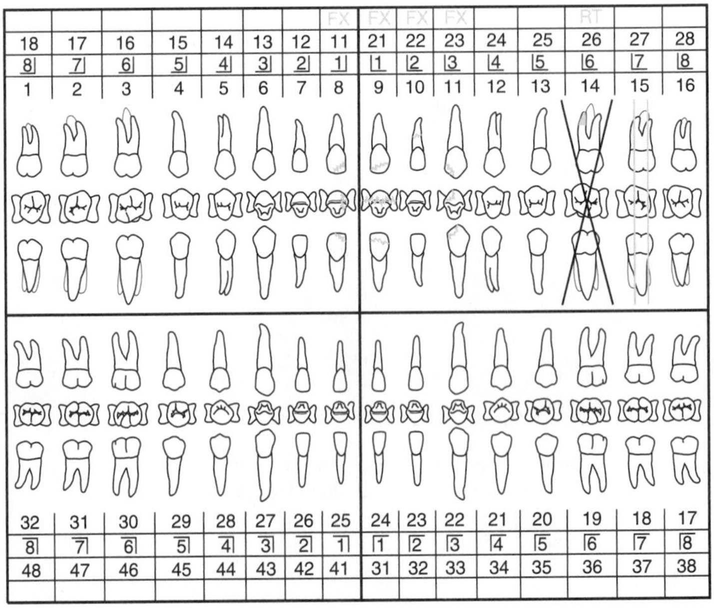

							FX	FX	FX	FX			RT		
18	17	16	15	14	13	12	11	21	22	23	24	25	26	27	28
8	7	6	5	4	3	2	1	1	2	3	4	5	6	7	8
1	2	3	4	5	6	7	8	9	10	11	12	13	14	15	16
32	31	30	29	28	27	26	25	24	23	22	21	20	19	18	17
8	7	6	5	4	3	2	1	1	2	3	4	5	6	7	8
48	47	46	45	44	43	42	41	31	32	33	34	35	36	37	38

Figure 14–5 Anatomic dental chart shown with Crown Fractures on teeth #8, #9, and #11, Root Fracture on tooth #10, Missing tooth #14 with a retained Root Tip, and tooth #15 is "To Be Extracted"

When a section of the tooth is Missing, it is necessary to draw the Fracture lines on all three views of the chart. In a situation where the tooth has an infraction or Fracture line, it is only necessary to draw the area on the view in which it appears on the tooth surface.

Figure 14–5 shows a Root Fracture on tooth #10. To chart a Root Fracture, locate the tooth number, and with a red pencil on the Facial view draw a zigzag line where the Fracture appears and print the letters "FX" in the designated box.

Charting Crown and Root Fractures on a Geometric Chart

To chart Crown Fractures on teeth #8, #9, and #11 on a geometric chart, locate the appropriate tooth numbers and with a red pencil draw a single zigzag line over the areas, which indicate the involved tooth surfaces for each tooth. Print the uppercase letters "FX" in the box above the designated tooth numbers (Figure 14–6).

To indicate superficial fissures and slight cracks in the enamel, draw them in red only on the surface in which they appear.

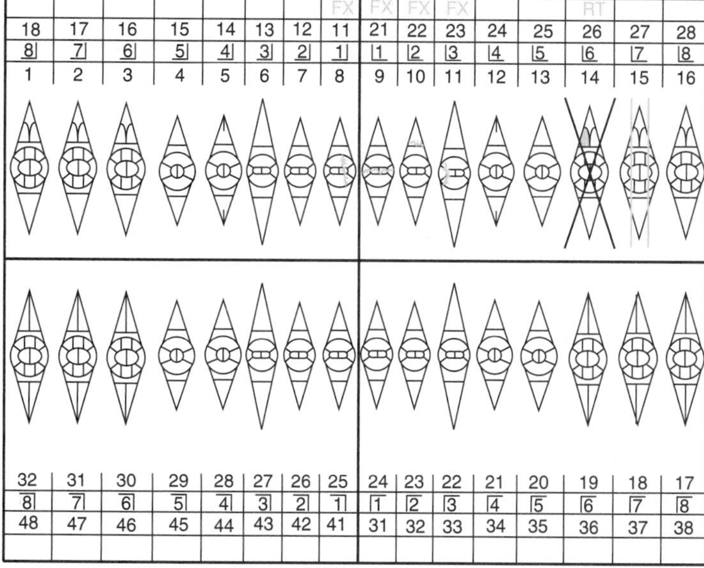

Figure 14–6 Geometric dental chart shown with Crown Fractures on teeth #8, #9, and #11, Root Fracture on tooth #10, Missing tooth #14 with a retained Root Tip, and tooth #15 is "To Be Extracted"

When a geometric chart without root diagrams is used to chart a Fractured root, draw in the root or roots next to the area that designates the Crown of the tooth, then indicate the Fracture line drawn in red and place the letters "FX" in the box.

Charting Crown and Root Fractures on a Numeric Coding System Chart

To chart Crown and Root Fractures on a numeric coding system chart, use a black pen to enter the date in the designated area. Locate the tooth notation numbers and with a red pen in the correct box, print the uppercase letters of the tooth surfaces involved or the word "Root" followed by a hyphen (-) and the uppercase letters "FX." Figure 14–7 is a numeric coding system chart, which shows tooth #8 as MIFL-FX, tooth #9 as MIDFL-FX, tooth #11 as MIFL-FX, and tooth #10 as Root-FX.

Charting a Residual Root Tip on an Anatomic, Geometric, and Numeric Coding System Chart

Due to the similar densities of bone and root structure, it is sometimes difficult to distinguish a retained Root Tip from the surrounding bone tissue.

To chart a residual Root Tip on anatomic and geometric charts, locate the tooth notation number and the tooth should already be charted with a blue "X" to indicate the tooth is Missing. With a red pencil draw a line on the involved root and fill in the area, which indicates the remaining Root Tip. In the box located above or below the designated tooth number, use the red pencil to place the uppercase letters "RT," which is the abbreviation for Root Tip.

4-2-97								MIFL-FX	MIDFL-FX	ROOT-FX	MIFL-FX			RT		
MAXILLA	1	2	3	4	5	6	7	8	9	10	11	12	13	14	15	16
				A	B	C	D	E	F	G	H	I	J			
				T	S	R	Q	P	O	N	M	L	K			
MANDIBLE	32	31	30	29	28	27	26	25	24	23	22	21	20	19	18	17

Figure 14–7 Numeric coding system dental chart shown with Crown Fractures on teeth #8, #9, and #11, Root Fracture on tooth #10, Missing tooth #14 with a retained Root Tip, and tooth #15 is "To Be Extracted"

To chart a retained Root Tip on a geometric chart without root diagrams, draw a small Root Tip and fill it in with red pencil; label the box provided with the letters "RT."

To indicate a retained Root Tip on the numeric coding system, locate the tooth number and in the designated box, which is marked as Missing, use a red pencil and print the uppercase letters "RT" on top of the blue "X." Figures 14–5, 14–6, and 14–7 show three different dental charts and the method used to chart a retained Root Tip for tooth #14.

Charting a Tooth as "To Be Extracted" on an Anatomic, Geometric, and Numeric Coding System Chart

To chart a tooth as "To Be Extracted" using the three different types of dental charts, use a red pencil and on the tooth diagrams for the anatomic and geometric charts and in the designated box used for a numeric coding system chart, draw two vertical lines "||." Figures 14–5, 14-6, and 14-7 show three different dental charts and the method used to chart tooth #15 as "To Be Extracted."

Review Questions

Matching

Directions: Place the uppercase letter(s) after the number to match each term with the statement that *best* defines it.

A Extraction
B Concussion
C Dislocation
D Fracture

1. ____ Composed of acrylic and wire
2. ____ Traumatic injury that results in the loss of a tooth
3. ____ A break in the tooth or root
4. ____ Displacement of a tooth
5. ____ The deliberate removal of a tooth
6. ____ Traumatic injury to the tooth that does not produce abnormal displacement

E Luxation	7.____	Traumatic injury to the tooth that does produce abnormal displacement
F Splint	8.____	Refers to the secondary code "FX"
G Tooth Avulsion	9.____	Indicated with two red vertical lines
	10.____	Indicated with a red zigzag line

Answers

1. **F,** 2. **G,** 3. **D,** 4. **E,** 5. **A,** 6. **B,** 7. **C,** 8. **D,** 9. **A,** 10. **D**

References

Brand, R. W., & Isselhard, D. E. (1994). *Anatomy of orofacial structures* (5th ed.). St. Louis: Mosby Year-Book, Inc.

Camp, J. H. (1991). Diagnosis and management of sports-related injuries to the teeth. *Dental Clinics of North America*, 35, 733.

Dorland's pocket medical dictionary (28th ed.). (1994). Philadelphia: W. B. Saunders Company.

Goaz, P. W., & White, S. C. (1994). *Oral radiology: Principles and interpretation* (3rd ed.). St. Louis: Mosby Year-Book, Inc.

Hovland, E. J. (1992). Horizontal root fractures: Treatment and repair. *Dental Clinics of North America*, 36, 509.

Thomas, C. L. (1997). *Taber's cyclopedic medical dictionary*. Philadelphia: F. A. Davis Company.

Woelfel, J. B., & Scheid, R. C. (1997). *Dental anatomy: Its relevance to dentistry* (5th ed.). Baltimore: Williams & Wilkins.

World Health Organization (1978). *Application of the international classification of diseases to dentistry and stomatology*, ICD-DA (2nd ed., pp. 88–89). Geneva: Author.

CHAPTER 15

The Oral Cavity and Periodontium: Manifestations of Soft and Hard Tissues

Key Terms

- Alveolar Cortical Plate Defects
- Col
- Dehiscence
- Fenestration
- Food Impaction
- Furcation
- Gingival Pocket
- Gingival Recession
- Gingivitis
- Horizontal Bone Loss
- Infrabony pocket
- Junctional Epithelium
- Lamina Propria
- Mobility
- Periodontal Ligament
- Periodontal Pocket
- Periodontitis
- Periodontium
- Suprabony Pocket
- Vertical Bone Loss

PERIODONTAL EXAMINATION CODES AND ABBREVIATIONS

Plaque and Calculus = + in red
Gingival inflammation = Papillary (P) Marginal (M) Attached (A) in red
Mobility = 0, N, 1, 1+, 2, 2+, 3 millimeters in red
Fremitis = N, +, ++, +++ in red
Probing depth is recorded in Arabic numerals in red
Attachment level = __________ in blue
Mucogingival junction = - - - - - - in blue
Bleeding = ⑥ a red circle around the probing depth

Suppuration (Exudate) = • a red dot above probing depth
Papillary hyperplasia = ∩ in red
Papilla loss = – in red
Furcation: Class I = /\ < 1 mm
Class II = △ (1) > 1 mm – < 3 mm (2) > 3 mm
Class III = ▲ through and through, covered by soft tissue
Class IV = ▲+ through and through, complete visualization

Introduction

The oral cavity begins at the lips and extends laterally to the cheeks. It is bound superiorly and inferiorly by the maxilla and mandible and its associated structures are composed of nerve, muscle, connective, and epithelial tissues. The osseous tissue that forms the sockets and surrounds the roots of the teeth in the maxilla and mandible is referred to as the alveolar process.

Oral Mucosa

The oral cavity is lined with oral mucosa, which consists of multiple layers of epithelial tissue known as stratified squamous epithelium. There are three types of mucous membranes that line the oral cavity and include the following:

- Masticatory mucosa. Covers the hard palate and gingiva but does not include the marginal (free) gingiva. Consists of keratinized stratified squamous epithelium that is firmly attached to the underlying connective tissues.
- Lining mucosa. Consists of nonkeratinized stratified squamous epithelium that covers the alveolar mucosa, lips, cheeks, soft palate, ventral surface of the tongue, and the floor of the mouth.
- Specialized mucosa. Consists of parakeratinized to keratinized stratified squamous epithelium that covers the dorsal surface of the tongue. There are four types of papillae located on the tongue and include the following:

- Filiform papillae. Projections of keratinized epithelial tissue that cover the anterior two thirds of the dorsal surface of the tongue. They provide a tactile function and are the most numerous of the papillae.
- Fungiform papillae. Consist of raised and rounded projections of epithelial tissue that are dispersed around the filiform papillae on the anterior two thirds of the dorsal surface of the tongue.
- Circumvallate papillae. Approximately ten to twelve large elevated circular projections that are encompassed by a channel. They form a V-shaped row on the posterior one third of the dorsal surface of the tongue with taste buds located along the sides.
- Foliate papillae. Vertical folds of stratified squamous epithelial tissue located on the posterior lateral border of the tongue containing taste buds.

Periodontium

The **periodontium** is made up of a group of structures that surround and support the teeth. These structures are the gingiva, periodontal ligament or membrane, cementum, and alveolar bone tissue (Figure 15–1A and B).

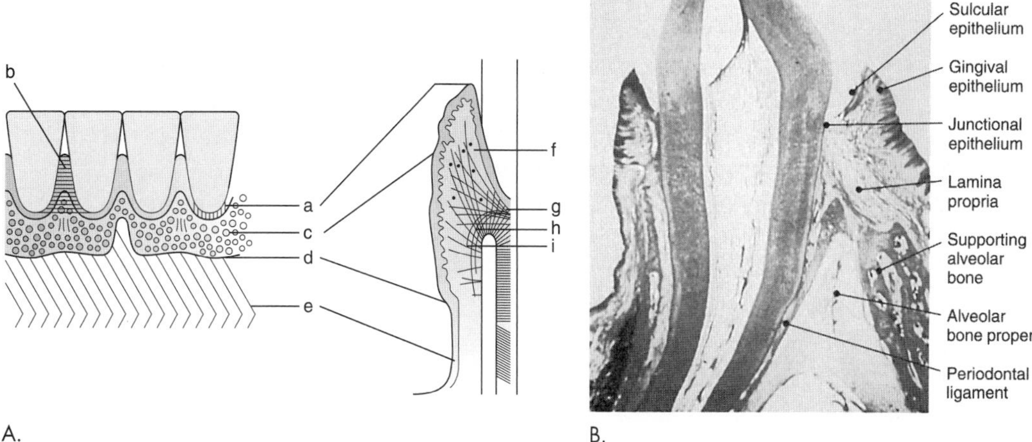

Figure 15–1 (A) Gingiva: *Diagram key*: (a) margin of the gingiva (b) interdental papilla (c) attached gingiva (d) mucogingival junction (e) alveolar mucosa; in cross section (f through I): fibers of the lamina propria (connective tissue); (f) circular fibers (g) dentogingival fibers (h) dentoperiosteal fibers (i) alveologingival fibers (Courtesy National Audiovisual Center) (B) Cross section of a tooth and the periodontium (Courtesy National Audiovisual Center)

Gingiva

The Gingiva consists of masticatory mucosa that surrounds the cervical region of the tooth and the alveolar processes of the maxilla and mandible (Plate 48) The following structures make up the gingiva:

- Marginal gingiva. Surrounds the cervical region of the tooth. It is not attached and forms the gingival sulcus.
- Free gingival groove. A shallow depression that separates the marginal gingiva from the attached gingiva.
- Attached gingiva. Parakeratinized or keratinized stratified squamous epithelium that extends from the free gingival groove to the mucogingival junction and is bound firmly to the underlying cementum and alveolar bone tissue.
- Mucogingival junction. Scalloped line between the keratinized gingival epithelium and the alveolar mucosa.
- Gingival epithelium (oral epithelium). The area of keratinized stratified squamous epithelium extending from the marginal gingiva to the mucogingival junction.
- Sulcular epithelium. The medial surface of the marginal gingiva descends inferiorly toward the cementoenamel junction region. This nonkeratinized tissue is not attached to the tooth surface and the area created between the tissue and the tooth forms a crevice referred to as the gingival sulcus.
- Junctional epithelium. Located at the base of the gingival sulcus, the sulcular epithelium joins this epithelial tissue and forms a band of nonkeratinized stratified squamous epithelium that encircles the tooth and forms an attachment on the cementum.
- Interdental papilla. An elevation of marginal free and attached gingival epithelial tissue, one located on the Facial and one on the Lingual surface, that extend interproximally between two teeth.
  - Col. A depression that consists of nonkeratinized epithelial tissue situated between the Facial and Lingual papillae (interdental papilla) that conforms to the contact area.
- Alveolar mucosa. Loosely attached nonkeratinized stratified squamous epithelial tissue located inferior to the attached gingiva.
- Frenum. A fold of mucous membrane tissue that connects an immobile part to a semi- or less mobile part and controls movement of the part.
  - Labial frenum. Attached from the base of the anterior vestibule, the inferior and medial surface of the lip, to the Labial surface of the attached

gingiva and the mucogingival junction at the midline on the maxilla and mandible.
- Buccal frena. Attached from the base of the posterior vestibule, the inferior and medial surface of the cheek, to the Labial surface of the attached gingiva and the mucogingival junction at the canine and premolar areas on the maxilla and mandible.
- Lingual frenum. Attached from the anterior region of the floor of the mouth to the ventral surface of the tongue.

The connective tissue structures located beneath the epithelium of the gingiva are referred to collectively as the **lamina propria**. At the base of the underlying gingival tissue is the basement membrane (basal lamina) that is comprised of a collagen-based acellular material.

Charting Attachment Level and Mucogingival Junction Level on a Periodontal Examination Record

Following the evaluation of probing depths, the attachment level is recorded on the periodontal examination record with a blue pencil. A continuous line is drawn across the Facial and Lingual surface views of each tooth to indicate the level of the junctional epithelium (epithelial attachment) as shown in Figure 15–2. Involvement of the mucogingival junction is represented when the attached gingiva is missing and the probe passes through the pocket directly into the alveolar mucosa. To indicate the mucogingival junction on the periodontal examination record, use a blue pencil and draw a continuous dashed line over the Facial and Lingual surface views of each tooth (see Figure 15–2).

Periodontal Ligament

The **Periodontal ligament** or membrane is collagen and fibrous connective tissues surrounded by an amorphous ground substance located in the periodontal space that encircle and attach the roots of the teeth to the alveolar bone tissue. The ends of the periodontal ligament that are embedded into the

PERIODONTAL EXAMINATION RECORD

Date	Maxillary	1	2	3	4	5	6	7	8	9	10	11	12	13	14	15	16
	Plaque = +			+ + +	+ + +	+ + +	+ + +	+ + +	+ +	+ + +							
	Gingival inflammation Papillary (P) Marginal (M) Attached (A)																
	Mobility = 0, N, 1, 1+, 2, 2+, 3																
	Calculus = +																
	Re-eval probing depth																
	Total loss of attachment																
	Recession/tissue-CEJ height																
	Baseline probing depth																

Occlusal examination:
Molar R Class I II Div. 1 2 III
L Class I II Div. 1 2 III
Canine R Class I II Div. 1 2 III
L Class I II Div. 1 2 III
Profile ______
Overbite ___ mm
Overjet ___ mm
Alignment ______ mm to R L
Open bite # ______
Cross bite # ______
Drift ______
Version ______

FACIAL / LINGUAL

Date	Maxillary	1	2	3	4	5	6	7	8	9	10	11	12	13	14	15	16
	Baseline probing depth																
	Recession/tissue-CEJ height																
	Total loss of attachment																
	Re-eval probing depth																
	Calculus = +																
	Gingival inflammation Papillary (P) Marginal (M) Attached (A)																
	Plaque = +																

Date	Mandibular	32	31	30	29	28	27	26	25	24	23	22	21	20	19	18	17
	Plaque = +			+ + +	+ + +	+ + +	+ + +	+ + +	+ + +	+ + +	+ + +	+ + +					
	Gingival inflammation Papillary (P) Marginal (M) Attached (A)																
	Calculus = +																
	Re-eval probing depth																
	Total loss of attachment																
	Recession/tissue-CEJ height																
	Baseline probing depth																

Attachment level = ______
Mucogingival junction = __ __ __
Bleeding = red circle around probing depth
Suppuration (Exudate) = red dot above probing depth
Papillary hyperplasia = red ⌒
Loss of Papilla = red —
Periodontal abscess = red ○

The Ramfjord teeth
Maxilla: #3, #9, #12
Mandible: #19, #25, #28

LINGUAL / FACIAL

Date	Mandibular	32	31	30	29	28	27	26	25	24	23	22	21	20	19	18	17
	Baseline probing depth																
	Recession/tissue-CEJ height																
	Total loss of attachment																
	Re-eval probing depth																
	Calculus = +								+ +	+ + +	+ + +	+ + +					
	Mobility = 0, N, 1, 1+, 2, 2+, 3																
	Gingival inflammation Papillary (P) Marginal (M) Attached (A)																
	Plaque = +																

Stain: Extrinsic ☐ Localized # ______ Generalized ☐
Intrinsic ☐ Localized # ______ Generalized ☐

Furcation: Class I = ⋀ < 1mm
Class II = △ (1) > 1mm - < 3mm (2) > 3mm
Class III = ▲ through-and-through, covered by soft tissue
Class IV = ▲+ through-and-through, complete visualization

*Record all abnormal conditions in red EXCEPT attachment level and mucogingival junction * All recorded in Arabic numerals * Mobility measurement is in millimeters

Figure 15–2 Periodontal examination record: Attachment level, mucogingival junction level, plaque, and calculus shown charted

cementum and alveolar bone are known as Sharpey's fibers. Also included are the two groups of connective tissue fibers that form the attachment apparatus: the gingival fiber apparatus (located within the gingival tissues) and the principal fiber apparatus (encompasses the root) as illustrated in Figure 15–1A and 15–3.

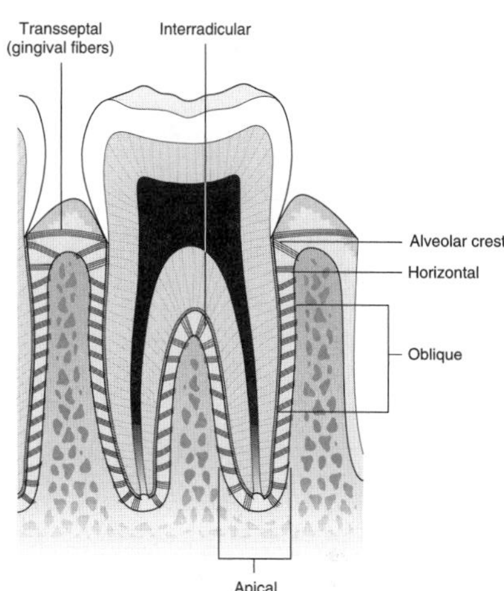

Figure 15–3 Principal fiber apparatus (Courtesy National Audiovisual Center)

- Gingival fiber apparatus:
  - Alveologingival fibers. Extend from the alveolar crest to the attached and free gingiva to provide support to the gingival tissue.
  - Dentogingival fibers. Extend from the cementum to the free gingiva to provide support to the gingival tissue.
  - Dentoperiosteal fibers. Extend from the cementum transversely to the alveolar crest.
  - Circular fibers. Extend around the cervical region of the tooth to provide stability.
  - Transseptal fibers. Extend from the cementum at the cervical region of one tooth across interproximally to an adjacent tooth.
- Principal fiber apparatus:
  - Alveolar crest fibers. Extend from the alveolar crest obliquely to the cementum just apical to the cementoenamel junction and the junctional epithelium to help counteract intrusive matter and forces.
  - Horizontal fibers. Extend from the cementum at the middle third of the root transversely to the adjacent alveolar bone tissue to help stabilize the tooth.
  - Oblique fibers. Extend from the cementum at the middle and apical thirds of the root in an oblique direction coronally attached to the alveolar bone tissue to help tolerate the stresses of mastication.
  - Apical fibers. Extend from the cementum around the root apex to the adjacent alveolar bone tissue to resist forces from a vertical direction. These fibers are formed following the complete formation of the root.
  - Interradicular fibers. Extend from the cementum throughout the furcation regions of maxillary and mandibular molar teeth to the adjacent alveolar bone tissue to prevent lateral and vertical stresses.

Cementum

The root of the tooth is covered by a bone-like connective tissue called cementum (described in Chapter 1). The function of cementum is to provide attachment sites for the gingival and principal fiber groups of the periodontal ligament, connecting the root of the tooth to the alveolar process.

Alveolar Bone

The alveolar process of the maxilla and mandible, also known as the alveolar bone, is the bone that supports the teeth and provides attachment for periodontal ligament fibers (see Figure 15–1 B).

- Alveolar bone proper (cribriform plate). Compact bone connective tissue that forms the inner lining of the alveoli (sockets) from which Sharpey's fibers of the periodontal ligament are attached. This area of cortical bone is referred to as the lamina dura and appears radiopaque on a dental radiograph.
- Supporting alveolar bone. Composed of cortical-compact bone and cancellous bone connective tissue providing support for the tooth.
  - Cortical-compact bone. The cortical bone comprises the Facial and Lingual plates of the alveolar bone of the maxilla and the Facial and Lingual plates, the lamina dura, alveolar crest, and the inferior border of the mandible. This bone appears as a dense radiopaque image on a dental radiograph.
  - Cancellous (spongy or trabecular). Located between the alveolar bone proper and the cortical-compact bone. This bone has numerous radiolucent interconnecting compartments called medullary spaces located within a honeycomb network that appear radiopaque and are referred to as trabeculae.

Etiology of Diseases of the Periodontium

The majority of the inflammatory diseases of the periodontium are caused primarily by microorganisms that colonize, proliferate, and release toxic byproducts on the tooth surface supragingivally and subgingivally. In addition, the combination of bacterial plaque, systemic, and/or local factors also contribute to the disease process.

Nonmineralized and Mineralized Deposits

- Nonmineralized deposits:
  - Acquired pellicle. A translucent thin layer composed of salivary glycoproteins that adhere to the teeth and other structures in the oral cavity. During the development of dental plaque, it provides the initial attachment site for microorganisms prior to colonization.
  - Bacterial plaque. A dense, nonmineralized mass of colonized microorganisms that adhere firmly to the acquired pellicle (Plate 17).
  - Materia alba. A white unstructured loosely adherent mass of desquamated epithelial cells, oral debris, and bacteria that lie on the surface of dental plaque.
  - Food debris. Loosely attached partially broken down food particles.
- Mineralized deposits:
  - Calculus. Mineralized bacterial plaque that forms a solid mass on the surfaces of teeth, restorations, and fixed and removable appliances, and is covered with plaque (Plate 18 and Figure 15–4).
  - Supragingival calculus. Occurs on the tooth surface coronal to the gingival margin.
  - Subgingival calculus. Occurs on the tooth surface apical to the gingival margin.

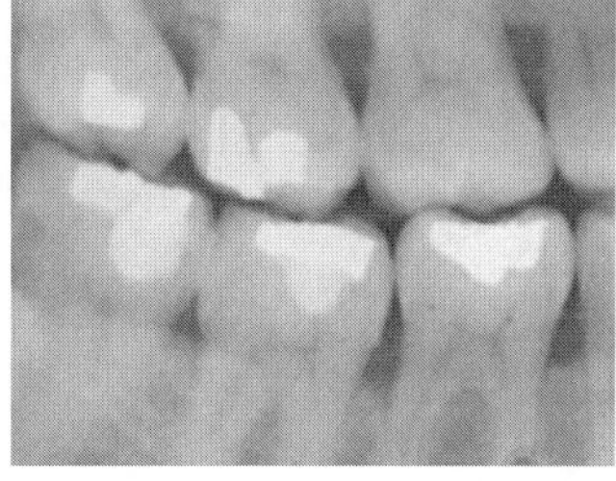

Universal System
#1 #2 #3 #4
#32 #31 #30 #29

Palmer System
8| 7| 6| 5|
8| 7| 6| 5|

ISO/FDI System
18 17 16 15
48 47 46 45

Figure 15–4 Subgingival calculus

Charting Bacterial Plaque and Calculus on a Periodontal Examination Record

To indicate the presence of the disclosed dental plaque shown in Plate 17 on the periodontal examination record, use a red pencil and on the Facial and Lingual surface views mark a (+) in the box that represents the Mesial, Facial or Lingual, and Distal surfaces, if plaque is present. The periodontal examination record in Figure 15–2 is shown with the dental plaque charted on teeth #3 to #9 and #22 to #30. The Labial surface in the middle and cervical third of tooth #8 is negative for plaque and does not show a (+) recorded. All of the remaining tooth surfaces have a recorded (+) and, therefore, indicate the presence of dental plaque. Other types of dental examination records may have a designated area on the chart where the examiner places a check in the appropriate box marked "Slight," "Moderate," or "Excessive," or the information is recorded in the progress notes section.

Pathogenesis of Periodontal Disease

Bacterial plaque is the primary etiologic factor in periodontal disease but the mere presence of oral microflora does not necessarily indicate disease will ensue. There are three stages involved in bacterial pathogenesis in the host: bacterial entry and colonization, invasion and proliferation with the production of toxic by-products, and the host response. In addition to bacterial plaque a combination of other factors can contribute to the development of periodontal infections such as an immunocompromised host, medications, endocrine imbalances, and hemotologic and genetic disorders.

The American Academy of Periodontology has developed a system of classifying types of inflammatory and degenerative diseases that affect the periodontium based on etiology and pathogenesis. The American Academy of Periodontology Classification System of Periodontal Disease includes the following:

- Gingival diseases
  - Gingivitis. Inflammation of the gingiva characterized by edema and redness due to bacterial plaque.
  - Chronic gingivitis. Gingival enlargement, redness, edema, bleeding, and loss of tissue shape, size, and surface texture due to the presence of bacterial plaque. The enlargement of the marginal gingiva may produce the formation of a pseudopocket without involvement of the alveolar bone tissue (Figure 15–5 and Plate 19).

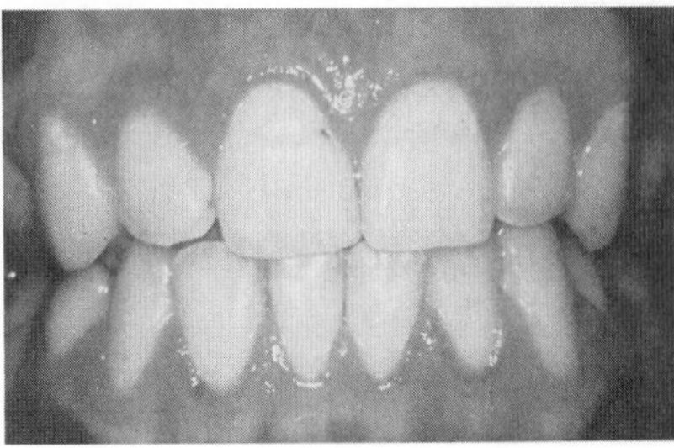

Figure 15–5 Marginal gingivitis

Universal System
#6 #7 #8 #9 #10 #11
#27 #26 #25 #24 #23 #22 #21

Palmer System
3| 2| 1| |1 |2 |3
3| 2| 1| |1 |2 |3 |4

ISO/FDI System
13 12 11 21 22 23
43 42 41 31 32 33 34

- Necrotizing ulcerative gingivitis (NUG) or formerly referred to as acute necrotizing ulcerative gingivitis (ANUG), trench mouth, or Vincent's infection. Severe inflammation of the gingiva, pain, and spontaneous bleeding. The interdental papilla becomes ulcerated and necrotic with the formation of craterlike defects and a pseudomembrane may form over the necrotic tissue. The breakdown of blood and debris produces a severe foul odor (Plate 20).

- Gingivitis associated with systemic diseases
  - Nutritional deficiency gingivitis. Inflammation of the gingiva in patients with scurvy (ascorbic acid deficiency).
  - Hormone-induced gingivitis. Inflammation of the gingiva associated with hormonal changes due to pregnancy, oral contraceptives, menstruation, puberty, and steroids (Plate 21).
  - Drug-influenced gingivitis. Gingival hyperplasia attributed to certain drugs that cause an increase in fibroblast activity, which in turn produces overgrowth of the connective tissue. The three most common drugs associated with gingival enlargement include phenytoin (dilantin), nifedipine, and cyclosporin A. The phenytoin shown in Plate 22 produces a generalized or more diffuse effect and the cyclosporin A typically causes a localized effect.
  - Linear gingival erythema (LGE) previously called HIV-gingivitis. Severely inflamed gingiva that appears as a red strip of tissue at the margin (Plate 23).

- Periodontal diseases
  - Periodontitis. Inflammation of the gingiva characterized by degeneration of the supporting connective tissue structures, alveolar bone, and apical migration of the junctional epithelium that produces loss of attachment (Plate 24).
  - Chronic adult periodontitis:
  - Early-onset periodontitis. A progressively slow disease that begins early in life but the clinical manifestations; attachment loss, periodontal pocket formation, and alveolar bone loss are evident by the middle to late thirties (Figure 15–6).
  - Moderate adult periodontitis. Characterized by increased levels of attachment loss, peri-

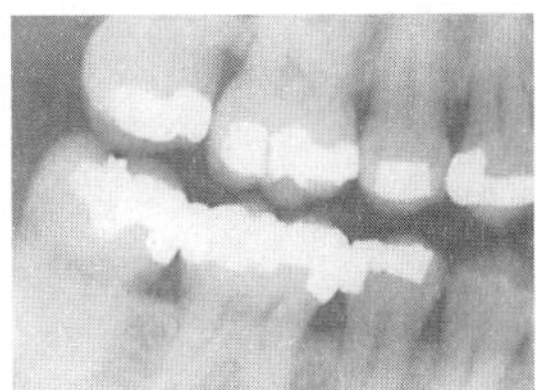

Universal System
#2 #3 #4 #5
#31 #30 #29 #28

Palmer System
7| 6| 5| 4|
7| 6| 5| 4|

ISO/FDI System
17 16 15 14
47 46 45 44

Figure 15–6 Early periodontitis; generalized loss of bone height

odontal pocket formation, and alveolar bone degeneration. Depending on the extent of bone loss, tooth mobility and furcation involvement may be evident (Figure 15–7).

- Advanced adult periodontitis. A rapid progression of alveolar bone loss accompanied by tooth mobility and furcation involvement (Figure 15–8).

- Early-onset periodontitis:
- Prepubertal periodontitis. Onset generally begins following the eruption of the primary dentition and may continue through the mixed dentition phase. The disease may be localized or generalized and is characterized by severe gingival inflammation, rapid loss of alveolar bone tissue, mobility, and tooth loss.
- Juvenile periodontitis. Occurs as a localized or secondary to untreated localized that affects adolescents. Appears to be a genetically based disease with familial distribution. Manifestations include severe bone loss around the permanent first molar and incisor teeth, mild inflammation,

Universal System
#2 #3 #4 #5
#31 #30 #29 #28

Palmer System
7| 6| 5| 4|
7| 6| 5| 4|

ISO/FDI System
17 16 15 14
48 47 46 45

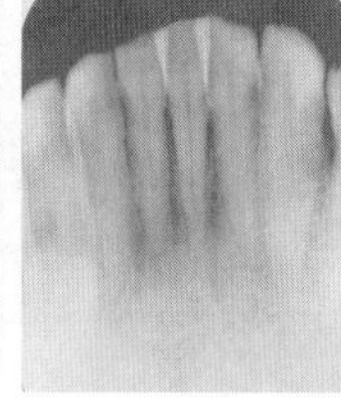

Universal System
#27 #26 #25 #24 #23 #22

Palmer System
3| 2| 1| |1 |2 |3

ISO/FDI System
43 42 41 31 32 33

Figure 15–7 Moderate periodontitis

Universal System
#2 #3 #4 #5 #6
#31 #30 #29 #28

Palmer System
7| 6| 5| 4| 3|
7| 6| 5| 4|

ISO/FDI System
17 16 15 14 13
48 47 46 45

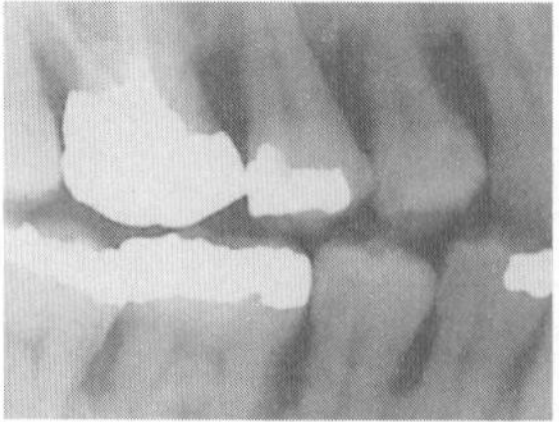

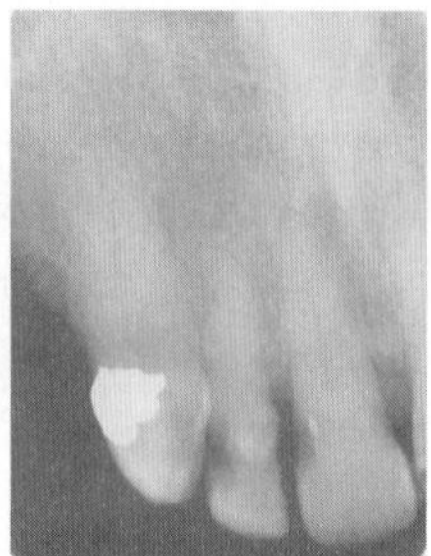

Universal System
#6 #7 #8

Palmer System
3| 2| 1|

ISO/FDI System
13 12 11

Figure 15–8 Advanced periodontitis

Universal System
#2 #3 #4 #5

Palmer System
7| 6| 5| 4|

ISO/FDI System
17 16 15 14

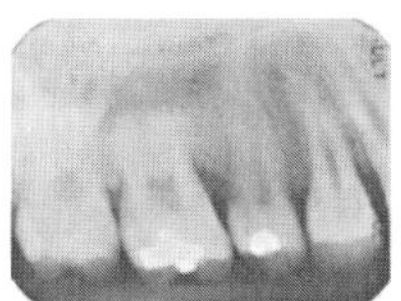

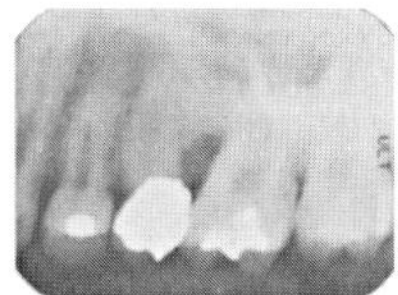

Universal System
#12 #13 #14 #15

Palmer System
|4 |5 |6 |7

ISO/FDI System
24 25 26 27

Figure 15–9 Juvenile periodontitis

and minimal quantities of bacterial plaque and calculus deposits. Abnormalities are frequently observed in phagocytic leukocyte counts demonstrated by decreased neutrophil chemotaxis (Figure 15–9).

- Rapidly progressive periodontitis. Onset is between puberty and the mid-thirties. The disease is characterized by generalized rapid loss of alveolar bone that affects a majority of the teeth.
- Refractory periodontitis. Characterized by multiple sites that exhibit progressive attachment loss and alveolar bone destruction. The involved areas are unresponsive to oral hygiene care and treatment due to the periodontal pathogens that continue to invade and infect the tissues.

- Periodontitis associated with systemic diseases and disturbances
  Early-onset periodontitis.
  Rapidly progressive periodontitis.
  Severe adult periodontitis.

- Necrotizing ulcerative periodontitis previously referred to as HIV-associated periodontitis (HIV-P). A severe and rapidly progressing disease that can be localized or generalized. The disease is characterized by erythematous soft tissue that rapidly degenerates to form extensive ulcerated and necrotic tissue accompanied by the severe loss of the periodontal attachment apparatus and alveolar bone.

The classification of periodontal diseases and the associated pathogenic microorganisms are represented in Table 15-1.

Table 15–1: Classification of Periodontal Diseases and Predominant Microorganisms

CLASSIFICATION	COMMON FORMS	MICROORGANISMS
Gingivitis	Chronic gingivitis	*Actinomyces* (species) *Fusobacterium nucleatum* *Veillonella parvula* *Prevotella intermedia* *Treponema* (species)
	Necrotizing ulcerative gingivitis	*Spirochetes* *Prevotella intermedia* *Fusobacterium* (species)
	Gingivitis associated with systemic diseases • Linear gingival erythema	• *Candida albicans* *Actinobacillus actinomycetemcomitans* *Fusobacterium nucleatum* *Camphylobacteria recta*
	• Scorbutic gingivitis	• No change in composition of microflora
	• Gingivitis associated with hormonal changes	• *Prevotella intermedia*
	• Gingivitis enlargement	• Increases in gingivitis-associated microorganisms increase the rate of overgrowth
Periodontitis	Adult periodontitis • Early • Moderate • Advanced	*Actinobacillus actinomycetemcomitans* *Porphoromonas gingivalis* *Prevotella intermedia* *Bacteriodes forsythus* *Eikenella corrodens* *Fusobacterium nucleatum* *Camphylobacteria rectus* *Treponema* (species)
	Early-onset periodontitis • Prepubertal periodontitis	• *Prevotella intermedia* *Actinobacillus actinomycetemcomitans* *Eikenella corrodens* *Caphocytophaga sputigena*
	• Juvenile periodontitis (localized/generalized) or rapidly progressive perodontitis	• *Actinobacillus actinomycetemcomitans* *Prevotella* (species)
	Refractory periodontitis	Three microbial complexes identified: • *Bacteriodes forsythus*, *Fusobacterium nucleatum*, *Camphylobacteria rectus* • *Streptococcus intermedius*, *Porphoromonas gingivalis*, *Peptostreptococcus micros* • *Streptococcus intermedius*, *Fusobacterium nucleatum* with and without *Porphoromonas gingivalis*
	Periodontitis associated with systemic diseases • Periodontitis related with systemic disturbances	• Periodontitis associated pathogens
	• Necrotizing ulcerative periodontitis	• Same as linear gingival erythema only or *Camphylobacteria recta* increases significantly

Manifestations of Soft Tissue

The examination of gingival tissues for signs of color, contour, and texture changes with or without bleeding and/or suppuration must all be considered to determine the presence of disease.

- Color:
  - Normal tissue. Generalized coral pink. Melanin pigmentation of light brown to black varies with race and complexion.
  - Abnormal tissue. Acute condition: erythematous, moderate to bright red. Chronic condition: cyanotic, bluish pink or red.
- Surface texture:
  - Normal tissue. Marginal free gingiva: smooth. Attached gingiva: stippled.
  - Abnormal tissue. Acute condition: shiny, glossy, and smooth. Chronic condition: fibrotic, hard with increased stippling; hyperkeratinization, firmness.
- Size:
  - Normal tissue. Tissue fits taut around the tooth.
  - Abnormal tissue. Acute and chronic: hypertrophied, bulbous, and enlarged.
- Shape:
  - Normal tissue. Marginal free gingiva: curved and flat. Interdental papillae: triangular, flat, and pointed.
  - Abnormal tissue. Marginal free gingiva: rolled and rounded. McCall's Festoon (rolled, prominent, and enlargement of the gingival margin). Interdental papillae: blunt, flat, bulbous, and cratered. Attached gingiva: Stillman's cleft (localized recession that appears as a V-shaped depression or Y-shaped slit that extends toward or past the mucogingival junction).
- Consistency:
  - Normal tissue. Marginal free gingiva: dense and firm. Attached gingiva: bound firmly in place.
  - Abnormal tissue. Marginal free gingiva: spongy, leaves an impression when pressed with a periodontal probe. Attached gingiva: firm, leaves no impression when pressed with a periodontal probe.
- Bleeding:
  - Normal tissue. No bleeding upon probing.
  - Abnormal tissue. Bleeding upon probing.

- Exudate and suppuration:
  - Normal tissue. No exudate/suppuration, formation and discharge of pus is expressed when pressure is applied to the area. Gingival crevicular fluid is an exudate (accumulated fluid) that is present in minimal quantities in normal healthy sulci.
  - Abnormal tissue. A periodontal abscess, an acute clinical manifestation, may develop when pus collects in the tissue due to a bacterial infection. Exudate/suppuration is expressed when pressure is applied to the area. The abscess is identified radiographically as a radiolucent area.

Charting Abnormal Tissue Manifestations on a Periodontal Examination Record

Changes in gingival health are evaluated and monitored by recording the extent and severity of gingival inflammation on the periodontal examination record shown in Figure 15–10. To indicate the gingival inflammation shown on teeth #7, #8, #9, and #10 (Plate 24) on the periodontal examination record, find the section called gingival inflammation and in the adjacent row of boxes locate the corresponding tooth designation numbers. Use the following abbreviations: Papillary (P), Marginal (M), and Attached (A) to classify the amount and severity of tissue involvement, and use a red pencil to print each letter that applies within the space provided. If two or more abbreviations are used, separate them with a front slash (/) (see Figure 15–10). The chart indicates (P/M) for teeth #7 and #10. This is read as: they have Papillary and Marginal inflammation on the Labial surfaces and teeth #8 and #9 (P/M/A) indicate that the attached gingiva is also involved on their Labial surfaces.

In addition, areas with marked papillary hyperplasia and loss of papilla are also depicted on the periodontal examination record. To indicate the hyperplasia of the papilla shown in Plate 23 between teeth #6, #7, #8, and #9, use a red pencil and draw a curved line "∩" on the chart located between the diagrams of the teeth to represent the affected papilla. The size of the curve that is drawn will also symbolize the extent of hyperplasia. To indicate the loss of papilla shown in Plate 20 between teeth #22, #23, #24, #25, and #26, use a red pencil and draw a straight line "–"on the chart between the corresponding tooth diagrams.

PERIODONTAL EXAMINATION RECORD

Date	Maxillary	1	2	3	4	5	6	7	8	9	10	11	12	13	14	15	16
	Plaque = +																
	Gingival inflammation Papillary (P) Marginal (M) Attached (A)							P/M	P/M/A	P/M/A	P/M						
	Mobility = 0, N, 1, 1+, 2, 2+, 3							F+1	2	2	1						
	Calculus = +																
	Re-eval probing depth																
	Total loss of attachment							1 1	555	565	545						
	Recession/tissue-CEJ height							232	131	131	121						
	Baseline probing depth	655	753	333	343	343	333	43④	42④	④34	42④	323	323	323	753	653	665

Occlusal examination:

Molar R Class I II Div. 1 2 III
L Class I II Div. 1 2 III

Canine R Class I II Div. 1 2 III
L Class I II Div. 1 2 III

Profile ______

Overbite ____ mm

Overjet ____ mm

Alignment ______ mm to R L

Open bite # ______

Cross bite # ______

Drift ______

Version ______

FACIAL / LINGUAL

Date	Maxillary	1	2	3	4	5	6	7	8	9	10	11	12	13	14	15	16
	Baseline probing depth	656	565														
	Recession/tissue-CEJ height																
	Total loss of attachment																
	Re-eval probing depth																
	Calculus = +																
	Gingival inflammation Papillary (P) Marginal (M) Attached (A)																
	Plaque = +																
Date	Maxillary	1	2	3	4	5	6	7	8	9	10	11	12	13	14	15	16

Date	Mandibular	32	31	30	29	28	27	26	25	24	23	22	21	20	19	18	17
	Plaque = +																
	Gingival inflammation Papillary (P) Marginal (M) Attached (A)																
	Calculus = +																
	Re-eval probing depth																
	Total loss of attachment																
	Recession/tissue-CEJ height																
	Baseline probing depth																

Attachment level = ______

Mucogingival junction = __ __ __

Bleeding = red circle around probing depth

Suppuration (Exudate) = red dot above probing depth

Papillary hyperplasia = red ⌒

Loss of Papilla = red —

Periodontal abscess = red ◯

The Ramfjord teeth
Maxilla: #3, #9, #12
Mandible: #19, #25, #28

LINGUAL / FACIAL

Date	Mandibular	32	31	30	29	28	27	26	25	24	23	22	21	20	19	18	17
	Baseline probing depth																
	Recession/tissue-CEJ height																
	Total loss of attachment																
	Re-eval probing depth																
	Calculus = +																
	Mobility = 0, N, 1, 1+, 2, 2+, 3																
	Gingival inflammation Papillary (P) Marginal (M) Attached (A)																
	Plaque = +																
Date	Mandibular	32	31	30	29	28	27	26	25	24	23	22	21	20	19	18	17

Stain: Extrinsic ☐ Localized # ______ Generalized ☐
Intrinsic ☐ Localized # ______ Generalized ☐

Furcation: Class I = △ < 1mm
Class II = △ (1) > 1mm - < 3mm (2) > 3mm
Class III = ▲ through-and-through, covered by soft tissue
Class IV = ▲+ through-and-through, complete visualization

*Record all abnormal conditions in red EXCEPT attachment level and mucogingival junction * All recorded in Arabic numerals * Mobility measurement is in millimeters

Figure 15–10 Periodontal examination record: Gingival inflammation, probing depth, loss of papilla, papillary hyperplasia, loss of attachment, bleeding, suppuration, mobility, and furcation involvement shown charted

Periodontal probing is used to assess periodontal tissue degeneration and pocket formation by measuring the depth of the sulcus from the marginal gingiva to the **junctional epithelium**. The sulcus around each tooth is divided into six sections—the Facial and Lingual surfaces each have three regions that are measured and the deepest millimeter probing depth measurement is recorded for each of the six regions.

To indicate the probing depths on the periodontal examination record, place the measurements adjacent to either the section marked "Baseline probing depth" if it is the initial appointment, or in the section designated as the "Re-evaluation probing depth" if it is a recall appointment. Use a red pencil to print the probing depth numbers in the boxes provided. When bleeding occurs during probing indicate this on the examination record. Use a red pencil and place a circle around the probing depth number "④." If suppuration appears during probing, use a red pencil and place a dot above the involved probing depth "•." To indicate a periodontal abscess that was detected as a radiolucent area on a dental radiograph on the periodontal examination record, use a red pencil and draw a circle around the involved region on the root. If the abscess has formed a fistula, draw a line extended from the circle that represents the abscess and the end of the line is marked with a dot. The chart indicates (see Figure 15–10) that tooth #3 has a periodontal abscess and tooth #2 has a periodontal abscess with a fistula. A periapical abscess and periodontal abscess with or without a fistula are charted the same on all charting forms.

In Figure 15–10, the chart indicates the baseline probing depths recorded for the Facial surfaces of the maxillary teeth. It shows that teeth #1, #2, #14, and #15 had a purulent discharge and in addition, teeth #7, #8, #9, and #10 also had bleeding upon probing.

The Clinical Attachment Level and Gingival Recession

The clinical attachment level is the relationship of the cementoenamel junction (CEJ) to the position of the attached epithelial tissues (junctional epithelium) at the base of the sulcus. The attachment level is measured with a probe from a fixed point of reference and differs from probing depth, which is measured without regard to a fixed point. Probing depths are measured from the free gingival crest to the epithelial attachment, which are both changeable points.

The stability of the epithelial attachment is a measure of health, and the apical migration of the attachment is evidence of disease progression. When the root surface is exposed because of apical migration of the epithelial attachment (junctional epithelium), it is referred to as **gingival recession**. Clinical attachment levels are measured and calculated in the following ways (Figure 15–11):

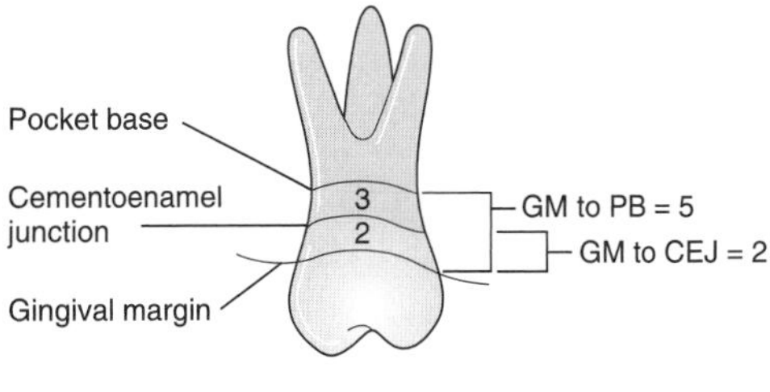

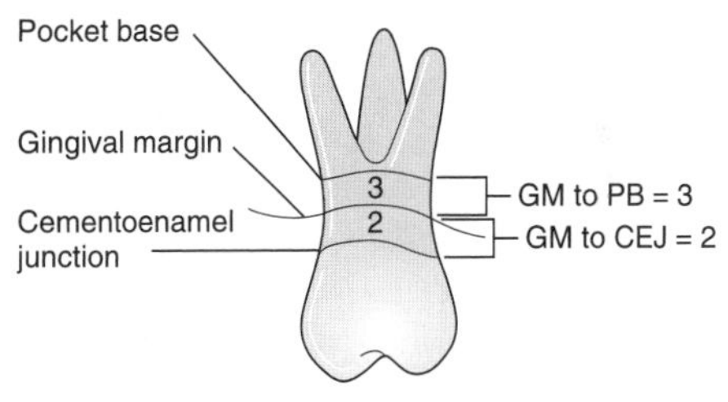

Figure 15–11 Calculation of attachment loss

Gingiva is coronal to the cementoenamel junction:

- Measure the pocket depth from the free gingival crest to the base of the pocket or sulcus.
- Measure from the cementoenamel junction to the free gingival crest.
- Subtract the second measurement (CEJ to free gingival crest) from the first measurement (free gingival crest to the pocket base) to obtain the attachment loss.

Gingival recession:

- Measure the pocket depth from the free gingival crest to the base of the pocket or sulcus.
- Measure from the cementoenamel junction to the free gingival crest.
- Add the two measurements together to obtain the attachment loss.

Charting Attachment Loss and Gingival Recession on a Periodontal Examination Record

To indicate attachment loss and gingival recession shown for teeth #7, #8, #9, and #10 in Plate 24 on the periodontal examination record, use a red pencil and in the designated area adjacent to the section marked "Recession/tissue-CEJ height" enter the measurements for the Labial surfaces (see Figure 15–10). To calculate and record attachment loss for tooth #7, subtract the tissue-to-CEJ height for the Disto-Labial, Labial, and Mesio-Labial regions from their corresponding probing depth, and enter the measurement in the column adjacent to the section indicated as "total loss of attachment." The loss of attachment for tooth #7 indicates 1 mm of loss on the Mesio-Labial and Disto-Labial surfaces and no attachment loss on the Labial surface. Teeth #8, #9, and #10 have gingival recession and, therefore, the probing depth and recession height are added together to determine the attachment loss. The total loss of attachment, beginning with the Mesio-Labial measurement recorded in millimeters, for tooth #8 = 555, tooth #9 = 565, and tooth #10 = 545.

In addition to recording recession measurements, recession levels on the Facial and Lingual surfaces are also illustrated on the tooth diagrams. To indicate the recession levels shown on teeth #8, #9, and #10 in Plate 24, use a red pencil to draw a curved line that corresponds with the 2 mm spaces adjacent to each tooth, and label the area with the recession level measurement. In Figure 15–10, teeth #8 and #9 are shown with curved lines that extend to the 3 mm region and are labeled accordingly, and tooth #10 is shown drawn and labeled as having 2 mm of recession.

Gingival and Periodontal Pockets

In the presence of infection, the gingival sulcus deepens and forms a pocket. A pocket is made up of the junctional epithelium, which forms the base of the pocket, bound together at the junction of the sulcular epithelium (outside wall) and the tooth surface (inside wall). Pockets are classified as gingival or periodontal and this is contingent upon whether or not there is apical migration of the epithelial attachment and loss of alveolar bone tissue (Figure 15–12). Pocket classifications are as follows:

Gingival pocket:

- Pocket formation due to an increase in the size of the gingiva without apical migration of the junctional epithelium or loss of alveolar bone.
- Gingival margin has migrated superiorly as a result of tissue enlargement.
- Presence of **suprabony pockets**; the base of the pocket is coronal to the alveolar bone crest (see Figure 15–12).

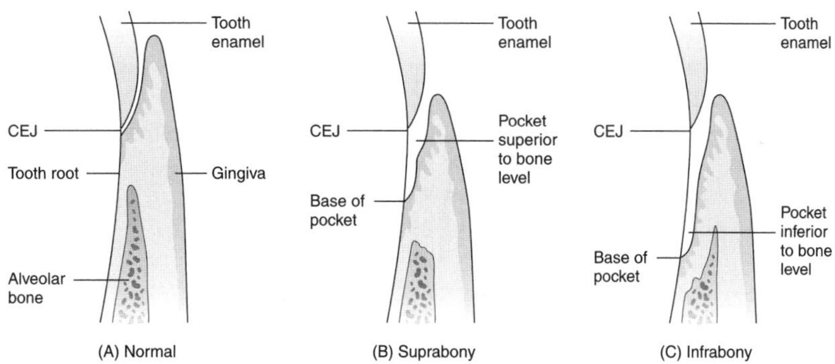

Figure 15–12 Types of bony pockets: (A) Normal (B) Suprabony (C) Infrabony

Periodontal pocket:

- Pocket formation due to tissue degeneration with apical migration of the junctional epithelium.
- Degeneration of the attachment apparatus and alveolar bone tissue.
- Formation of suprabony pockets; the base of the pocket is coronal to the alveolar bone crest or **infrabony pockets** (intrabony pockets); the base of the pocket is apical to the alveolar bone crest (see Figure 15–12).

Horizontal and Vertical Alveolar Bone Loss and Defects of the Alveolar Cortical Plate

In healthy alveolar bone tissue, the cementoenamel junction is located approximately 1 to 2 mm from the alveolar crest. The lamina dura forms the bony wall of the tooth socket that consists of cortical bone and surrounds the periodontal ligament space. Radiographically, it appears as a radiopaque line (Figure 15–13).

The assessment of diseased alveolar bone and diagnosis of periodontal disease is determined through a clinical examination performed in conjunction with an evaluation of dental radiographs. In response to inflammation, the alveolar bone is resorbed, the height of the bone is reduced, and the crest of the lamina dura appears radiographically as an indistinct and radiolucent area. The direction and pattern of bone degeneration varies and the

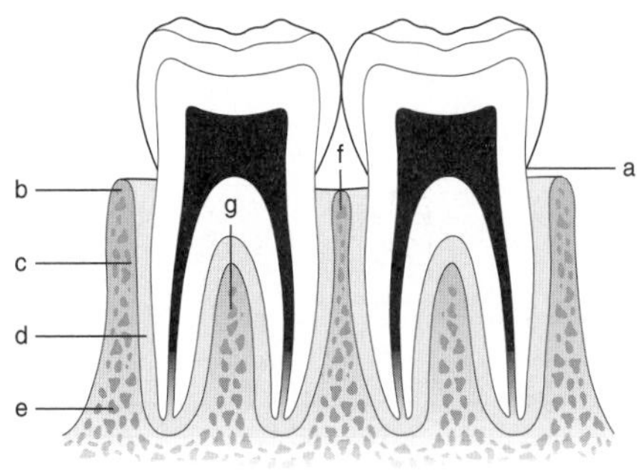

A. Diagram of the radiographically visible features

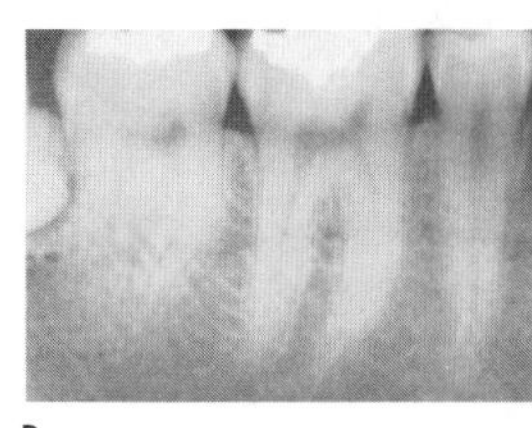
B.

Universal System
#31 #30 #29

Palmer System
7| 6| 5|

ISO/FDI System
47 46 45

Figure 15–13 Normal appearance of periodontal structures: *Diagram key:* (a) cementoenamel junction (CEJ) (b) alveolar crest (c) lamina dura (d) periodontal ligament (PDL) space (e) supporting bone (f) interproximal bone (g) interradicular bone

following lists explain the two types of bone loss patterns and the defects of the alveolar cortical plate.

Horizontal bone loss:

- Reduction in the height of bone tissue in an apical direction perpendicular to the long axis of the tooth.
- The crest of the alveolar bone is parallel with an imaginary line that extends between the cementoenamel junction of two adjacent teeth.
- Reduction of 1.0 to 1.5 mm from the CEJ.
- Observed with a suprabony pocket.
- Localized loss of bone tissue occurs in a specific region or generalized loss of bone is present in all regions (Figure 15–14).

Universal System
#3 #4 #5 #6
#30 #29 #28 #27

Palmer System
6| 5| 4| 3|
6| 5| 4| 3|

ISO/FDI System
16 15 14 13
46 45 44 43

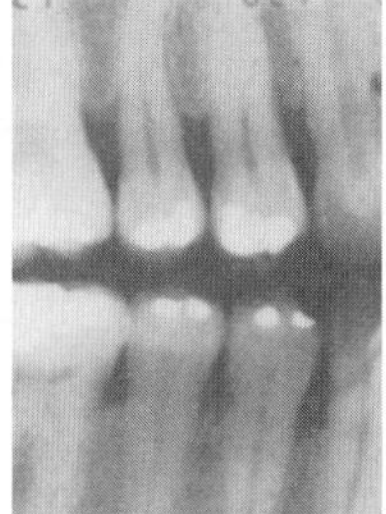

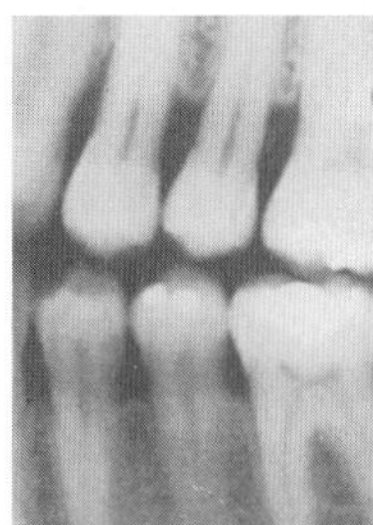

Universal System
#11 #12 #13 #14
#22 #21 #20 #19

Palmer System
|4 |5 |6 |7
|4 |5 |6 |7

ISO/FDI System
23 24 25 26
33 34 35 36

Figure 15–14 Vertical and horizontal bone loss

Vertical or angular **bone loss:**

- Reduction in the height of the crestal bone at an angle.
- The crest of the alveolar bone is not parallel with an imaginary line that extends between the cementoenamel junction of two adjacent teeth.
- Bone loss is greater on the Mesial surface of one tooth than it is on the Distal surface of the adjacent tooth or vice versa.
- Observed with an infrabony pocket.
- The occurrence is generally localized on the Mesial tooth surface of the second and third molar teeth.
- Results from traumatic occlusion and disease.

Alveolar cortical plate defects:

- **Dehiscence**. Absence of the alveolar cortical plate and the formation of a cleftlike defect in the bone accompanied by soft tissue recession and exposure of the root surface.
- **Fenestration**. A spherical-shaped defect in the alveolar cortical plate formed inferior to the remaining intact cortical bone that exposes the root on either the Facial or Lingual surface.

Mobility

The periodontal membrane that surrounds and supports the teeth accommodates the teeth by allowing them to move slightly, giving them mobility. A small degree of mobility is considered normal. **Mobility** is considered pathologic when a greater degree of movement that exceeds normal is observed. The degeneration of epithelial tissue, connective tissue, alveolar bone tissue, and traumatic occlusion will increase mobility. Mobility can be measured in two ways: when the teeth are not in functional occlusion with the use of instrumental evaluation performed with two blunt-ended instruments, and digital assessment and direct observation of the maxillary teeth when they are in occlusion. The systems for classifying mobility and fremitus include the following:

Mobility:

- 0 = Ankylosis
- N = Normal, physiologic
- 1 = Slight mobility, greater degree of movement than normal

- 1+ = Slightly greater mobility than a mobility of 1 mm
- 2 = Moderate mobility, displacement is greater than 1 mm
- 2+ = Slightly greater mobility than a mobility of 2 mm
- 3 = Severe mobility, displacement may be in all directions, horizontal as well as vertical.

Fremitus:

- N = Normal (no detectable vibration or movement)
- + = One-degree fremitus, detection of a slight vibration
- + + = Two-degree fremitus, palpable vibration with minimal observable movement
- + + += Three-degree fremitus, clearly observable movement

Furcation Involvement

The anatomical region of multirooted teeth where the roots separate is referred to as the **furcation**. Periodontally involved multirooted teeth with loss of attachment and alveolar bone are inclined to have furcation involvement. The degree of furcation involvement is determined by how much bone tissue has been destroyed and by the degree to which a probe can or cannot be engaged in the area. The extent of furcations is measured by whether or not a probe can be engaged in the area. The following is a summary of the classifications and charting symbols for furcation involvement:

- Class I = /\ Early involvement: < 1 mm
- Class II = △ Moderate involvement: (1) > 1 mm – < 3 mm, (2) > 3 mm
- Class III = ▲ Severe involvement: Through and through, covered by soft tissue
- Class IV = ▲+ Severe involvement: Through and through, complete visualization

Charting Mobility, Fremitus, and Furcation Involvement on a Periodontal Examination Record

To indicate mobility and fremitus on teeth #7, #8, #9, and #10 shown in Plate 24 on the periodontal examination record, locate the section called "Mobility" and in the row adjacent to it locate the tooth designation numbers. Use a red pencil and print the level of mobility in the appropriate space. To indicate fremitus, use a red pencil and print an uppercase "F" followed by either "+," "++," or "+++" in the same space that is used for mobility (see Figure 15–10).

Figure 15–10 indicates that tooth #7 has one-degree fremitus and slight mobility, teeth #8 and #9 show moderate mobility, and tooth #10 has slight mobility.

To indicate furcation involvement on the periodontal examination record, use a red pencil and on the involved furcation site draw the designated symbol that represents the level of furcation involvement. Figure 15–10 shows early furcation development on tooth #19, moderate involvement on tooth #30, and severe involvement with complete visualization of the furcation on tooth #31.

Contributing Factors in Disease Progression

There are a variety of factors that predispose the development of gingival and periodontal diseases. Tooth irregularities, dental anomalies, and congenital defects are factors that influence the accumulation of bacterial plaque and are discussed further in Chapters 17 and 21.

The effect of tooth position (plunger cusp) and an open contact area can cause food particles to be forced into the gingival sulcus and this condition is referred to as **food impaction** (Plate 25 and Figure 15–15). Open contact areas can be a result of a natural space located between adjacent teeth in the same arch called diastema, pathologic frenum attachment, or undercontoured restorations with faulty interproximal margins (Plate 26). These circumstances can produce tissue trauma that will render the area more prone to disease.

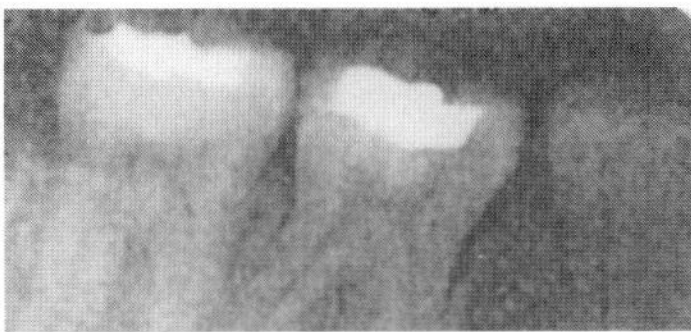

Figure 15–15 Open contact

Universal System
#31 #30 #29

Palmer System
7⏋ 6⏋ 5⏋

ISO/FDI System
47 46 45

Charting Open Contact, Poor Contact, Food Impaction Area, and Pathologic Frenum

To indicate the open contact area between teeth #29 and #30 (see Figure 15–15) on the periodontal examination record, use a red pencil and locate the tooth designation numbers. Draw two vertical lines adjacent to each other "||" located between teeth #29 and #30. Each line will extend from the interproximal area at the level of the CEJ on the Facial surface view and past the Occlusal or Incisal view to the CEJ on the Lingual surface view (see Figure 15–10).

To indicate an area with poor contact, follow the procedure previously mentioned for open contact with the exception of the placement of a single zigzag line through the interproximal region. The area between teeth #26 and #27 is shown charted with a poor contact area (see Figure 15–15).

To indicate the region of food impaction between teeth #30 and #31 shown in Plate 25 and Figure 15–15, use a red pencil and locate the region between teeth #30 and #31. Draw an arrow "↓" that extends from the interproximal surface of either the Facial or Lingual surface side and direct it toward the Occlusal or Incisal tooth surface view (see Figure 15–10).

To indicate the presence of a pathologic frenum on the periodontal examination record, use a red pencil and on the Facial surface view between the diagrams that represent the central incisor teeth place a large triangle filled in completely with horizontal lines (see Figure 15–10).

These four procedures can be charted on the anatomic and geometric charts in the same ways that were previously mentioned. To indicate an area of open contact on a numeric coding system chart, follow the previously mentioned procedure and place each red vertical line directly adjacent to the black line that separates the two diagrams that represent the teeth. To show areas of poor contact, food impaction, and pathologic frenum on a numeric chart, place the red zigzag line, arrow, or triangle directly on the black vertical line located between the diagrams that represent the involved teeth.

Review Questions

Multiple Choice

Directions: Select the letter of the choice that *best* answers the question.

1. Periosteal fibers that attach the periodontal ligament to the cementum are called:
   a. circular fibers. b. Von Ebner's fibers.
   c. Tomes' fibers. d. Sharpey's fibers.
2. The difference between a periodontal pocket and a pseudopocket is:
   a. bleeding upon probing.
   b. visible inflammation of the gingiva.
   c. proliferation of the gingiva in a coronal direction.
   d. apical migration of the junctional epithelium.
3. The epithelial attachment is made up of:
   a. cuboidal epithelium with slight keratinization.
   b. cuboidal epithelium with extensive amounts of keratinization.
   c. stratified squamous epithelium with no keratinization.
   d. stratified squamous epithelium with extensive amounts of keratinization.
4. Subgingival calculus is usually darker in color because:
   a. as the blood breaks down, pigments are incorporated into the deposit.
   b. of the higher amount of calcium phosphate found within the deposit.
   c. its location prevents the washing action of the saliva.
   d. none of the above.
5. Periodontal disease differs from gingivitis in:
   a. etiology.
   b. pathogenesis.
   c. reaction of the tissues.
   d. amount of tissue involvement.
   e. types of injurious agents seen in tissue.
6. During an episode of gingivitis, poor tissue tone is associated with:
   a. bleeding.
   b. dilation of the blood vessels in the tissue.
   c. destruction of the collagen fibers found in the area.
   d. large numbers of inflammatory cells invading the area.

7. The pellicle found on the surface of the dental enamel initially is derived from:
   a. saliva.
   b. tooth structure.
   c. dietary components.
   d. bacterial byproducts.
8. Which of the bacteria listed below are most frequently associated with necrotizing ulcerative gingivitis?
   a. Cocci and rods
   b. Filaments and rods
   c. Fusiforms and spirochetes
   d. Gram-positive forms and spirochetes
9. Which of the following changes in papillary contour is found with a previous infection of necrotizing ulcerative gingivitis?
   a. Enlargement
   b. Cratering
   c. Atrophy
   d. Recession
10. Which of the following is described as inflammation extending from the gingiva into the supporting structures with loss of attachment?
    a. Gingivitis
    b. Periodontal disease
    c. Secondary occlusal trauma
    d. Hyperkeratinization of gingiva
11. A healthy periodontal ligament surrounding a normal tooth appears as ____________________ on a radiograph.
    a. an unbroken radiopaque line around the root of the tooth
    b. a radiopaque line only on the lateral sides of the root of the tooth
    c. an unbroken radiolucent line around the root of the tooth
    d. a radiolucent line only on the lateral sides of the root of the tooth
12. Which of the following are similar in localized juvenile periodontal disease and adult periodontal disease?
    a. Age of onset
    b. Rate of attachment loss
    c. Formation of periodontal pockets
    d. Composition of microbial flora
    e. Amount and distribution of bone loss
13. In pregnancy gingivitis, the part of the gingiva most susceptible to enlargement or formation of a pregnancy tumor is the:
    a. alveolar mucosa.
    b. marginal gingiva.
    c. attached gingiva.
    d. interdental papilla.

Answers

1. **d,** 2. **d,** 3. **c,** 4. **a,** 5. **d,** 6. **c,** 7. **a,** 8. **c,** 9. **b,** 10. **b,** 11. **c,** 12. **c,** 13. **d**

References

American Academy of Periodontology. (1989a). *Proceedings of the world workshop in clinical periodontics* (pp. 11–13). (Consensus Report, Discussion Section II). Chicago: Author.

American Academy of Periodontology. (1989b). *Proceedings of the world workshop in clinical periodontics* (pp. IX, 24–26). (Consensus Report, Discussion Section IX). Chicago: Author.

American Academy of Periodontology. (1989c). *Proceedings of the world workshop in clinical periodontics* (pp. IX-27). (Consensus Report, Discussion Section IX). Chicago: Author.

American Academy of Periodontology, Department of Scientific, Clinical, and Educational Affairs. (1993, June). *Guidelines for periodontal therapy* (pp. 1–5). Chicago: Author.

Rosental I. M., Abrams, H., & Kopczyk, R. A. (1988). The relationship of inflammatory periodontal disease to diabetic status in insulin-dependent diabetes mellitus. *Journal of Clinical Periodontology*, 15, 425.

Watanabe, K. (1990). Prepubertal periodontitis: A review of diagnostic criteria, pathogenesis, and differential diagnosis. *Journal of Clinical Periodontal Research*, 25, 31.

CHAPTER 16

Endodontics

Key Terms

Acute Apical Abscess
Acute Apical Periodontitis
Apicoectomy
Chronic Apical Abscess
Chronic Apical Periodontitis
Chronic Pulpitis
Endodontics
Fistula
Gutta-Percha
Hemisection
Irreversible Acute Pulpitis
Periapical Radiolucency
Pulpectomy
Pulpitis
Pulpotomy
Retrofilling
Reversible Pulpitis
Root Amputation
Temporary Restoration

PRIMARY CODE

M = Mesial
I = Incisal (#6–#11 and #22–#27)
O = Occlusal (#1–#5, #12–#16, #17–#21, and #27–#32)
D = Distal
F = Facial (#6–#11 and #22–#27)
B = Buccal (#1–#5, #12–#16, #17–#21, and #27–#32)
L = Lingual

SECONDARY CODE

-A = Anomaly
-G = Gold (blue diagonal lines)
-H = Porcelain
-N = Non-precious (blue cross-hatch)
-E = Resin (blue outline)
-S = Silver Amalgam (solid blue)
-R = Root Canal (blue vertical line)
△ = Apicoectomy (blue outline)
△S = Silver Amalgam Retrofilling (blue outline)
• = and also
(-A) = Periapical radiolucency (red outline)

PRIMARY CODE	SECONDARY CODE
X = Missing	(A)↘ = Periapical radiolucency with fistula (red outline)
C = Crown	FX = Fracture (red zigzag line)
	• p = Retention Post (blue)
	-Z = Temporary Restoration (blue)

Introduction

The branch of dentistry concerned with the diagnosis and treatment of diseases of the dental pulp and the periapical tissues is called **endodontics**. Circumstances that contribute to the injury and death of the dental pulp are extensive dental caries, traumatic injury, mechanical pulp exposure, and chemical and thermal irritants.

Diseases of the Dental Pulp and Periapical Tissues

The diseases of the dental pulp and periapical tissues include the following:

- **Pulpitis**. Inflammation of the pulp tissue. Associated with the previously mentioned factors that cause injuries to the dental pulp.
  - **Reversible pulpitis**. Carious lesions that progress into the dentin and produce pain of short duration. Radiographically, Carious lesions involve the dentin adjacent to the pulp tissue.
  - **Irreversible acute pulpitis**. Associated with severe pain that becomes progressively more intense. Radiographically, there is no evidence of bone loss.
  - **Chronic pulpitis**. Generally asymptomatic, with little or no discomfort. Radiographically, may note resorption in the pulp canal.
- **Acute apical periodontitis**. The rapid onset of inflammation of the apical region that is associated with severe pain caused by pressure between the alveolar process and the tooth. The tooth becomes slightly elevated (supraversion) in the alveolar socket and is sensitive to touch and closure.

Radiographically, no detectable **periapical radiolucency** or dark area is seen in the periapical tissues that surround the tooth.

- **Acute apical abscess**. Moderate pain is associated with inflammation caused by bacterial invasion and necrosis of the infected pulp canal. The gradual development of necrotic tissue by-products destroys the alveolar bone tissue. Radiographically, a widened periodontal space or large periapical alveolar radiolucency may be visible.
- **Chronic apical periodontitis** (granuloma). The invasion and proliferation of bacteria and their by-products results in a region of chronic inflammatory tissue that may become encapsulated. Significant bone loss can occur with little or no pain. Radiographically, a periapical alveolar radiolucency is visible (Figure 16–1A and B).
- **Chronic apical abscess**. The inflammatory pulpal response to a bacterial infection that progresses slowly. Generally asymptomatic, but the involved region may at one time have given the patient discomfort. The abscess forms a **fistula**, a passageway from the apical region through the bone to the gingiva. This tract allows the toxic exudate and liquid by-products produced from inflammation to drain from the area. Radiographically, the presence of a more diffuse periapical radiolucency that may include external resorption of the root apex is visible.

Nonsurgical and Surgical Treatments of the Dental Pulp and Periapical Tissues

Following the diagnostic evaluation of the pulp and periapical tissues, the definitive diagnosis will determine whether a nonsurgical or surgical therapy is required. The nonsurgical treatments include the following:

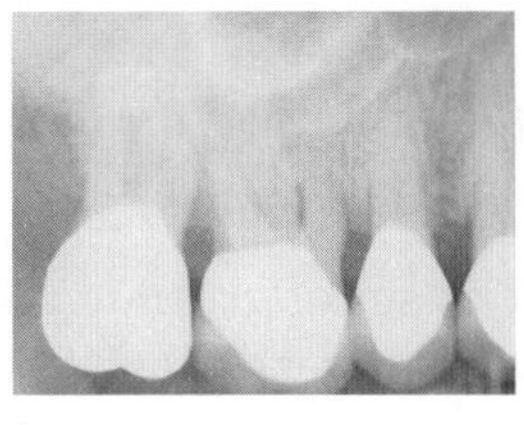

A.

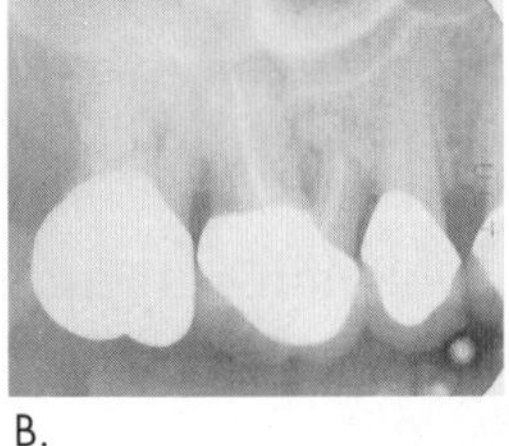

B.

Universal System
#2 #3 #4 #5

Palmer System
7| 6| 5| 4|

ISO/FDI System
17 16 15 14

Figure 16-1 (A) Periapical radiograph shown with a periapical radiolucency on tooth #3 (B) Periapical radiograph shown of tooth #3 with a gutta-percha Root Canal filling

- **Pulpotomy**. Pulp extirpation from the coronal portion of the tooth.
- **Pulpectomy**. Pulp extirpation from the coronal and root portions of the tooth (see Figure 16–1B).

Endodontic surgery is performed to resolve problems of an endodontically treated, pulpless, or periodontally involved tooth and includes the following:

- Surgical incision and drainage. Emergency procedures for acute lesions that exhibit pain and swelling.
  - –Trephination. A procedure utilized to drain the toxic exudate from within the cancellous bone tissue that is trapped behind the cortical plate of the alveolar process, and to alleviate periapical pain.
- Radicular surgery. Surgery that pertains to the root and the surrounding tissues.
  - – **Apical** and corrective surgery. Curette the apical region, foramen, and periapical tissues and mechanically repair the damaged tissues.
  - – **Apicoectomy.** Resection of the apical portion of the root (Figure 16–2).
  - – **Retrofilling.** A restorative procedure used to place a filling into the apical portion of the resected root to seal the canal (see Figure 16–2).
  - – **Root amputation.** Resection of a diseased root from a multirooted tooth where it joins the crown (Figure 16–3A, B, C, and D).

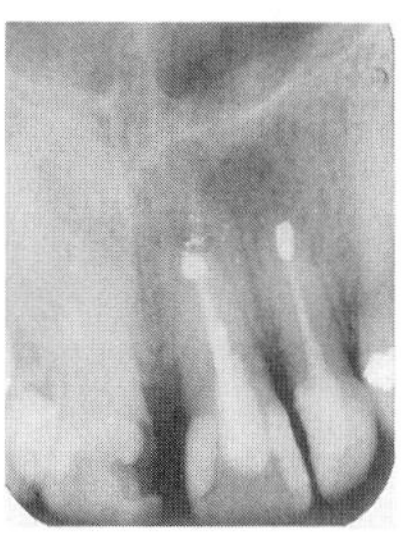

Universal System
#7 #8 #9 #10

Palmer System
2| 1| |1 |2

ISO/FDI System
12 11 21 22

Figure 16-2 Periapical radiograph of teeth #9 and #10 each shown with a Lingual Resin restoration, an Apicoectomy, and Silver Amalgam Retrofilling; tooth #9 is also shown with a Retention Post and Mesio-Lingual and Disto-Lingual Resin restorations. (Courtesy Peter J. Schindelholz, D.D.S., S.C.)

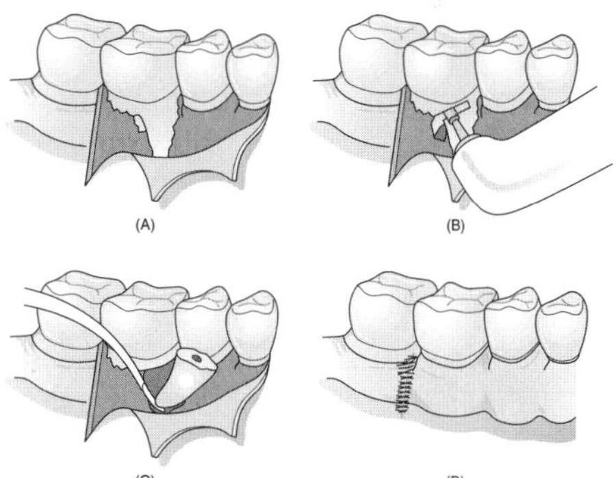

Figure 16-3 Root amputation: (A) The Mesial root is accessed through a full thickness flap. (B) The Mesial root is resected with a high-speed rotary handpiece. (C) The resected root is elevated and removed. (D) The bone and surrounding tissues in the area recover.

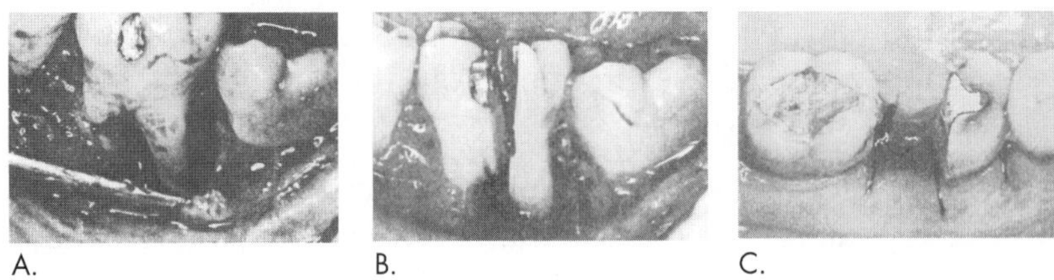

Figure 16-4 Hemisection: (A) A severe osseous defect that involves the Distal root of the mandibular first molar. (B) The mandibular first molar is hemisectioned. (C) The Mesial half of the hemisectioned tooth remains

- **Hemisection.** Resection of an entire half of a tooth. Maxillary molars and premolars are resected from Mesial to Distal and from Buccal to Lingual in mandibular molars (Figure 16–4A, B, and C).

Charting a Periapical Radiolucency, Fistula, Root Canal Filling, Apicoectomy, Silver Amalgam Retrofilling, and Retention Post on an Anatomic Chart

To chart the periapical radiolucency shown on tooth #3 in Figure 16–1A on an anatomic chart, locate the tooth notation number and use a red pencil to draw an outline of the area around the involved root apex on the Facial surface view (Figure 16–5).

To chart a fistula, follow the same procedure previously mentioned that describes a periapical radiolucency. Draw a red line attached to the outlined area and extend it up toward the Crown to the middle third of the root and mark the end with a large red dot. In Figure 16–5, tooth #4 is shown charted with a fistula.

In Figure 16–1 B, a periapical radiograph of tooth #3 is shown with a Root Canal filling made of **gutta-percha** that appears radiopaque. To indicate that tooth #3 has a Root Canal filling on an anatomic chart, locate the tooth number and with a blue pencil on both the Buccal and Lingual tooth surface views in each root draw a line that extends from the CEJ to the root apex (see Figure 16–5). If the Root Canal is underfilled, indicate this by not extending the line to the end of the root apex. Indicate an overfilled canal by extending the line past the root apex.

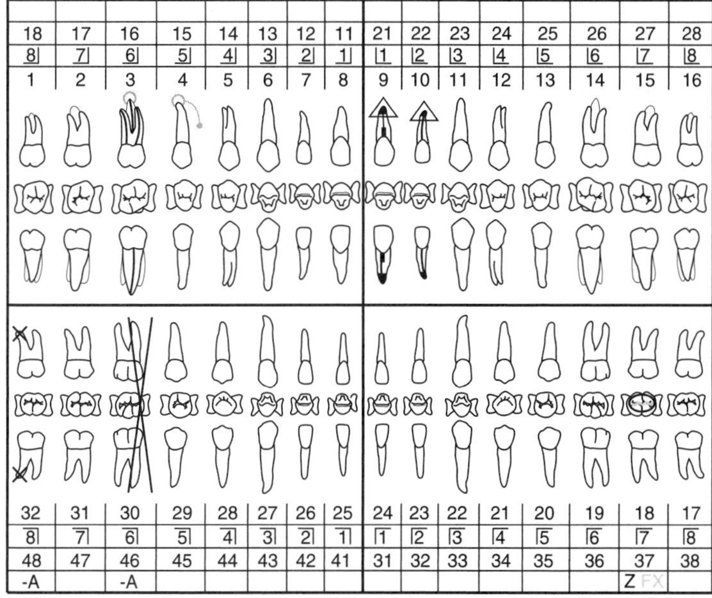

Figure 16-5 Anatomic chart shown with a periapical radiolucency and Root Canal filling on tooth #3; tooth #4 is shown charted with a periapical radiolucency and fistula; teeth #9 and #10 are each shown with a Root Canal filling, an Apicoectomy, a Silver Amalgam Retrofilling; tooth #9 is also shown with a stainless steel Retention Post; tooth #18 has a Temporary Restoration with an Occlusal surface Fracture; tooth #30 has been hemisected and the Distal Crown and root remains; tooth #32 indicating the Distal root has been amputated

To indicate that teeth #9 and #10 in Figure 16–2 each have a Root Canal filling, an Apicoectomy, and a Silver Amalgam Retrofilling, first indicate each Root Canal filling as previously described. To show that each tooth has had an Apicoectomy with a Silver Amalgam Retrofilling, use only the Facial surface views. At the region where the portions of the root apices have been removed, use a blue pencil to draw a triangle with the point directed away from the apex. To indicate the Silver Amalgam Retrofillings, use both the Facial and Lingual surface views, and at the end of each root use a blue pencil to outline the restored area then completely fill it in (see Figure 16–5).

Tooth #9 in Figure 16–2 is shown with a Retention Post, which appears as a radiopaque image, inserted into the Crown and root. A Retention Post is used on endodontically treated teeth to strengthen the retention capabilities of the tooth. It can be prefabricated out of stainless steel or custom made from Gold and Non-precious metals and can either be used in conjunction with or without a retention core. The core is made of Silver Amalgam, silver-impregnated glass ionomer, or Resin restorative materials, and is used to reconstruct and replace lost tooth structure. Custom-fabricated Gold Retention Post and core is another approach that is used to restore endodontically treated teeth that require a full cast dental Crown.

To indicate the stainless steel Retention Post on tooth #9 on an anatomic chart, locate the tooth notation number. On both the Facial and Lingual surface views, use a blue pencil to draw a small rectangle that begins at the CEJ and extends down to the middle portion of the root. To indicate that the Retention Post is made from stainless steel, completely fill in the rectangular areas (see Figure 16–5). To indicate a Gold Retention Post, completely fill in the rectangular area with diagonal lines, and to show a Non-precious metal Retention Post, cross-hatch the entire area.

Charting a Periapical Radiolucency, Fistula, Root Canal Filling, Apicoectomy, Silver Amalgam Retrofilling, and Retention Post on a Geometric Chart

To show the periapical radiolucency and Root Canal filling seen on tooth #3 in Figure 16–1A and B on a geometric chart, locate the tooth designation number and on the Buccal surface view around the involved root apex use a red pencil to outline the area (Figure 16–6).

To chart a periapical lesion with a fistula on a geometric chart, the same procedure that was previously described using an anatomic chart is followed, and is shown charted on tooth #4 in Figure 16–6.

18	17	16	15	14	13	12	11	21	22	23	24	25	26	27	28
8	7	6	5	4	3	2	1	1	2	3	4	5	6	7	8
1	2	3	4	5	6	7	8	9	10	11	12	13	14	15	16

32	31	30	29	28	27	26	25	24	23	22	21	20	19	18	17
8	7	6	5	4	3	2	1	1	2	3	4	5	6	7	8
48	47	46	45	44	43	42	41	31	32	33	34	35	36	37	38
-A		-A												Z FX	

Figure 16-6 Geometric chart shown with a periapical radiolucency and Root Canal filling on tooth #3; tooth #4 is shown charted with a periapical radiolucency and fistula; teeth #9 and #10 are each shown with a Root Canal filling, an Apicoectomy, and a Silver Amalgam Retrofilling; tooth #9 is also shown with a stainless steel Retention Post; tooth #18 has a Temporary Restoration with an Occlusal surface Fracture; tooth #30 has been hemisected and the Distal Crown and root remains; tooth #32 indicates the Distal root has been amputated

To show the Root Canal filling on tooth #3, the Root Canal filling, Apicoectomy, and the Silver Amalgam Retrofilling on teeth #9 and #10, and stainless steel Retention Post on tooth #9 on a geometric chart, follow the procedures previously referred to for charting these conditions on an anatomic chart.

Charting a Periapical Radiolucency, Fistula, Root Canal Filling, Apicoectomy, Silver Amalgam Retrofilling, and Retention Post on a Numeric Coding System Chart

To indicate the periapical radiolucency located on tooth #3 in Figure 16–1A on a numeric coding system chart, use a black pen to enter the date, 5-9-93. In the column adjacent to the date in the box located above the tooth notation number, use a red pencil to draw a circle and inside the circle print a hyphen (-) followed by the secondary code "A" for Anomaly (-A). In addition to this entry, the examiner may also prefer to enter a more detailed description of the periapical radiolucency in the progress notes (Figure 16–7).

In Figure 16–1B, tooth #3 is shown with a Root Canal filling and Porcelain-covered Non-precious metal Crown. To indicate this on a numeric coding system chart, use a black pen and enter the date in the appropriate column.

6-25-94				-A					-S	-S						
5-21-93			C-NHR						L-ER •P	L-ER						
5-9-93			-A						ML-E DL-E							
MAXILLA	1	2	3	4 A	5 B	6 C	7 D	8 E	9 F	10 G	11 H	12 I	13 J	14	15	16
MANDIBLE	32	31	30	T 29	S 28	R 27	Q 26	P 25	O 24	N 23	M 22	L 21	K 20	19	18	17
5-9-93															O-E O-FX	
5-21-93															O-Z	
6-25-94	-A		-A													

Figure 16-7 Numeric coding system chart shown with a periapical radiolucency and Root Canal filling on tooth #3; tooth #4 is shown charted with a periapical radiolucency and fistula; teeth #9 and #10 are each shown with a Root Canal filling, an Apicoectomy, and a Silver Amalgam Retrofilling; tooth #9 is also shown with a stainless steel Retention Post; tooth #18 has a Temporary Restoration with an Occlusal surface Fracture; tooth #30 has been hemisected and the Distal Crown and root remain; tooth #32 indicates the Distal root has been amputated

Locate the box above the tooth designation number and enter the primary code "C" followed by the secondary codes "NHR" (C-NHR).

This chart is read as: on 5-9-93 a periapical radiolucency was detected on tooth #3. On 5-21-93 tooth #3 received a Root Canal filling and Porcelain-covered Non-precious metal Crown (see Figure 16–7).

The presence of a red circle with the secondary code "-A" inside is always representative of an Anomaly, specifically, a periapical lesion. A red circle with a red line that extends from it and terminates in a dot with the secondary code "-A" inside is always indicative of an Anomaly, specifically, a fistula. In Figure 16–7, the chart indicates that on 6-25-94 a periapical radiolucency with a fistula was detected on tooth #4.

To indicate the endodontic treatment on teeth #9 and #10 on the numeric coding system chart, use a black pen to enter the date then in the box located above the tooth notation numbers, enter the primary code "L" followed by the secondary codes "ER" (L-ER). On tooth #10 follow the secondary codes with a "•," a superscript dot "•," and a lowercase "p" to indicate a Retention Post (L-ER••p).

To show that teeth #9 and #10 each have an Apicoectomy with a Silver Amalgam Retrofilling" enter the date in the appropriate column. In the boxes located above the tooth numbers, draw a triangle "△" to represent the Apicoectomy and inside the triangle, print a hyphen followed by the secondary code "S" (-S) to indicate the Silver Amalgam Retrofilling (△-S) (see Figure 16–7).

The chart is read as: on 5-9-93 tooth #9 was restored with a Mesio-Lingual Resin and also a Disto-Lingual Resin. On 5-21-93 tooth #9 received a Root Canal filling and Lingual Resin restoration with a Retention Post, and tooth #10 was also treated endodontically and received a Lingual Resin restoration. On 6-25-94 teeth #9 and #10 each had an Apicoectomy with Silver Amalgam Retrofillings (see Figure 16–7).

Temporary Restorations

When the prognosis of a tooth is questionable, an intermediate or **Temporary Restoration** that contains eugenol will help to sedate the tooth and further protect it from mechanical and thermal injury. The formulation of zinc oxide and eugenol, an obtundent, as a temporary restorative material will reduce irritability and deaden sensibility of the dental pulp.

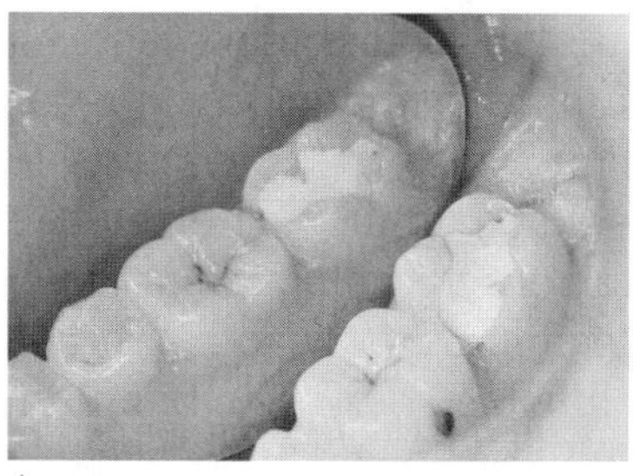

A.

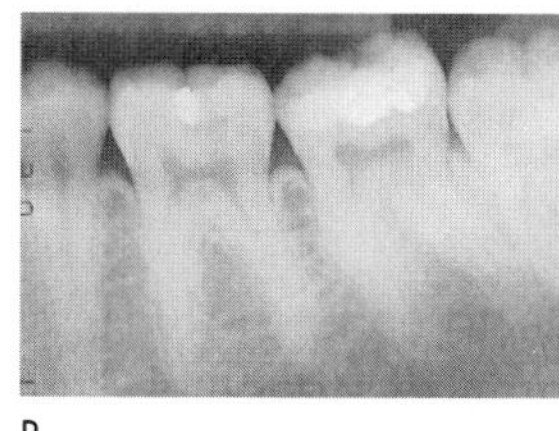

B.

Universal System
#20 #19 #18 #17

Palmer System
┌5 ┌6 ┌7 ┌8

ISO/FDI System
35 36 37 38

Figure 16-8 (A) Photograph of tooth #18 shown with a Temporary Restoration on the Occlusal surface and an Occlusal surface Fracture (B) Periapical radiograph shown of tooth #18 in which the Temporary Restoration appears as a radiopaque image

In Figure 16–8A, tooth #18 is shown with a Temporary Restoration adjoined to the original remaining Resin restoration that shows an Occlusal surface Fracture and marginal breakdown. The periapical radiograph of this area in Figure 16–8B shows the Temporary Restoration appear as a radiopaque image, and the region of the radiograph where the Resin restoration is also appears radiopaque, with the same degree of white. Therefore, it is difficult to distinguish the two types of restorations from a radiograph alone.

Charting a Temporary Restoration on an Anatomic Chart

To indicate the Temporary Restoration on tooth #18 in Figure 16–8A and B on an anatomic chart, locate the tooth designation number. Use a blue pencil to outline the restoration on only the Occlusal surface view as it appears clinically. In the box located above or below the tooth number, use a blue pencil and print the secondary code "Z" to indicate Temporary Restoration. To indicate the Fractured Occlusal surface, with a red pencil place a zigzag line over the involved area and print "FX" in the designated box (as described in Chapter 22). The Temporary Restoration and Fractured restoration on tooth #18 are shown charted on the anatomic chart in Figure 16–5.

Charting a Temporary Restoration on a Geometric Chart

To chart the Temporary Restoration and Fractured restoration on a geometric chart, follow the same procedures previously described when using an anatomic chart (see Figure 16–6).

Charting a Temporary Restoration on a Numeric Coding System Chart

To indicate a Temporary Restoration on a numeric coding system chart, use a black pen to enter the date. Locate the tooth notation number and beneath it in the designated box, use a blue pencil to print the primary code "O" of the tooth surface involved and a hyphen (-) followed by the secondary code "Z" (O-Z). To indicate the Fractured restoration, use a red pencil and print the primary code "O" followed by the uppercase letters "FX" (O-FX) (as described in Chapter 22).

In Figure 16–7 the chart is read as: on 5-9-93 there was an Occlusal Resin restoration with a Fracture on the Occlusal surface. On 5-21-93 a Temporary Restoration was placed on the Occlusal tooth surface.

Charting a Root Amputation and a Hemisection on an Anatomic Chart

To show a root amputation on an anatomic chart, locate the tooth number and use a blue pencil to place the symbol "x" over the resected root. Begin the lines at the furcation and end them at the root apex on both the Facial and Lingual surface views. In the designated box, print a hyphen followed by the secondary code "A" (-A) for Anomaly. Then in the progress notes describe which root was amputated. Figure 16–5 is shown with a Distal root amputation on tooth #32.

To show a tooth with a hemisection on an anatomic chart, follow the procedure for a root amputation except place the symbol "x" over the Missing half of the tooth and cover all three tooth surface views. Print the secondary code "-A" in the designated box and in the progress notes describe the side of the tooth that was removed. In Figure 16–5, tooth #30 is shown with the Mesial side of the tooth removed.

Charting a Root Amputation and a Hemisection on a Geometric Chart

To show a root amputation on a geometric chart, follow the procedures previously described when charting on the anatomic chart except when indicating a Mesial or Distal amputation on a maxillary molar only the Facial view is used. Tooth #32 is shown in Figure 16–6 with a Distal root amputation.

To show a hemisection on a geometric chart, follow the procedures previously mentioned when charting on an anatomic chart (see Figure 16–6).

Charting a Root Amputation and a Hemisection on a Numeric Coding System Chart

To indicate a root amputation on a numeric coding system chart, use a black pen to enter the date. In the designated box beneath the tooth notation number, use a blue pencil to print a hyphen followed by the secondary code "A" (-A). In the progress notes, describe which root was amputated (see Figure 16–7). The chart indicates that teeth #30 and #32 each have an Anomaly. The progress notes indicate that on 6-25-94, tooth #30 had a hemisection with the Mesial portion of the tooth removed and tooth #32 had the Distal root amputated.

Review Questions

Multiple Choice

Directions: Select the letter of the choice that *best* answers the question.

1. This symbol "△" drawn in blue represents:
   a. a hemisection. b. a root amputation.
   c. an Apicoectomy. d. all of the above.

2. The term that refers to inflammation of the pulp is
   a. pulpectomy. b. fistula.
   c. pulpotomy. d. pulpitis.
3. Severe pain and sensitivity to touch are the symptoms of:
   a. acute apical abscess. b. acute apical periodontitis.
   c. chronic apical abscess. d. chronic apical periodontitis.
4. The disorder that is generally symptom-free is:
   a. acute apical abscess. b. acute apical periodontitis.
   c. chronic apical abscess. d. chronic apical periodontitis.
5. The material used for a Root Canal filling is:
   a. Retrofilling. b. gutta-percha.
   c. Retention Core. d. none of the above.
6. Which of the following appears as a radiopaque image on a radiograph?
   a. Temporary Restoration b. Gutta-percha
   c. Retention Post d. All of the above
7. The procedure that is generally performed following an Apicoectomy is:
   a. Retrofilling. b. endodontics.
   c. root amputation. d. Temporary Restoration.
8. Drawn as a red circle with a line extended from it is a/an:
   a. fistula. b. acute apical abscess.
   c. root amputation. d. acute apical periodontitis.
9. Which of the following appears as a radiolucent area on a dental radiograph?
   a. Retrofilling b. Gutta-percha
   c. Acute apical abscess d. All of the above
10. A blue "X" placed over an entire root indicates a/an:
   a. hemisection. b. root amputation.
   c. Apicoectomy. d. Root Canal.

Answers

1. **c,** 2. **d,** 3. **b,** 4. **c,** 5. **b,** 6. **d,** 7. **a,** 8. **a,** 9. **c,** 10. **b**

References

Besner, E., & Michanowicz, A. E. (1994). *Practical endodontics: A clinical atlas*. St. Louis: Mosby.

Dorland's pocket medical dictionary (28th ed.). (1994). Philadelphia: W. B. Saunders Company.

Finkbeiner, B. L., & Johnson, C. S. (1995). *Mosby's comprehensive dental assisting: A clinical approach*. St. Louis: Mosby.

Thomas, C. L. (1997). *Taber's cyclopedic medical dictionary*. Philadelphia: F. A. Davis Company.

CHAPTER 17

Mechanical, Chemical, and Idiopathic Causes of the Loss and Discoloration of Tooth Structure

Key Terms

- Abrasion
- Attrition
- Demineralization
- Endogenous
- Erosion
- Exogenous
- Extrinsic Stain
- Fluorosis
- Hypocalcification
- Intrinsic Stain

ABBREVIATIONS AND CHARTING SYMBOLS

"abr" = abrasion, lowercase "x" in blue
"att" = attrition, horizontal line "—" in blue
"demin" = demineralization, back slash lines "\\\\" in blue
"ero" = erosion, single bracket "⌣" in blue

Introduction

The loss of tooth structure can occur as a result of wear from normal tooth-to-tooth contact, exposure to chemical agents, improperly utilized oral hygiene devices, and dental caries. The use of fluorides strengthens the enamel tooth structure and aids in the prevention of dental caries. However, when excessive quantities of fluoride are ingested and absorbed during tooth development and mineralization it can result in **fluorosis** (Plate 30). This causes deficient calcification of the enamel tooth structure referred to as **hypocalcification**. The affected teeth are marked with mottled enamel that can vary in appearance from small white spots to extensive brown regions. The white spots are the areas that appear on the enamel tooth structure in contrast to the remaining tooth surface, and can occur as the result of either an area of fluorosis or an area of **demineralization** (decalcification). Demineralized areas are formed as a result of acid byproducts released by dental plaque that break down the enamel and cause a loss of minerals in the subsurface structure (Figure 17–1 and Plate 27).

Attrition is the wearing away of tooth structure as a result of mastication. It occurs on the Incisal edges of anterior teeth and the Occlusal surfaces of posterior teeth. A wear facet is a worn and flattened area on a tooth surface that occurs as a result of attrition, bruxism, or malocclusion (Figure 17–2 and Plate 28).

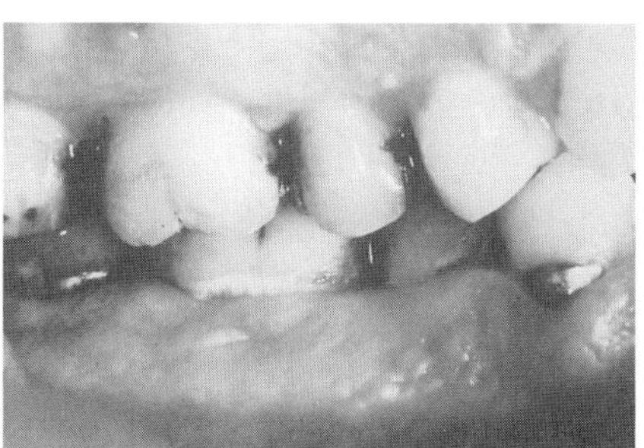

Universal System
#2 #3 #4 #5 #6
#31 #30 #29 #28

Palmer System
7| 6| 5| 4| 3|
7| 6| 5| 4|

ISO/FDI System
17 16 15 14 13
47 46 45 44

Figure 17–1 Demineralization shown on the cervical third of tooth #30

Universal System
#3 #4 #5 #6 #7 #8 #12 #13
#31 #30 #29 #28 #27 #26 #25 #24 #23 #22 #21 #20 #19

Palmer System
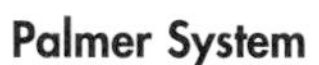
6| 5| 4| 3| 2| 1| |4 |5
7| 6| 5| 4| 3| 2| 1| |1 |2 |3 |4 |5 |6

ISO/FDI System
16 15 14 13 12 11 24 25
47 46 45 44 43 42 41 31 32 33 34 35 36

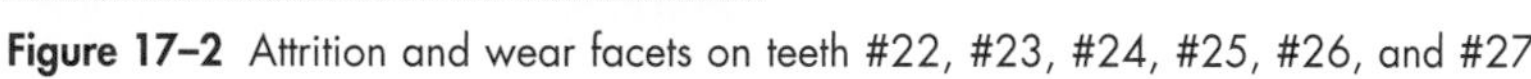

Figure 17–2 Attrition and wear facets on teeth #22, #23, #24, #25, #26, and #27

The mechanical wearing away of tooth structure other than that associated with mastication is called **abrasion**. The forceful strokes of a toothbrush accompanied by an abrasive dentifrice or inanimate objects place against the enamel tooth structure and exposed root surfaces can produce wear. The root surfaces on the maxillary anterior and posterior teeth and mandibular posterior teeth are shown with extensive abrasion in Plate 31.

The loss of tooth structure caused by a chemical process is referred to as **erosion**. When the acidic contents of the stomach are retained on the surface of the tongue because of recurrent episodes of regurgitation, they cause the chemical erosion of the smooth palatal surfaces of the teeth, which is seen in individuals with the eating disorder bulimia nervosa. The Facial surfaces of the anterior teeth are most often affected by frequent use of carbonated beverages and by sucking lemons and other citrus fruits (Figure 17–3 and Plate 29).

Dental stains or discolorations occur on the teeth in three ways: (1) they adhere directly to the acquired pellicle; (2) they are contained within mineralized (calculus) and nonmineralized (dental plaque, materia alba, and food debris) deposits; and (3) they are incorporated within the tooth structure. The etiology of tooth discoloration is due to chromogenic bacteria, exposure to environmental agents, organic substances, and inorganic elements.

Stains are classified according to location and source. The following are types of stains according to their location:

- **Extrinsic stain**. Occurs on the external tooth surface and may be removed by scaling, polishing, and toothbrushing procedures.
- **Intrinsic stain**. Incorporated within the tooth structure and cannot be removed by scaling, polishing, and toothbrushing procedures.

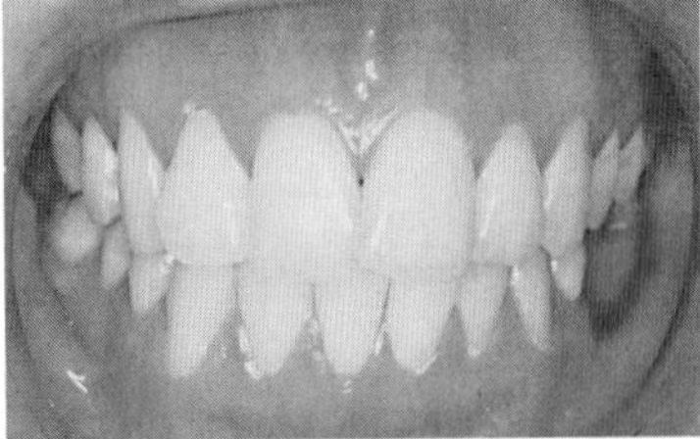

Universal System
#3 #4 #5 #6 #7 #8 #9 #10 #11 #12 #13
#30 #29 #28 #27 #26 #25 #24 #23 #22

Palmer System
6┘ 5┘ 4┘ 3┘ 2┘ 1┘ └1 └2 └3 └4 └5
6 5┐ 4┐ 3┐ 2┐ 1┐ ┌1 ┌2 ┌3

ISO/FDI System
16 15 14 13 12 11 21 22 23 24 25
46 45 44 43 42 41 31 32 33

Figure 17–3 Erosion on teeth #23, #24, #25, and #26

Stains are also classified according to their source and include the following:

- **Exogenous**. Originates outside the tooth from exposure to environmental agents.
  - Exogenous extrinsic. Originates from the outside and remains on the external tooth surface.

    Green stain. Discoloration of bacterial plaque
    Yellow stain. Discoloration of bacterial plaque
    Orange stain. Chromogenic bacteria discolor dental plaque
    Black line stain. Inorganic elements embedded in bacterial plaque
    Gray/green stain. Marijuana resin and pigments
    Tobacco stain. Tobacco tars and pigments
    Brown stain. Chlorhexidine antimicrobial agent
  - Exogenous intrinsic. Originates from the outside and is incorporated within the tooth surface.

    Gray-black stain. Silver Amalgam and copper amalgam, silver nitrate, and iodine
    Brown-black stain. Tin sulfide formation from stannous fluoride and ammoniacal silver nitrate
- **Endogenous**. Originates within the tooth from systemic disturbances
  - Endogenous intrinsic. Originates from inside and is incorporated within the tooth surface.

    Yellow-brown to gray stain. Tetracycline antibiotics (Plate 32), pulpless teeth, and developmental defects

Charting Abrasion, Attrition, Erosion, and Demineralization on an Anatomic Chart

To indicate the regions of abrasion on the maxillary and mandibular teeth shown in Plate 31 on an anatomic chart, locate the tooth designation numbers of the involved teeth. On the tooth diagrams in the areas on the root surfaces where the abrasion appears, use a blue pencil and place a lowercase "x." In the designated box located above or beneath the tooth diagram, print the lowercase letters "abr." In Figure 17–4, teeth #3, #4, #5, #6, #7, #8, #9, #10, #11, #12, #13, #14, #28, #29, and #30 are shown charted with abrasion on the Facial root surfaces.

Figure 17–4 Anatomic chart shown with abrasion charted on teeth #3, #4, #5, #6, #7, #8, #9, #10, #11, #12, #13, #14, #28, #29, and #30; attrition involving teeth #22, #23, #24, #25, #26, and #27; erosion on teeth #23, #24, #25, and #26; and demineralization on tooth #30

		abr	abr	abr	abr	abr	abr	abr	abr	abr	abr	abr	abr		
18	17	16	15	14	13	12	11	21	22	23	24	25	26	27	28
8	7	6	5	4	3	2	1	1	2	3	4	5	6	7	8
1	2	3	4	5	6	7	8	9	10	11	12	13	14	15	16

ero

32	31	30	29	28	27	26	25	24	23	22	21	20	19	18	17
8	7	6	5	4	3	2	1	1	2	3	4	5	6	7	8
48	47	46	45	44	43	42	41	31	32	33	34	35	36	37	38
		demin abr	abr	abr	att	att	att	att	att	att					

To indicate the areas with attrition shown in Figure 17–2 and Plate 28 on an anatomic chart, locate the tooth notation numbers of the involved teeth and on the Facial surface diagrams use a blue pencil to draw a continuous horizontal line through the Incisal third of each tooth "—." Locate the designated box below each tooth number and print the lowercase letters "att." The chart in Figure 17–4 indicates that teeth #22, #23, #24, #25, #26, and #27 have attrition.

To indicate the erosion shown on the Labial surfaces of teeth #23, #24, #25, and #26 shown in Figure 17–3 and Plate 29 on an anatomic chart, locate the tooth designation numbers. On the Labial surface view below the diagrams of the roots, use a blue pencil to draw a bracket "⏟," placed horizontally, that will encompass the involved teeth. At the tip of the bracket, print the lowercase letters "ero." The chart in Figure 17–4 shows erosion on the Labial surfaces of the mandibular central and lateral incisors.

To show the demineralization located on the cervical third of tooth #30 shown in Figure 17–1 and Plate 27 on an anatomic chart, locate the tooth designation number and use a blue pencil to draw short diagonal lines in the involved area and label it "demin" (see Figure 17–4).

Charting Abrasion, Attrition, Erosion, and Demineralization on a Geometric Chart

To indicate the teeth with abrasion shown in Plate 31 on a geometric chart, follow the procedure previously mentioned for charting abrasion on an anatomic chart. The geometric chart in Figure 17–5 shows abrasion charted on the Facial root surfaces of teeth #3, #4, #5, #6, #7, #8, #9, #10, #11, #12, #13, #14, #28, #29, and #30.

To show the areas of attrition shown in Figure 17–2 and Plate 28 on a geometric chart, follow the procedure previously mentioned. The horizontal line is drawn through the circle that represents the Incisal or Occlusal surface located in the center of each diagram. The chart shown in Figure 17–5 indicates teeth #22, #23, #24, #25, #26, and #27 have attrition.

To show the erosion present on teeth #23, #24, #25, and #26 shown in Figure 17–3 and Plate 29 on a geometric chart, follow the previously mentioned procedure for charting erosion on an anatomic chart. Figure 17–5 indicates erosion on the Labial tooth surfaces of the mandibular central and lateral incisors.

To indicate the demineralized area on tooth #30 shown in Figure 17–1 and Plate 27 on a geometric chart, follow the procedures previously mentioned. In addition, completely fill in each tooth surface section with diagonal lines that extend from the top to the bottom of each box (see Figure 17–5).

		abr	abr	abr	abr	abr	abr	abr	abr	abr	abr	abr	abr		
18	17	16	15	14	13	12	11	21	22	23	24	25	26	27	28
8	7	6	5	4	3	2	1	1	2	3	4	5	6	7	8
1	2	3	4	5	6	7	8	9	10	11	12	13	14	15	16

ero

32	31	30	29	28	27	26	25	24	23	22	21	20	19	18	17
8	7	6	5	4	3	2	1	1	2	3	4	5	6	7	8
48	47	46	45	44	43	42	41	31	32	33	34	35	36	37	38
		demin abr	abr	abr	att	att	att	att	att	att					

Figure 17–5 Geometric chart shown with abrasion charted on teeth #3, #4, #5, #6, #7, #8, #9, #10, #11, #12, #13, #14, #28, #29, and #30; attrition involving teeth #22, #23, #24, #25, #26, and #27; erosion on teeth #23, #24, #25, and #26; demineralization on tooth #30

Charting Abrasion, Attrition, Erosion, and Demineralization on a Numeric Coding System Chart

To indicate abrasion, attrition, erosion, and demineralization on a numeric coding system chart, enter the date with black ink in the designated area. Locate the tooth notation numbers of the involved teeth, and in the box located above or below them use a blue pencil to print the appropriate abbreviation. The numeric coding system chart in Figure 17–6 is read as: on 3-10-94 abrasion is present on teeth #3, #4, #5, #6, #7, #8, #9, #10, #11, #12, #13, #14, #28, #29, and #30. On 5-1-95 the chart indicates attrition involving teeth #22, #23, #24, #25, #26, and #27 and erosion is present on teeth #23, #24, #25, and #26. During the 1-23-96 appointment, demineralization was detected on tooth #30.

Charting Extrinsic and Intrinsic Stains

To indicate extrinsic or intrinsic stains on an anatomic chart, geometric chart, numeric coding system chart, or periodontal examination record, locate the designated area marked "Stain" at the bottom of each chart. Use a blue pencil and place a check in the box that most accurately describes the type and amount of stain present. Additional comments that pertain may be written in the examination progress notes.

1-23-96																
5-1-95																
3-10-94			abr	abr	abr	abr	abr	abr	abr	abr	abr	abr	abr	abr		
MAXILLA	1	2	3	4 A	5 B	6 C	7 D	8 E	9 F	10 G	11 H	12 I	13 J	14	15	16
MANDIBLE	32	31	30	T 29	S 28	R 27	Q 26	P 25	O 24	N 23	M 22	L 21	K 20	19	18	17
3-10-94			abr	abr	abr											
5-1-95						att	ero att	ero att	ero att	ero att	att					
1-23-96			demin													

Figure 17–6 Numeric coding system chart shown with abrasion charted on teeth #3, #4, #5, #6, #7, #8, #9, #10, #11, #12, #13, #14, #28, #29, and #30; attrition involving teeth #22, #23, #24, #25, #26, and #27; erosion on teeth #23, #24, #25, and #26; and demineralization on tooth #30

Review Questions

Matching

Directions: Place the uppercase letter(s) after the number to match each term with the statement that *best* defines it.

A Abrasion
B Attrition
C Demineralization
D Endogenous
E Erosion
F Exogenous
G Extrinsic stain
H Fluorosis
I Hypocalcification
J Intrinsic stain

1. ____ Incorporated into the tooth
2. ____ Often seen in individuals with bulimia nervosa
3. ____ White spots may form in the enamel tooth structure
4. ____ A deficient calcification of the enamel tooth structure
5. ____ Caused by forceful toothbrushing
6. ____ Caused by a loss of minerals
7. ____ Originates outside the mouth from environmental agents
8. ____ Produced by tooth-to-tooth contact
9. ____ Removed with toothbrushing
10. ____ Originates within the tooth from systemic disturbances

Answers

1. **J,** 2. **E,** 3. **H,** 4. **I,** 5. **A,** 6. **C,** 7. **F,** 8. **B,** 9. **G,** 10. **D**

References

Bevenius, J., L'Estrange, P., & Angmar-Mansson, B. (1988). Erosion: Guidelines for the general practitioner. *Australian Dental Journal*, 33, 407.

Cutress, T. W., & Suckling, G. W. (1990). Differential diagnosis of dental fluorosis. *Journal of Dental Research*, 69, 714.

Den Besten, P. K., & Thariani, H. (1992). Biological mechanisms of fluorosis and level and timing of systemic exposure to fluoride with respect to fluorosis. *Journal of Dental Research*, 71, 1238.

Dorland's pocket medical dictionary (28th ed.). (1994). Philadelphia: W. B. Saunders Company.

Fejerskov, O., Manji, F., & Baelum, V. (1990). The nature and mechanisms of dental fluorosis in man. *Journal of Dental Research*, 69, 692.

Haring, J. I., & Ibsen, O. A. C. (1992). *Oral pathology for the dental hygienist* (pp. 267–269). Philadelphia: W. B. Saunders Company.

Harrison, J. L., & Roeder, L. B. (1991). Dental erosion caused by cola beverages. *General Dentistry*, 39, 23.

Ishii, T., & Suckling, G. (1991). The severity of dental fluorosis in children exposed to water with a high fluoride content for various periods of time. *Journal of Dental Research*, 70, 952.

Jarvinen, V. K., Rytomaa, I. I., & Heinonen, O. P. (1991). Risk factors in dental erosion. *Journal of Dental Research*, 70, 942.

Krutchkoff, D. J., Eisenberg, E., O'Brien, J. E., and Ponzillo J. J. (1990). Cocaine-induced dental erosions (Correspondence). *New England Journal of Medicine*, 322, 408.

Rytomaa, I., Meurman, J. H., Koskinen, J., Laakso, T., Gharazi, L., & Turunen, R. (1988). In vitro erosion of bovine enamel caused by acidic drinks and other foodstuffs. *Scandinavian Journal of Dental Research*, 96, 324–333.

Thomas, C. L. (1997). *Taber's cyclopedic medical dictionary*. Philadelphia: F. A. Davis Company.

VanDette, J. M., & Cornish, L. A. (1989). Medical complications of illicit cocaine use. *Clinical Pharmacology*, 8, 401–411.

Villa, Vigil M. A., Arenal, A. A., and Gonzalez, M. A. R. (1989). Notation of numerical abnormalities by an addition to the F.D.I. System. *Quintessence International*, 20, 299–302.

CHAPTER 18

Malpositions of Individual Teeth

Key Terms

Buccoversion
Drift
Extrusion
Intrusion
Labioversion
Linguoversion
Malpositioned
Supraerupt
Tilt
Torsiversion

ABBREVIATIONS AND CHARTING SYMBOLS

buccoversion "BV" and labioversion "LaV" = "↑" from the center of the Occlusal or Incisal surface directed toward the Buccal or Labial surface in blue

linguoversion "LV" = "↓" from the center of the Occlusal or Incisal surface directed toward the Lingual surface in blue

drift (Mesial) = "→D" from the center of the Occlusal or Incisal surface directed toward the midline in blue

drift (Distal) = "D←" from the center of the Occlusal or Incisal surface directed away from the midline in blue

tilt (Mesial) = " ⇙crosses from the Distal over the Occlusal to the Mesial surface in blue

tilt (Distal) = "⇙" crosses from the Mesial over the Occlusal to the Distal surface in blue

torsiversion = "◯" centered on the Occlusal surface to indicate the clockwise rotation Buccal to Lingual in blue

ABBREVIATIONS AND CHARTING SYMBOLS

torsiversion = "↺" centered on the Occlusal surface to indicate the counter clockwise rotation Lingual to Buccal in blue
extrusion = "↓" directed toward the root tip on the Facial surface view in blue
intrusion = "↑" directed away from the root tip on the Facial surface view in blue
(IMP) = Impacted in blue
(U) = Unerupted in blue

Introduction

When a tooth erupts and there is a lack of adequate space, the tooth generally becomes **malpositioned**. When compared to the other teeth in the same arch that are in normal alignment, the improperly aligned tooth is identified according to the structure it is positioned toward. An anterior tooth positioned toward the lip, Labial to normal, is referred to as **labioversion** and a posterior tooth positioned toward the cheek, Buccal to normal, is called **buccoversion**. An anterior or posterior tooth positioned toward the tongue, Lingual to normal, is referred to as **linguoversion**, and any tooth that is rotated or turned is called **torsiversion**.

A tooth can also assume a position that is inferior or superior to normal position. As a result of disease or trauma, a tooth can become depressed in the alveolar bone and be positioned below the line of occlusion (**intrusion**), or it may **supraerupt** and extend above the line of occlusion (**extrusion**).

Charting Teeth in Labioversion and Buccoversion on an Anatomic Chart

Figure 18–1 is a photograph that shows teeth #22 and #27 in labioversion, which means the teeth are in a position Labial to normal. To chart these teeth on an anatomic chart, locate the ADA tooth designation numbers #22 and #27 then locate the diagram that represents the Incisal edge. With a blue pencil, draw an arrow from the center of the Incisal edge and extend it out toward the Labial view (Figure 18–2).

Universal System

#2 #3 #4 #5 #6 #7 #8 #9 #10 #11 #12 #13 #14 #15
#31 #30 #29 #28 #27 #26 #25 #24 #23 #22 #21 #20 #19 #18

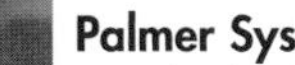

Palmer System

7| 6| 5| 4| 3| 2| 1| |1 |2 |3 |4 |5 |6 |7
7| 6| 5| 4| 3| 2| 1| |1 |2 |3 |4 |5 |6 |7

ISO/FDI System

17 16 15 14 13 12 11 21 22 23 24 25 26 27
47 46 45 44 43 42 41 31 32 33 34 35 36 37

Figure 18–1 Anterior photograph showing malpositioned teeth

Figure 18–2 Anatomic chart showing malpositions of individual teeth charted

Tooth #14 is a posterior tooth shown in buccoversion, which means the tooth is aligned in a position that is Buccal to normal (see Figure 18–1). A posterior tooth in buccoversion is charted the same way an anterior tooth is charted in Labioversion. The arrow is drawn so that it begins in the center of the Occlusal surface view and extends out toward the Buccal surface view (see Figure 18–2).

Charting Teeth in Labioversion and Buccoversion on a Geometric Chart

To chart teeth #22 and #27 in labioversion and #14 in buccoversion on a geometric chart, locate the tooth numbers and the areas that represent the Incisal edges and Occlusal surfaces. With a blue pencil begin at the center of these areas and draw an arrow out toward the edge of the outside circle, which indicates the Labial and Buccal surfaces (Figure 18–3).

Charting Teeth in Labioversion and Buccoversion on a Numeric Coding System Chart

To chart teeth #22 and #27 in labioversion and tooth #14 in buccoversion on a numeric coding system chart, begin by using a black pen and enter the date in the appropriate spaces above the words "Maxilla" and "Mandible." On the same line as the date below teeth #22 and #27, draw an arrow that extends from the top of the box to just before the bottom of the box with a blue pencil and label it with the letters "LaV" (labioversion). The arrow drawn in this direction indicates that the tooth is positioned toward the Labial surface. On

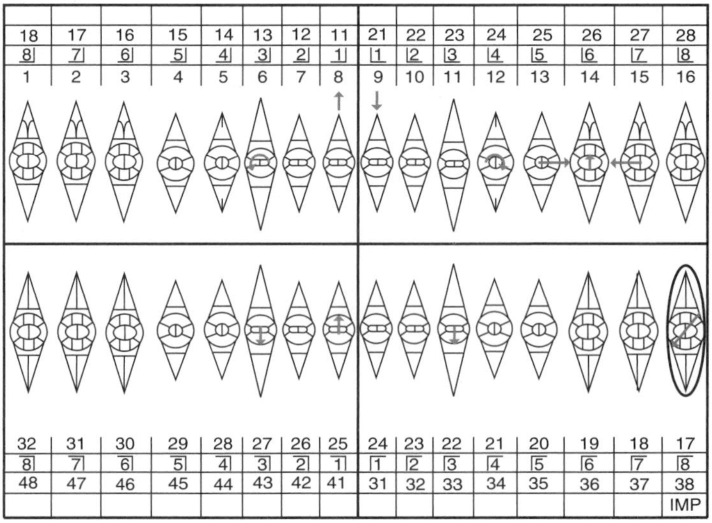

Figure 18–3 Geometric chart showing malpositions of individual teeth charted

4-23-98						↶ T		I ↑	↓ E			↷ T	→ D	BV ↑	D ←	
MAXILLA	1	2	3	4	5	6	7	8	9	10	11	12	13	14	15	16
				A	B	C	D	E	F	G	H	I	J			
				T	S	R	Q	P	O	N	M	L	K			
MANDIBLE	32	31	30	29	28	27	26	25	24	23	22	21	20	19	18	17
4-23-98						↓ LaV		LV ↑			↓ LaV					IMP

Figure 18–4 Numeric coding system chart showing malpositions of individual teeth charted

the same line above tooth #14, draw the arrow and label it with the uppercase letters "BV" (buccoversion) to indicate that the tooth is positioned toward the Buccal surface (Figure 18–4).

Charting a Tooth in Linguoversion on an Anatomic Chart

Figure 18–5 is shown with the mandibular anterior tooth #25 in linguoversion, which means the tooth is aligned in a position that is Lingual to normal. To indicate tooth #25 is in linguoversion on an anatomic chart, locate the tooth number and the diagram that represents the Incisal edge. With a blue pencil begin at the center of the diagram and draw an arrow that extends from the Incisal edge to the Lingual surface view (see Figure 18–2).

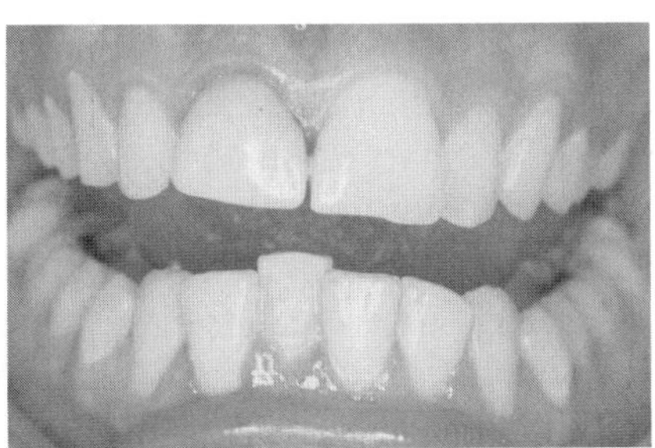

Universal System

#3 #4 #5 #6 #7 #8 #9 #10 #11 #12 #13 #14

#31 #30 #29 #28 #27 #26 #25 #24 #23 #22 #21 #20 #19 #18

Palmer System

6⌋ 5⌋ 4⌋ 3⌋ 2⌋ 1⌋ ⌊1 ⌊2 ⌊3 ⌊4 ⌊5 ⌊6

7⌉ 6⌉ 5⌉ 4⌉ 3⌉ 2⌉ 1⌉ ⌈1 ⌈2 ⌈3 ⌈4 ⌈5 ⌈6 ⌈7

ISO/FDI System

16 15 14 13 12 11 21 22 23 24 25 26

47 46 45 44 43 42 41 31 32 33 34 35 36 37

Figure 18–5 Anterior photograph shown with tooth #25 in linguoversion

Charting a Tooth in Linguoversion on a Geometric Chart

Figure 18–3 shows tooth #25 charted in linguoversion on a geometric chart. To chart tooth #25 locate the tooth number and the area that represents the Incisal edge. With a blue pencil begin at the center of this area and draw an arrow that extends out toward the edge of the outside circle, which indicates the Lingual tooth surface.

Charting a Tooth in Linguoversion on a Numeric Coding System Chart

To chart tooth #25 in linguoversion on a numeric coding system chart, begin by using a black pen and enter the date in the appropriate spaces above the words "Maxilla" and "Mandible." On the same line as the date below tooth #25, draw an arrow that extends from the bottom of the box to just before the top with a blue pencil and label it with uppercase letters "LV" (linguoversion). The placement of the arrow pointed in the proper direction is very important in addition to labeling labioversion and linguoversion (see Figure 18–4).

Charting a Tooth in Torsiversion on an Anatomic Chart

Shown in Figure 18–6, tooth #6 is rotated in a counterclockwise direction and Figure 18–7 shows tooth #12 rotated in a clockwise direction. Torsiversion is the term that applies to turned or rotated teeth. To chart teeth #6 and #12 in torsiversion on an anatomic chart, locate the tooth numbers on the diagram that represents the Incisal edge and Occlusal surface. With a blue pencil draw a curved arrow on both diagrams in the direction in which the teeth are rotated. Tooth #6 shows the arrow curved in a counterclockwise direction and tooth #12 is shown with the arrow directed in a clockwise direction (see Figure 18–2).

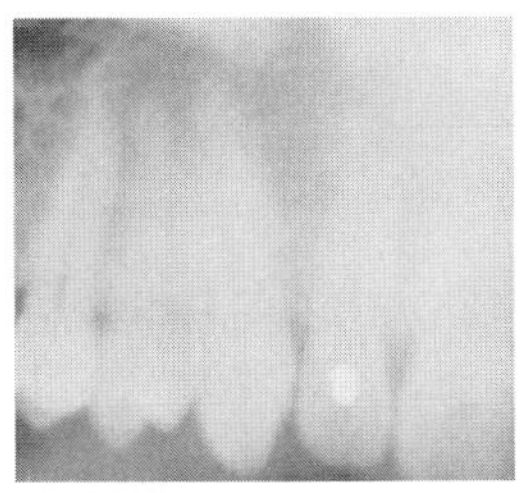

Universal System
#4 #5 #6 #7 #8

Palmer System
5┘ 4┘ 3┘ 2┘ 1┘

ISO/FDI System
15 14 13 12 11

Figure 18–6 Periapical radiograph showing torsiversion of tooth #6

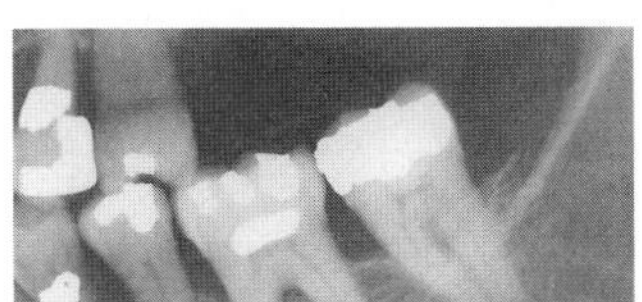

Universal System
H #12
#21 #20 #19 #18

Palmer System
└C └4
┌4 ┌5 ┌6 ┌7

ISO/FDI System
63 24
34 35 36 37

Figure 18–7 Bitewing radiograph showing torsiversion of tooth #12

Charting a Tooth in Torsiversion on a Geometric Chart

To chart teeth #6 and #12 in torsiversion on a geometric chart, locate the tooth notation numbers and depending on the direction each tooth is turned, either begin on the right or left side between the two circles and draw a curved arrow with a blue pencil. Tooth #6 shows the arrow beginning on the right side and it extends around beyond the left side to indicate a counterclockwise direction. Tooth #12 shows the arrow pointed in the opposite direction to indicate a clockwise rotation (see Figure 18–3).

Charting a Tooth in Torsiversion on a Numeric Coding System Chart

To chart teeth #6 and #12 in torsiversion on a numeric coding system chart, locate the tooth notation numbers adjacent to the date (see Figure 18–4). Use a blue pencil to draw the curved arrows in each of the boxes located above the tooth numbers. Depending on the direction the tooth is rotated, draw the arrow to extend either to the left, to indicate a counterclockwise rotation, or to the right, to show a clockwise rotation. Print an uppercase letter "T" at the tip of the arrow.

Charting Extrusion and Intrusion on an Anatomic Chart

Figure 18–8 is a periapical radiograph, which shows tooth #9 as extruded. The tooth has migrated past the line of occlusion in response to a traumatic injury. Because the Crown has been restored, the extrusion is not obvious at the line of occlusion but rather it is apparent from the area that surrounds the root apex. Tooth #9 is considerably lower than tooth #8 when the root apices are compared. The terms *supraversion*, *supraerupted*, and *extruded* are synonymous with the condition referred to as extrusion.

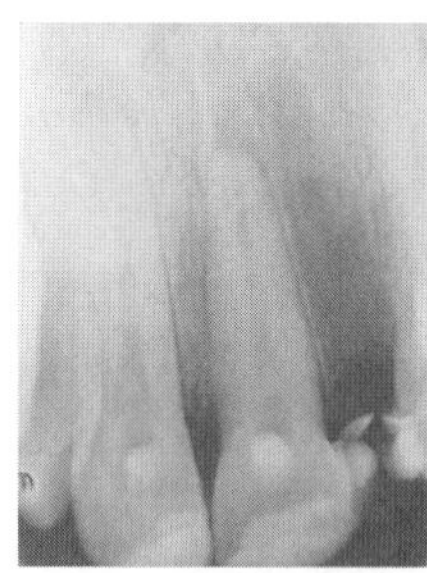

Universal System
#7 #8 #9 #11

Palmer System
2| 1| |1 |3

ISO/FDI System
12 11 21 23

Figure 18–8 Anterior periapical radiograph shown with tooth #9 extruded

To chart tooth #9 as extruded, locate the tooth designation number and above the Facial view of the tooth diagram draw an arrow with a blue pencil to extend and point toward the Root Tip (see Figure 18–2).

The apical migration of a tooth is referred to as intrusion (intruded or infraversion). Intrusion is the term that describes a tooth depressed below the line of occlusion; for example, a primary tooth that becomes ankylosed.

To chart intrusion of tooth #8 on an anatomic chart, draw an arrow to extend out and away from the root area on the Facial view of the chart as shown in Figure 18–2.

Charting Extrusion and Intrusion on a Geometric Chart

To show intrusion and extrusion charted on a geometric chart, with a blue pencil place an arrow facing either inward or outward from the root tip. Figure 18–3 shows tooth #9 charted as being extruded and tooth #8 as intruded.

Charting Extrusion and Intrusion on a Numeric Coding System Chart

To chart tooth #8 as intruded and tooth #9 as extruded on a numeric coding system chart, locate the tooth notation numbers adjacent to the date. Use a blue pencil to draw vertical arrows in each of the boxes located above the tooth numbers. Draw the point of the arrow so it is directed upward from the bottom of the box for intrusion and downward from the top of the box for extrusion and print an uppercase letter "I" or "E" at the tip of the arrow (see Figure 18–4).

Mesial and Distal Drift and Tilt

When teeth are lost, such as following an extraction of a tooth or the premature loss of a primary tooth, the surrounding teeth **drift** out of position. Figure 18–9 shows that tooth #14 is Missing and teeth #13 and #15 have drifted into the space. The migration of tooth #13 in a Distal direction is referred to as Distal drift and the movement of tooth #15 in a Mesial direction is called Mesial drift.

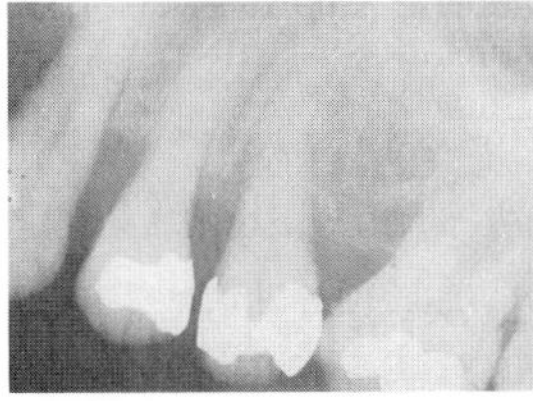

Universal System
#11 #12 #13 #15

Palmer System
⌊3 ⌊4 ⌊5 ⌊7

ISO/FDI System
23 24 25 27

Figure 18–9 Posterior periapical radiograph shown with Mesial drift of tooth #15 and Distal drift of tooth #13

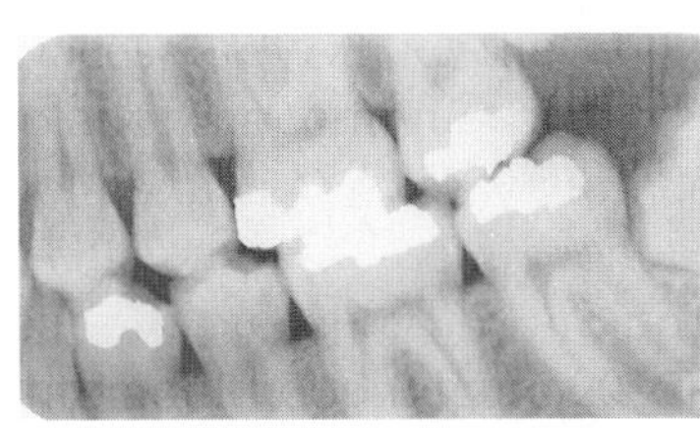

Universal System
#12 #13 #14 #15
#22 #21 #20 #19 #18 #17

Palmer System
⌊4 ⌊5 ⌊6 ⌊7
⌈3 ⌈4 ⌈5 ⌈6 ⌈7 ⌈8

ISO/FDI System
24 25 26 27
33 34 35 36 37 38

Figure 18–10 Bitewing radiograph showing Mesial tilt of Impacted tooth #17

The term **tilt** is used to indicate the direction of Unerupted or Impacted teeth. Figure 18–10 shows tooth #17 as Impacted in a Mesial direction. An Impacted tooth positioned in a Distal direction is called Distal tilt.

Figure 18–11 represents the malpositions of individual teeth due to the loss of a tooth.

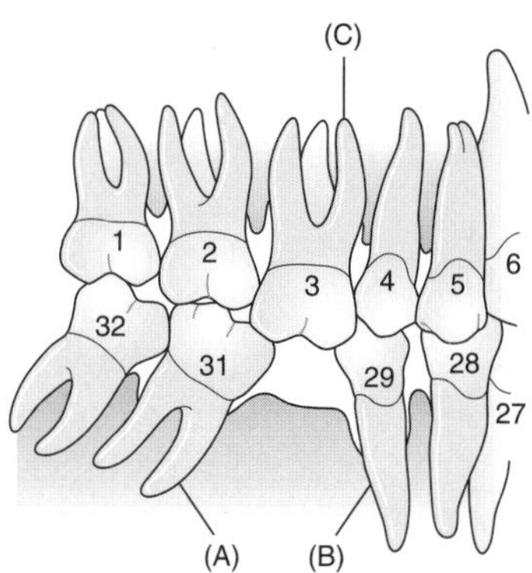

Figure 18–11 Malpositions of individual teeth: (A) Tooth #31, Mesial drift (B) Tooth #29, Distal drift (C) Tooth #3, extrusion

Charting the Drift and Tilt of a Tooth on an Anatomic Chart

To chart tooth #13 as Distal drift and tooth #15 as Mesial drift on an anatomic chart, find teeth #13 and #15 on the dental chart then locate the diagrams that represent the Occlusal surface views. With a blue pencil, draw an arrow from the center of the Occlusal surface on tooth #12 and extend it out toward the edge of the Distal surface view. On the Occlusal surface view of tooth #15, draw and extend the arrow out from the center to the edge of the Mesial surface (see Figure 18–2).

To chart tooth #17 as an Impacted third molar with Mesial tilt, locate tooth #17 and with a blue pencil circle the entire tooth diagram and label it "IMP." To indicate the direction of the tilt on the Facial surface view, draw a diagonal arrow that starts at the upper right side of the diagram and angles downward and points to the opposite side. An arrow that points to the Mesial tooth surface indicates Mesial tilt, and an arrow that points to the Distal tooth surface indicates Distal tilt. Figure 18–2 shows tooth #17 charted as Impacted with Mesial tilt.

Charting the Drift and Tilt of a Tooth on a Geometric Chart

To chart the Distal drift of tooth #13 and Mesial drift of tooth #15 on a geometric chart, locate the tooth numbers and the surface area views that represent the Occlusal surfaces. With a blue pencil begin at the center of the Occlusal surfaces and draw an arrow to extend out toward the edge of the outside circles, which represents the Distal and Mesial tooth surfaces (see Figure 18–3).

To chart tooth #17 as an Impacted third molar with Mesial tilt on a geometric chart, draw and label the Impacted tooth (#17) as it is done when using an anatomic chart. To indicate Mesial tilts, draw a diagonal arrow that begins at the upper right side of the diagram and ends at the lower left side. To illustrate Distal tilt, draw the arrow from the upper left side of the diagram and extend it diagonally to point at the lower right side. An arrow that is pointed toward the Mesial tooth surface indicates Mesial tilt and a diagonal arrow directed at the Distal tooth surface indicates Distal tilt (see Figure 18–3).

Charting the Drift and Tilt of a Tooth on a Numeric Coding System Chart

To chart tooth #13 as Distal drift and #15 as Mesial drift on a numeric coding system chart, locate the tooth notation numbers adjacent to the date. Use a blue pencil to draw horizontal arrows in each of the boxes located above the tooth numbers. Draw the point of the arrow so it is aimed toward the direction the tooth has drifted and label it with the uppercase letter "D" for drift (see Figure 18–4).

To indicate tooth #17 as an Impacted tooth with Mesial tilt on a numeric coding system chart, enter the date in the designated area and locate the tooth notation number. Draw a circle in the appropriate box below and place the uppercase letters "IMP" inside. Place a diagonal arrow over the top of the circle to the left to indicate Mesial tilt, and to the right to indicate Distal tilt (see Figure 18–4).

Review Questions

Matching

Directions: Place the uppercase letter(s) after the number to match each term with the statement that *best* defines it.

A Buccoversion	1. ____ Positioned toward the lips
B Distal drift	2. ____ Rotated or turned
C Distal tilt	3. ____ Above the line of occlusion
D Extrusion	4. ____ An Impacted tooth tipped toward the Mesial surface

E Intrusion
F Labioversion
G Linguoversion
H Mesial drift
I Mesial tilt
J Torsiversion

5. ____ Below the line of occlusion
6. ____ Migration of a tooth in a Distal direction
7. ____ Positioned toward the tongue
8. ____ An Unerupted tooth tipped toward the Distal surface
9. ____ Positioned toward the cheek
10. ____ Migration of a tooth in a Mesial direction

Answers

1. **F,** 2. **J,** 3. **D,** 4. **I,** 5. **E,** 6. **B,** 7. **G,** 8. **C,** 9. **A,** 10. **H**

References

Brand, R. W., & Isselhard, D. E. (1994). *Anatomy of orofacial structures*. St. Louis: Mosby Year-Book.

Dorland's pocket medical dictionary (24th ed.). (1989). Philadelphia: W. B. Saunders Company.

Schulte, W., d'Hoedt, B., Lukas, D., Maunz, M., & Steppeler, M. (1992). Periotest for measuring periodontal characteristics—correlation with periodontal bone loss. *Journal of Periodontal Research*, 24, 184–190.

Thomas, C. L. (1997). *Taber's cyclopedic medical dictionary*. Philadelphia: F. A. Davis Company.

Wang, H. L., Burgett, F. G., Shyr, Y., & Ramfjord, S. (1994). The influence of molar furcation involvement and mobility on furture clinical periodontal attachment loss. *Journal of Periodontology*, 65, 25–29.

Woelfel, J. B., & Scheid, R. C. (1997). *Dental anatomy: Its relevance to dentistry* (5th ed.). Baltimore: Williams & Wilkins.

CHAPTER 19

Dental Indices

Key Terms

Assessment
Dean's Classification of Fluorosis
Epidemiologic Indices
Indices
Irreversible
Ramjford Teeth
Reliability
Reproducibility
Reversible
Variability

Introduction

Although there are many **indices** for recording and quantitating dental disease, only the two major indices are included in this chapter. The first are the **reversible** indices. These measure conditions that can be reversed, for example, gingivitis. The second type of index is **irreversible**. These indices measure cumulative conditions that cannot be reversed. An example of this type of index would measure dental caries.

In the context of **epidemiologic indices**, the term **reliability** means the ability of a dental index to measure a condition in the same subject repeatedly, obtaining the same score results each time. The definition implies that reliability is a matter of degree because all measurements are subject to error (method and observer) or **variability**.

The most obvious implications of unreliable measures are that prevalence estimates become questionable when comparisons are made between groups. This means that measurements from longitudinal studies may no longer reveal the differences between treatment and control groups. Reliability is considered a more general term than **reproducibility** or repeatability, the latter of which is usually restricted to repeat examination data.

There are two classifications of dental indices. They are reversible and irreversible. A reversible index is one that can change, for example, the Plaque

Free Score. The individual being scored can change the score by improving his or her plaque removal. In contrast is the **Dean's Classification of Fluorosis**. Once a tooth has been overexposed to high levels of fluoride, the tooth will always have fluorosis.

The use of indices in dentistry is important for assessing individual patients and populations. An index helps the dental professional with the **assessment**, planning, and implementation of either individual dental care or dental programs for large groups of people.

Indices Used to Measure Plaque Accumulation

Most plaque indices used to measure plaque accumulation utilize a numerical scale to measure the extent of the surface area of a tooth covered by plaque. For these purposes, plaque is defined as a soft, nonmineralized tooth deposit, which includes debris and materia alba.

Simplified Oral Hygiene Index (OHI-S)

The Simplified Oral Hygiene Index is a reversible index that measures oral hygiene status. As outlined in Table 19–1, the OHI-S measures the surface area of the tooth that is covered by debris and calculus. The imprecise term *debris* was used because it was not practical to distinguish among plaque, debris, and materia alba. In addition, the practicality of determining the weight and thickness of the soft deposits prompted the assumption that the dirtier the mouth is, the greater the tooth surface area covered by debris. This also implied a time factor because the longer oral hygiene practices are neglected, the greater the likelihood the surface area of the tooth will be covered by debris. The OHI-S consists of two components: a Simplified Debris Index (DI-S) and a Simplified Calculus Index (CI-S). Each component is assessed on a scale of 0 to 3.

The importance of the OHI-S is that, like the Periodontal Index (PI), it has been used extensively throughout the world and has contributed greatly to the understanding of periodontal disease. The high degree of correlation between the OHI-S and the PI makes it possible, if one of the two scores is known, to calculate the other score. The major strength of the OHI-S is its use in epidemiologic surveys and in evaluation of dental health education programs and longitudinal studies.

Table 19-1: Simplified Oral Hygiene Index

INSTRUMENTS AND EQUIPMENT:
Mouth mirror, adequate light, periodontal probe or explorer

PROCEDURE:

- Select the tooth with the most debris in each sextant.

DI-S:

- Run the side of the tip of a probe or explorer across the surface of the tooth to estimate the surface area covered by debris.

CI-S:

- Use the explorer to estimate the surface area of the tooth covered by supragingival calculus.
- Identify subgingival deposits by exploring or probing.
- Record on definite deposits of hard calculus.

CRITERIA:

DI-S:

0 = No debris or stain present
1 = Soft debris covering not more than one third of the tooth surface being examined, or the presence of extrinsic stains without debris, regardless of surface area covered
2 = Soft debris covering more than one third but not more than two thirds of the exposed tooth surface
3 = Soft debris covering more than two thirds of the exposed tooth surface

CI-S:

0 = No calculus present
1 = Supragingival calculus covering not more than one third of the tooth of the exposed surface
2 = Supragingival calculus covering more than one third but not more than two thirds of the exposed tooth surface, or the presence of individual flecks of subgingival calculus around the cervical portion of the tooth
3 = Supragingival calculus covering more than two thirds of the exposed tooth surface or a continuous heavy band of subgingival calculus around the cervical portion of the tooth, or both

SCORING:

DI-S *and* CI-S:

Divide the total scores by the number of sextants. Scores will range from 0 to 3.

Excellent	0
Good	0.1–0.6
Fair	0.7–1.8
Poor	1.9–3.0

OHI-S:

Combine the DI-S and the CI-S scores. OHI-S score will range from 0 to 6.

Excellent	0
Good	0.1–1.2
Fair	1.3–3.0
Poor	3.1–6.0

Turesky-Gilmore-Glickman Modification of the Quigley-Hein Plaque Index

Quigley and Hein reported a plaque measurement that focused on the gingival third of the tooth. Only Facial surfaces of the anterior teeth were examined, using a basic disclosing agent and a numerical scoring system of 0 to 5. The modification was designed to increase the objectivity of the Quigley-Hein index by redefining the scores of the gingival third area. Plaque is assessed on the Facial and Lingual surfaces of all of the teeth after disclosing. See Table 19–2 for a complete breakdown of the criteria used for this index. The strength of this plaque index is its application to longitudinal studies and clinical trials of preventive and therapeutic agents. The Turesky-Gilmore-Glickman Modification of the Quigley-Hein Plaque Index is considered one of the two indices of choice when assessing plaque in clinical trials.

Plaque Index (PLI)

The Plaque Index is unique among indices because it ignores the coronal extent of plaque on the tooth surface area and concentrates assessment only

Table 19-2: Turskey-Gilmore-Glickman Modification of the Quigley-Hein Plaque Index

INSTRUMENTS AND EQUIPMENT:
Adequate source of lighting, disclosing agent, air

PROCEDURE:
- Disclose plaque, rinse.
- Dry teeth with air.
- Buccal and Lingual surfaces are scored.

CRITERIA:
0 = No plaque
1 = Separate flecks or a discontinuous band of plaque at the gingival margin
2 = A thin, continuous band of plaque (up to 1 mm) at the gingival margin
3 = A band of plaque wider than 1 mm but covering less than one third of the gingival third of the tooth surface
4 = Plaque covering at least one third but less than two thirds of the tooth surface
5 = Plaque covering two thirds or more of the tooth surface

SCORING:
Scores are totaled and divided by the number of surfaces examined.

on the thickness of plaque at the gingival area of the tooth. The criteria for this index can be found in Table 19–3. It was developed to parallel the Gingival Index (GI) of Loe and Silness. It examines the same scoring units of the teeth used for the GI.

Unlike most indices, the PLI does not exclude or substitute for teeth with gingival restorations or Crowns. Either all or only selected teeth may be used in the PLI. The strength of the PLI is in its application to longitudinal studies and clinical trials.

Modified Navy Plaque Index

The Modified Navy Plaque Index records the presence or absence of plaque with a score of 1 or 0 for each tooth to include the designated areas of each

Table 19-3: The Plaque Index (PLI)

INSTRUMENTS AND EQUIPMENT:
Air, adequate light, mouth mirror, probe or explorer, disclosing agent as needed

PROCEDURE:

- Dry the teeth.
- Evaluate bacterial plaque on the cervical third only.
- Use a disclosing agent to distinguish between 0 and 1 scores.
- Include plaque on the surface of calculus and restorations.

CRITERIA:

0 = No plaque
1 = A film of plaque adhering to the free gingival margin and adjacent area of the tooth; the plaque may be recognized only after application of disclosing agent or by running the explorer across the tooth surface
2 = Moderate accumulation of soft deposits within the gingival pocket that can be seen with the naked eye on the tooth and gingival margin
3 = Abundance of soft matter within the gingival pocket and/or on the tooth and gingival margin

SCORING:
Each area is assigned a score. Scores are totaled and divided by 4. Scores for individual teeth may be grouped and totaled and divided by the number of teeth examined.

Excellent	0
Good	0.1–0.9
Fair	1.0–1.9
Poor	2.0–3.0

tooth surface of the six Ramfjord Index Teeth. This index is of value in assessing health education programs and the ability of individuals to perform oral hygiene practices.

Distal Mesial Plaque Index (DMPI)

The Distal Mesial Plaque Index is a variation of the Modified Navy Plaque Index. The DMPI places more emphasis on the gingival and interproximal areas of a tooth.

Irritants Index

Plaque is one of the two factors measured in the Irritants Index, which is a component of the Gingival Periodontal Index (GPI). The presence and coronal extent of plaque are scored on a scale of 0 to 3. Other factors that contribute to the Irritants Index are supragingival and subgingival calculus and subgingival irritants, such as overhanging or deficient restorations.

Patient Hygiene Performance Index

The Patient Hygiene Performance Index (PHP) was the first index developed for the sole purpose of assessing a patient's individual performance in removing debris after oral hygiene instruction. It records the presence or absence of debris as 1 or 0, respectively. The six surfaces of the six OHI-S teeth are used. The PHP Index is more sensitive than the OHI-S because it divides each tooth surface into five areas: three longitudinal thirds, with the middle third subdivided horizontally into thirds. Specific criteria for the PHP can be found in Table 19–4. The value of the PHP is chiefly its application to individual patient education.

Shick-Ash Modification of Plaque Criteria

The Shick-Ash Modification of Plaque Criteria excluded consideration of the interproximal areas of the teeth. Scoring of plaque present was limited to the gingival half of the Facial and Lingual surfaces of the Ramfjord Index teeth. The criteria for the Shick-Ash Modification of Plaque Criteria are shown in Table 19–5.

Table 19-4: Patient Hygiene Performance Index

INSTRUMENTS AND EQUIPMENT:
Disclosing agent, mouth mirror, adequate light source

PROCEDURE:

- Apply disclosing agent, rinse.
- Divide each tooth surface into five sections:
  - Vertically: Mesial, middle, and Distal.
  - Horizontally: middle third is subdivided into gingival, middle, and Occlusal or Incisal.
- Score each five sections.

CRITERIA:

0 = No debris, or questionable
1 = Debris definitely present

SCORING:
Add five scores for each tooth, each score will range from 0 to 5.
Total scores from individual teeth and divide by the number of teeth examined.

Excellent	0
Good	0.1–1.7
Fair	1.8–3.4
Poor	3.5–5.0

Table 19-5: Shick-Ash Modification Plaque Criteria

INSTRUMENTS AND EQUIPMENT:
Air, adequate lighting, disclosing agent

PROCEDURE:

- Disclose teeth and rinse.
- Examine.

CRITERIA:

0 = Absence of dental plaque
1 = Dental plaque in the interproximal area or at the gingival margin covering less than one third of the gingival half of the Facial or Lingual surface of the tooth
2 = Dental plaque covering more than one third but less than two thirds of the gingival half of the Facial or Lingual surface of the tooth
3 = Dental plaque covering two thirds or more of the gingival half of the Facial or gingival surface of the tooth

SCORING:
Score is totaled and divided by the number of teeth examined.

The plaque score per person is obtained by totaling all of the individual tooth scores and dividing by the number of teeth examined. These modified plaque criteria are suitable for clinical trials of preventive or therapeutic agents.

Plaque Free Score

The Plaque Free Score was designed to identify the location and number of plaque-free surfaces. The use of the Plaque Free Score is outlined in Table 19–6. This index is excellent for individual patient motivation.

Plaque Control Record

The Plaque Control Record was developed to count tooth surfaces with plaque present. This index scores four areas of each tooth. The criteria for scoring plaque with this index can be found in Table 19–7.

Modified Plaque Control Record

The Modified Plaque Control Record uses the same criteria as the Plaque Control Record. In the modification, six surfaces are scored instead of the four scored in the original index. The complete outline of the Modified Plaque Control Record can be found in Table 19–8.

Table 19-6: Plaque Free Score

INSTRUMENTS AND EQUIPMENT:
Disclosing agent, mouth mirror, adequate light

PROCEDURE:
- Apply disclosing agent, rinse.
- Examine each tooth for plaque, record four surfaces per tooth—Lingual, Facial, Mesial, and Distal.

CRITERIA:
Plaque is present or absent.

SCORING:
Total teeth present and total surfaces with plaque. Multiply the number of teeth present by 4 (total surfaces available) then subtract the number of surfaces with plaque from the total number of available tooth surfaces (number of plaque-free surfaces). Finally, divide the number of plaque-free surfaces by the total surface available and multiply by 100 (percent plaque-free surfaces).

Table 19–7: Plaque Control Record

INSTRUMENTS AND EQUIPMENT:
Disclosing agent, mouth mirror, adequate light

PROCEDURE:
- Apply disclosing agent, rinse.
- Examine each tooth.
- Record the presence or absence of plaque for four surfaces: Facial, Lingual, Mesial, and Distal.

CRITERIA:
Record areas of plaque only.

SCORING:
Total the number of teeth present; multiply by 4 to obtain the number of available surfaces. Multiply the number of plaque-stained surfaces by 100 and divide by the total number of available surfaces to derive the percent of surfaces; the lower the percentage of stained surfaces the better.

Table 19–8: Modified Plaque Control Record

INSTRUMENTS AND EQUIPMENT:
Disclosing agent, mouth mirror, adequate light

PROCEDURE:
- Apply disclosing agent, rinse.
- Examine each tooth.
- Record presence or absence of plaque for six surfaces: Facial, Lingual, Mesio-Lingual, Disto-Lingual, Disto-Buccal, and Mesio-Buccal.

CRITERIA:
Record areas of plaque only.

SCORING:
Total the number of teeth present; multiply by 6 to obtain the number of available surfaces. Multiply the number of plaque-stained surfaces by 100 and divide by the total number of available surfaces to derive the percent of surfaces; the lower the percentage of stained surfaces the better.

Ramfjord Plaque Index

The Ramfjord Plaque Index scores plaque on teeth using a range of 0 to 3. The complete criteria and use of the Ramfjord Plaque Index can be found in Table 19–9.

Table 19–9: The Ramfjord Plaque Index

INSTRUMENTS AND EQUIPMENT:
Adequate lighting, disclosing agent, air

PROCEDURE:
- Apply disclosing agent, rinse.
- Examine teeth #3, #9, #12, #19, #25, and #28.
- Score four surfaces per tooth: Facial, Lingual, Mesial, and Distal.

CRITERIA:

0 = No plaque

1 = Plaque present on some but not all interproximal, Facial, and Lingual surfaces of the tooth

2 = Plaque present on all interproximal, Facial, and Lingual surfaces, but covering less than one half of these surfaces

3 = Plaque extends over all interproximal, Facial, and Lingual surfaces, and covering more than one half of these surfaces

SCORING:
Add the plaque scores for each tooth and divide by the number of teeth examined.

Plaque Accumulation Scoring System (PASS)

The Plaque Accumulation Scoring System was designed as a more efficient, time-saving plaque evaluation tool. The tool was designed to be evaluated and scored by one person. The plaque system evaluates plaque both supragingivally and subgingivally. PASS evaluates four surfaces on five teeth (Table 19–10).

Indices Used to Assess Gingival Inflammation

Papillary-Marginal-Attached Gingival Index (P-M-A)

Thought to be the oldest reversible index, the Papillary-Marginal-Attached Index measures the extent of gingival changes in large groups of patients. This index is used to count the number of areas affected by gingivitis. It is thought the number of areas affected will directly correlate to the severity of gingivitis present in the mouth. The Buccal and Lingual gingiva around each tooth is divided into three scoring units. The method for completing the P-M-A Index can be found in Table 19–11. The value of this index lies in its broad application to epidemiological surveys and clinical trials and its capacity for use with individual patients.

Table 19-10: The Plaque Assessment Scoring System

INSTRUMENTS AND EQUIPMENT:
Light, periodontal probe

PROCEDURE:

- Five teeth are selected for examination: four first molars and one maxillary incisor. If one of the list teeth is Missing examine the next tooth to the Distal; if that tooth is also Missing, a Mesial tooth is considered.
- Each quarter of the tooth is swept with the probe approximately 1mm into the sulcus. Any plaque visible on the probe is considered a positive.

CRITERIA:
Plaque is present or absent.

SCORING:
Twenty scoring surfaces are available. The number of plaque surfaces are counted and divided by 20.

Table 19–11: Papillary-Marginal-Attached Gingival Index

INSTRUMENTS AND EQUIPMENT:
Mouth mirror, periodontal probe for pressing on gingival tissue

PROCEDURE:

- Use a routine order from the maxillary left second molar around to the maxillary right second molar and proceed to the mandibular right second molar around to the mandibular left second molar. Third molars are excluded.

CRITERIA:

Gingival Area	*Score*	*Criteria*
Papillary	P	0 = Normal, no inflammation
		1+ = Mild papillary engorgement, slight increase in size
		2+ = Obvious increase in size of gingival papilla; bleeding on pressure
		3+ = Excessive increase in size with spontaneous bleeding
		4+ = Necrotic papilla
		5+ = Atrophy and loss of papilla through inflammation
Marginal	M	0 = Normal, no inflammation
		1+ = Engorgement, slight increase in size; no bleeding
		2+ = Obvious engorgement; bleeding on pressure

Continues

Table 19–11: Continued

CRITERIA:

Gingival Area	*Score*	*Criteria*
Marginal		
		3+ = Swollen collar; spontaneous bleeding beginning infiltration into attached gingiva
		4+ = Necrotic gingiva
		5+ = Recession of the free marginal gingiva below the cementoenamel junction due to inflammatory changes
Attached	A	0 = Normal, pale pink; stippled
		1+ = Slight engorgement with loss of stippling; change in color may or may not occur
		2+ = Obvious engorgement of attached gingiva; marked increase in redness; pocket formation present
		3+ = Advanced periodontitis; deep pockets present

SCORING:

Mild gingivitis	1–4 papilla 0–2 margins
Moderate gingivitis	4–8 papilla 2–4 margins
Severe gingivitis	more than 8 papilla more than 4 margins

Periodontal Index (PI)

The Periodontal Index is intended to estimate the extent of deeper periodontal disease than the PMA Index could measure. This is done by determining the presence or absence and severity of gingival inflammation, pocket formation, and masticatory function. See Table 19–12 for an outline of the PI. Because the PI measures both reversible and irreversible aspects of periodontal disease, it is an excellent choice as an epidemiological index.

Gingival Index (GI)

The Gingival Index was developed solely for assessing the severity of gingivitis. As can be seen in Table 19–13, this index can be used to evaluate a segment of the mouth or a group of teeth. The numerical scores of the

Table 19-12: The Periodontal Index

INSTRUMENTS AND EQUIPMENT:
Mouth mirror, explorer, and periodontal probe

PROCEDURE:
- Each tooth is scored based on the condition of the surrounding tissue.

CRITERIA:

Score	Condition	Description
0 =	Negative	Neither obvious inflammation in the investing tissues nor the loss of function caused by destruction of supporting tissue
1 =	Mild Gingivitis	Overt area of inflammation in the free gingiva that does not circumscribe the tooth
2 =	Moderate Gingivitis	Inflammation completely circumscribes the tooth but there is no apparent break in the epithelial attachment
4 =	Severe Gingivitis	(Used when radiographs are available.) There is early notch-like resorption of the alveolar crest
6 =	Gingivitis with pocket formation	Epithelial attachment has been broken and there is a pocket, not merely a deepened gingival crevice caused by swelling in the free gingiva. There is no interference with normal masticatory function; the tooth is firm and has not drifted
8 =	Advanced destruction with loss of masticatory function	The tooth may be loose; may have drifted length of the tooth root or a definite infrabony pocket with widening of the PDL; may sound dull on percussion with a metallic instrument; may be depressible in its socket

Rule: When is doubt, assign the lesser scores.

SCORING:
Add scores for each tooth and divide by the number of teeth examined to obtain the individual's score.

Condition	Score
Clinically normal supportive tissues	0–0.2
Simple Gingivitis	0.3–0.9
Beginning destructive periodontal disease	1.0–1.9
Established destructive periodontal disease	2.0–4.9
Terminal disease	5.0–8.0

GI can be associated with various degrees of gingivitis. This index can be used to determine the prevalence and severity of gingivitis. The GI is the index of choice in controlled clinical trials of preventive or therapeutic agents.

Table 19-13: Gingival Index

INSTRUMENTS AND EQUIPMENT:
Adequate light, mouth mirror, probe

PROCEDURE:
- Four gingival areas are examined: Distal, Facial, Mesial, and Lingual.
- Dry teeth and gingiva, press probe on gingiva to determine degree firmness; use the probe to run along near the entrance on the gingival sulcus to evaluate bleeding.

CRITERIA:
0 = Normal gingiva
1 = Mild inflammation; slight change in color, slight edema; no bleeding on palpation
2 = Moderate inflammation; redness, edema, and glazing; bleeding on probing
3 = Severe inflammation; marked redness and edema; ulceration; tendency to spontaneous bleeding

SCORING:
Scores are totaled and divided by the number of teeth assessed.

Excellent (healthy tissue)	0
Good	0.1–1.0
Fair	1.1–2.0
Poor	2.1–3.0

Modified Gingival Index (MGI)

The Modified Gingival Index was created after eliminating the bleeding criterion, making the MGI noninvasive. Redefining the criteria for mild and moderate inflammation, the MGI increases sensitivity in the lower portion of the scoring scale. For use of the MGI, see Table 19–14.

Periodontal Disease Index (PDI)

The Periodontal Disease Index is similar to the PI because both are used to measure the presence and severity of periodontal disease. The PDI does this by combining the assessments of gingivitis and gingival sulcus depth on six selected teeth (#3, #9, #12, #19, #25, and #28). This group of teeth, referred to as the **Ramfjord teeth**, have been tested as reliable indicators for other regions of the mouth. Calculus and plaque are examined to produce a comprehensive assessment of periodontal status. Details of the PDI can be found in Table 19–15. The PDI has been used in epidemiologic surveys, longitudinal studies of periodontal disease, and clinical trials of therapeutic or preventive procedures.

Table 19–14: Modified Gingival Index

INSTRUMENTS AND EQUIPMENT:
Adequate light source, mouth mirror, periodontal probe

PROCEDURE:

- The periodontal probe is drawn horizontally along the soft tissue wall of the entrance to the gingival sulcus.

CRITERIA:

0 = Absence of inflammation
1 = Mild inflammation; slight change in color, little change in texture of any portion of the marginal or papillary gingival unit
2 = Mild inflammation; criteria as above but involving the entire marginal or papillary gingival unit
3 = Moderate inflammation; glazing, redness, edema, and/or hypertrophy of the marginal or papillary gingival unit
4 = Severe inflammation; marked redness, edema, and/or hypertrophy of the marginal or papillary gingival unit, spontaneous bleeding, congestion, or ulceration

SCORING:
Scores are totaled and divided by the number of teeth assessed.

Excellent (healthy tissue)	0
Good	0.1–1.0
Fair	1.1–2.0
Poor	2.1–3.0

Table 19–15: Periodontal Disease Index

INSTRUMENTS AND EQUIPMENT:
Standardized light source, Cotton roll for drying gingival tissue, calibrated periodontal probe

PROCEDURE:

Gingival status:

- Dry the gingival tissue, observe color and form. Apply gentle pressure with probe to determine consistency.

Crevice depth:

- Two measurements are made at the middle of the Facial surface and at the Facial aspect of the Mesial contact. The side of the probe should be held touching both teeth.
- If the gingival margin is on the enamel, measure from the gingival margin to the cementoenamel junction (CEJ) and record the measurement. If the epithelial attachment is on the Crown and the (CEJ) cannot be felt by the probe, record the depth of the gingival sulcus on the Crown. Then record the distance from the gingival margin to the bottom of the pocket if the probe can be moved apically to the CEJ without resistance or pain. The distance from the CEJ to the bottom of the pocket can then be found by subtracting the first from the second measurement.

Continues

Table 19–15: Continued

- If the gingival margin is on the cementum, record the distance from the CEJ to the gingival margin as a minus value. Then record the distance from the CEJ to the bottom of the gingival sulcus as a plus value. Both loss of attachment and actual sulcus depth can easily be assessed from the scores.

Calculus status:

- A subgingival explorer may be used to locate and determine the extent of a calculus deposit.

Plaque status:

- Apply disclosing solution, rinse with water. Use mouth mirror to observe areas with plaque.

CRITERIA:

Gingival status:

0 = Absence of signs of inflammation
1 = Mild to moderate inflammatory gingival changes, not extending around the tooth
2 = Mild to moderately severe gingivitis extending all around the tooth
3 = Severe gingivitis characterized by marked redness, swelling, tendency to bleed, and ulceration, not necessarily extending around the tooth

Crevice depth:

0–3 = When the gingival crevice or pocket in one of the measured areas extends apical to the CEJ
4 = When the crevices (pockets) of any two recorded areas extend apical to the CEJ not more than, but including 3 mm; the gingivitis score is then disregarded
5 = When the crevices (pockets) of any two recorded areas extend apical to the CEJ from 3 mm to 6 mm inclusive; the gingivitis score is then disregarded
6 = When the crevices (pockets) extend more than 6 mm apical to the CEJ in any two measured areas; the gingivitis score is then disregarded

Calculus status:

0 = No calculus
1 = Supragingival calculus extending only slightly below the free gingival margin (not more than 1 mm)
2 = Moderate amount of supragingival and subgingival calculus, or subgingival calculus only
3 = Abundance of supragingival and subgingival calculus

Plaque status:

0 = No plaque on the gingival half
1 = Plaque covering less than one third of the gingival half
2 = Plaque covering one third or less than two thirds of the gingival half
3 = Plaque covering two thirds or more of the Facial or Lingual surfaces of the gingival half

Continues

Table 19–15: Continued

SCORING:

Gingival status and crevice depth:

Add scores for individual teeth and divide by the number of teeth examined.

0–3 = Gingivitis (0 = no disease, 3.9 = severe gingivitis)

4–6 = Periodontitis (4 = early disease; 6 advanced disease)

Calculus status:

Add scores for each surface and divide by the number of surfaces.

Plaque status:

Add the scores for each tooth and divide by the number of teeth examined.

Indices of Gingival Bleeding

The use of gingival bleeding indices is desirable because bleeding is thought to be a more objective indicator of disease than early gingival color changes, while providing evidence of recent plaque exposure. In general, the indices utilizing palpation or interproximal cleaning aids are more suitable for the diagnosis of gingivitis and evaluation of a patient's progress in plaque control programs. Indices utilizing apical probing are more suitable for diagnosing periodontitis and for assessing the effects of subgingival pocket therapy.

Sulcus Bleeding Index (SBI)

The Sulcus Bleeding Index measures sulcular bleeding on probing. This is the first criterion for indicating gingival inflammation. The complete method can be seen in Table 19–16.

Papillary Bleeding Index (PBI)

The Papillary Bleeding Index uses a scale of 0 to 4. A timing component was added to the PBI in an effort to make the PBI more sensitive than the GI in assessing gingival changes (Table 19–17).

Bleeding Points Index

The Bleeding Points Index was developed to assess a patient's oral hygiene. It determines the presence or absence of gingival bleeding interproximally and on Facial and Lingual surfaces of each tooth (Table 19–18).

Table 19–16: Sulcus Bleeding Index

INSTRUMENTS AND EQUIPMENT:
Periodontal probe, adequate source of light

PROCEDURE:
- Hold probe parallel with the long axis of the tooth for M units and direct probe toward the col for P units. Wait 30 seconds after probing before scoring.
- Dry gingiva, if needed, to observe color changes clearly.

CRITERIA:
0 = Healthy appearance of P and M, no bleeding on sulcus probing
1 = Apparently healthy P and M showing no change in color and no swelling, but bleeding from sulcus on probing
2 = Bleeding on probing and change of color caused by inflammation. No swelling or macroscopic edema
3 = Bleeding on probing and change in color and slight edematous swelling
4 = (1) Bleeding on probing and change in color and obvious swelling
(2) Bleeding on probing and obvious swelling
5 = Bleeding on probing and spontaneous bleeding and change in color, marked swelling with or without ulceration

SCORING:
Each of the four gingival units (M, P) is scored. The scores are totaled and divided by 4 to obtain the score for each tooth. The individual tooth scores are added together and divided by the number of teeth scored to obtain a score for the mouth.

Gingival Bleeding Index (GBI)

The Gingival Bleeding Index assesses the presence or absence of gingival bleeding at the interproximal spaces. It is suitable for assessment of patient progress with a plaque control program. This index is useful when the patient is instructed to perform self-evaluation in a plaque control program (Table 19–19).

Interdental Bleeding Index

The Interdental Bleeding Index is also referred to as the Eastman Interdental Bleeding Index. This index measures the presence or absence of interproximal bleeding. A specific stimulus permits the dentist and, perhaps more important, the patient to monitor interproximal gingival health (Table 19–20).

Table 19–17: Papillary Bleeding Index

INSTRUMENTS AND EQUIPMENT:
Periodontal probe, adequate light source

PROCEDURE:
- The mouth is divided into quadrants.
- The maxillary right and mandibular left are probed Lingually.
- The maxillary left and mandibular right are probed Buccally.
- The papillary sulcus is swept on the Mesial and Distal aspects of the tooth.

CRITERIA:
0 = No bleeding after probing
1 = Only one point of bleeding after probing
2 = Several points of bleeding after probing
3 = Interdental triangle fills with blood after probing
4 = Blood flows immediately along the gingival groove after probing

SCORING:
Each papilla is scored according to the criteria. The scores are totaled and divided by the number of papilla examined.

Table 19–18: The Bleeding Points Index

INSTRUMENTS AND EQUIPMENT:
Adequate source of light, mirror, periodontal probe

PROCEDURE:
- The probe is gently inserted into the sulcus and walked along the length of the tooth, both on the Buccal and Lingual.
- The operator removes the probe and waits for 3 seconds and then scores six areas per tooth.
- Scores are recorded for the Distal, Mesial from both the Buccal and Lingual aspects along with the direct Buccal and direct Lingual.

CRITERIA:
Bleeding is either present or absent.

SCORING:
The individual patient score is determined by dividing the number of bleeding points by the total number of areas scored (number of teeth × 6 sites/tooth) and multiplied by 100 to obtain a percentage of bleeding points for the patient.

Table 19–19: Gingival Bleeding Index

INSTRUMENTS AND EQUIPMENT:
Unwaxed dental floss

PROCEDURE:
- Pass floss interproximally, first on one side of the papilla and then on the other.
- Curve the floss around the adjacent tooth and bring the floss below the gingival margin.
- Move the floss up and down for one stroke, taking care not to lacerate the gingiva.
- Adapt floss to provide controlled, consistent pressure.
- Use a new length of clean floss for each area.
- Retract for visibility of bleeding from both Facial and Lingual aspects.
- Allow 30 seconds for reinspection of an area that does not show bleeding immediately either in the area or on the floss.

CRITERIA:
Bleeding indicates disease. No attempt is made to quantify the severity of disease.

SCORING:
The number of bleeding areas and scorable units are recorded.

Table 19–20: Interdental Bleeding Index

INSTRUMENTS AND EQUIPMENT:
Wooden interdental cleaners

PROCEDURE:
- Interdental cleaner is inserted between the teeth from the Facial aspect, depressing the papilla 1 mm to 2 mm.
- Repeat process 4 times; wait 15 seconds before scoring bleeding.

CRITERIA:
0 = No bleeding
1 = Bleeding

SCORING:
Number of papilla with bleeding are counted.

Indices Used to Measure Periodontal Destruction

The destruction of bone is still the most important criterion for assessing the severity of periodontal disease.

Gingival Recession Index

The Gingival Recession Index is used in epidemiologic surveys.

Extent and Severity Index (ESI)

The Extent and Severity Index was developed because of a lack of satisfaction with previous indices for periodontal disease and the emergence of a newer conceptual model of periodontal disease pathogenesis. The older model, the PI, was based on the concept of periodontal disease as a slowly progressing, continuous disease process. In the newer model, periodontal disease is viewed as a chronic process with intermittent periods of activity and remission, affecting individual teeth and sites around the teeth at different rates. Unlike the PI, which uses a mouth mirror only, the ESI uses the National Institute for Dental Research (NIDR) now called NIDCR (National Institute of Dental and Craniofacial Research) periodontal probe to determine attachment levels (Table 19–21).

Table 19–21: Extent and Severity Index (ESI)

INSTRUMENTS AND EQUIPMENT:

Periodontal probe, mouth mirror, adequate light

PROCEDURE:

- Measurements are completed in contralateral quadrants (i.e., upper right and lower left, or upper left and lower right). A maximum of fifty-six sites should be measured.
- For each site, probe the distance from the gingival margin to the sulcus.
- Subtract the first measurement from the second. This number indicates the severity of the disease.

CRITERIA:

By the adopted rule, a site is diseased if the attachment loss exceeds 1 mm.

SCORING:

Severity (S) = the mean loss of attachment (in excess of 1 mm)
Extent (E) = the percent of site that exhibits disease; E is rounded to the nearest whole number
The ESI is expressed as (E, S)

Indices Used to Measure Calculus

In general, the indices used to assess calculus may be divided into three categories: the indices most appropriate to epidemiologic surveys; those that are appropriate to longitudinal studies, with an examination every 3 to 6 months; and those that are used in short-term clinical studies, usually no longer than 6 weeks.

Volpe-Manhold Probe Method of Calculus Assessment (VM)

The Volpe-Manhold Probe Method of Calculus Assessment was developed for longitudinal studies of the quantity of supragingival calculus formed. A periodontal probe graduated in millimeter divisions is used to measure the deposits of calculus on the Lingual surfaces of the six mandibular anterior teeth. The Volpe-Manhold Probe Method of Calculus Assessment has been shown to possess a high degree of inter- and intraexaminer reproducibility. Criteria used for the VM index can be found in Table 19–22.

Calculus Surface Index (CSI)

The Calculus Surface Index is one of two indices that are used in short-term (e.g., < 6 weeks) clinical trials of calculus-inhibiting agents. The objective of

Table 19–22: The Volpe-Manhold Probe Method of Calculus Assessment

INSTRUMENTS AND EQUIPMENT:
Adequate light, periodontal probe with millimeter markings

PROCEDURE:
- Bisect the Lingual aspect of the tooth into three segments.
- Measure the height and width of supragingival calculus deposits. Measurements are made in three planes: (1) bisecting Lingual surface, (2) diagonally through the greatest area of calculus, (3) diagonally through the Disto-Incisal angle.

CRITERIA:
Obtain millimeter measurements for calculus deposit present in the mouth.

SCORING:
Tooth scores are averaged to provide calculus height and to give a score for the individual.

this type of study is to determine rapidly whether a specific agent has any effect on reducing or preventing supragingival or subgingival calculus. The CSI assesses the presence or absence of supragingival and/or subgingival calculus on the four mandibular incisors. The index has also been applied to the six mandibular anterior teeth. The presence or absence of calculus is determined by visual examination or by tactile examination using a mouth mirror and a sickle-type dental explorer.

Calculus Surface Severity Index (CSSI)

A companion index to the CSI is the Calculus Surface Severity Index. The CSSI measures the quantity of calculus present on the surfaces examined for the CSI.

Marginal Line Calculus Index (MLCI)

A second index that is frequently used in short-term clinical trials of anti-calculus agents is the Marginal Line Calculus Index. This index was developed to assess the accumulation of supragingival calculus on the gingival third of the tooth or, more specifically, supragingival calculus at the gingival margin.

Indices Used to Assess Treatment Needs

Interpretations of the indices described in this section are to be viewed with caution because of existing difficulty concerning the estimation of treatment needs. Without knowing the response of the periodontal tissues to periodontal therapy, any estimate of treatment needs may be subject to over- or underestimation of what is clinically prudent.

Gingival Periodontal Index

The Gingival Periodontal Index (GPI) is a modification of the PDI of Ramfjord for the purpose of screening persons to determine who needs periodontal treatment. The primary objective in using the index is to determine the tooth or surrounding tissues with the severest condition within each of the six segments. Each segment is assessed for each of the three components of periodontal disease as described in Table 19–23.

Table 19–23: The Gingival Periodontal Index

INSTRUMENTS AND EQUIPMENT

Periodontal probe, light source

PROCEDURE:

- The maxillary and mandibular arches are each divided into three segments: the six anterior teeth, the left posterior teeth, and the right posterior teeth. Assess each segment for each of the three components of periodontal disease described previously.

CRITERIA:

0 = Tissue tightly adapted to the teeth; firm consistency with physiologic architecture
1 = Slight to moderate inflammation indicated by changes in color and consistency involving one or more teeth in the same segment but not completely surrounding any one tooth
2 = Above changes either singly or combined completely encircling one or more teeth in a segment
3 = Marked inflammation, as indicated by loss of surface continuity (ulceration), spontaneous hemorrhage, loss of Facio-Lingual continuity or any interdental papilla, marked deviation from normal contour (such as thickening or enlargement covering more than one third of the tooth recession and clefts)

SCORING:

The area with the highest score determines the gingival score for the entire segment. The gingival status for the mouth is obtained by dividing the sum of the gingival scores by the number of segments.

The GPI has been used extensively in military populations. Unlike the traditional indices used in epidemiology (which attempt primarily to assess the status of a specific disease condition with only the crudest suggestion of determining treatment needs), the GPI was developed for the specific purpose of detecting periodontal disease early, allowing for early treatment.

Periodontal Treatment Need System

The Periodontal Treatment Need System (PTNS) was the next index to evolve with the purpose of assessing treatment needs. This index has been used with interesting results. The PTNS attempts to place individuals into one of four classes based on treatment procedures relative to time requirements. See Table 19–24 for the specific treatment classes.

The index also considers the presence or absence of gingivitis, plaque, and the presence of pockets 5 mm or greater in each quadrant.

Table 19–24: The Periodontal Treatment Need System

INSTRUMENTS AND EQUIPMENT:
Adequate source of light, periodontal probe, explorer

PROCEDURE:
- Examine the mouth or quadrant for presence of plaque, calculus and/or overhangs, inflammation, and pocket depths.

CRITERIA:

Classification	Unit	Plaque	C/Over	Inflam.	Pocket depth
Class 0	Mouth	No	No	No	Not considered
Class A	Mouth	Yes	No	Yes	< 5 mm
Class B	Quadrant	Yes	Yes	Yes	< 5 mm
Class C	Quadrant	Yes	Yes	Yes	> 5 mm

SCORING:

Class O	No treatment
Class A	Oral hygiene instruction
Class B	Class A and scaling and/or removal of overhang
Class C	Class B and complex periodontal treatment

Community Periodontal Index of Treatment Needs

The World Health Organization (WHO) appointed an expert committee to review the methods available to assess periodontal status and treatment needs. The resulting index, after extensive field testing by investigators from the WHO and the International Dental Federation, was called the Community Periodontal Index of Treatment Needs (CPITN). The CPITN was designed to assess periodontal treatment needs rather than periodontal status. The CPITN assesses the presence or absence of gingival bleeding on gentle probing; the presence or absence of supragingival or subgingival calculus; and the presence or absence of periodontal pockets, subdivided into shallow and deep. A specially designed periodontal probe with a 0.5 mm ball tip and gradations corresponding to shallow and deep pockets was developed to probe for bleeding and calculus and to determine pocket depth in epidemiologic surveys. The criteria for the CPITN can be seen in Table 19–25.

The value of the CPITN is that it permits rapid examination of a population to determine periodontal treatment needs. However, much effort is expended and a great deal of useful information is lost when only the worst score

Table 19–25: Community Periodontal Index of Treatment Needs

INSTRUMENTS AND EQUIPMENT:
Adequate lighting, World Health Organization (WHO) probe

PROCEDURE:
- Probe each tooth using the WHO probe.
- Record the deepest code for the sextant.

CRITERIA:

Code 0 = Healthy periodontal tissue
Code 1 = Bleeding after gentle probing
Code 2 = Supragingival and/or subgingival calculus or defective margin of filling or Crown
Code 3 = 4 mm or 5 mm pocket
Code 4 = 6 mm or deeper pathologic pocket

SCORING:
The highest code found in the sextant is recorded for that sextant.

per sextant is recorded. It has been found that the CPITN underestimated the number of pockets larger than 6 mm in older age groups and overestimated the need for scaling in younger age groups.

Periodontal Screening and Recording (PSR)

The American Academy of Periodontology (AAP) has proposed the use of the CPITN for individual patients as a periodontal screening and recording (PSR) tool for general practitioners. The use of this index has become an integral part of many private dental practices in the United States. The PSR criteria can be found in Table 19–26.

Indices of Dental Caries

Decayed-Missing-Filled Teeth Index (DMFT)

There are several variations of the DMFT index for assessing the caries experience of an individual. The DMFT is an irreversible index that can evaluate

Table 19–26: The Periodontal Screening and Recording Index

INSTRUMENTS AND EQUIPMENT:
Adequate lighting source, World Health Organization (WHO) probe

PROCEDURE:
- Probe each tooth using the WHO probe.
- Record the deepest code for the sextant.

CRITERIA:

Code 0 = Colored area of probe completely visible in the deepest probing depth of the sextant
Code 1 = Colored area of probe completely visible in the deepest probing depth of the sextant; no calculus, no defective margins, no bleeding after gentle probing
Code 2 = Colored area of probe completely visible in the deepest probing depth; supragingival and/or subgingival calculus; defective margins of restorations
Code 3 = Colored area of probe only partly visible in the deepest probing depth; requirements for codes 1 and 2 may be present
Code 4 = Colored area of probe completely disappears; probing depth greater than 5.5 mm
Code 1*, 2*, 3*, 4* = (Clinical Abnormality) Any notable feature such as furcation involvement, mobility, mucogingival problem, and/or marked area of recession

SCORING:
The highest code found in the sextant is recorded for that sextant.

both past and present caries experience. Tables 19–27 through 19–30 show the use of the variations of this index. This is an important index in longitudinal studies as well as shorter studies.

Indices Used to Measure Fluorosis

Fluorosis is the hypomineralization of the enamel caused by excessive exposure to fluoride during tooth development. The amount of fluorosis is dependent on the amount of fluoride the individual has been exposed to over time. Several indices have been developed to assess the amount of change in the enamel following the exposure to high levels of fluoride.

Dean's Classification of Dental Fluorosis

Dean developed his index around 1939. The original classification had a seven-point ordinal scale. After working with this scale for several years, Dean revised his ordinal scale to five points. The classification of dental fluorosis developed by Dean is found in Table 19–31.

Table 19–27: Decayed, Missing, and Filled Permanent Teeth

INSTRUMENTS AND EQUIPMENT:
Adequate lighting, mouth mirror, explorer

PROCEDURE:
- Teeth are observed by visual means and with the explorer.

CRITERIA:
Identification of dental caries:
- The lesion is clinically visible and obvious.
- The explorer tip can penetrate into soft yielding material.
- Discoloration or loss of translucency typical of undermined or demineralized enamel is apparent.
- Explorer tip in a pit or fissure resists removal after moderate-to-firm pressure on insertion.

Recording: Each tooth is recorded once.
- D recordings:
  - When both dental caries and a restoration are present, the tooth is listed as D.
  - When a Crown is broken down as a result of dental caries, the tooth may be recorded as D.
- M recordings:
  - When the tooth has been extracted because of dental caries, the tooth is recorded as M.
  - When it is carious, nonrestorable, and indicated for extraction, the tooth is recorded as M.
- F recordings:
  - Permanent and temporary fillings are recorded as F.
  - A tooth with a defective filling but without evidence of dental caries is recorded as F.

SCORING:
Total each component separately (D, M, F), then total D + M + F = DMF.

Table 19–28: Decayed, Missing, and Filled Permanent Tooth Surfaces

INSTRUMENTS AND EQUIPMENT:
Adequate lighting, mouth mirror, explorer

PROCEDURE:
- Tooth surfaces are observed by visual means and with the explorer.

CRITERIA:
Identification of dental caries:
- The lesion is clinically visible and obvious.
- The explorer tip can penetrate into soft yielding material.
- Discoloration or loss of translucency typical of undermined or demineralized enamel is apparent.
- Explorer tip in a pit or fissure resists removal after moderate-to-firm pressure on insertion.

Continues

Table 19–28: Continued

CRITERIA:

Recording: Each tooth is recorded once.

- D recordings:
  - When both dental caries and a restoration are present, the tooth is listed as D.
  - When a Crown is broken down as a result of dental caries, the tooth may be recorded as D.
- M recordings:
  - When the tooth has been extracted because of dental caries, the tooth is recorded as M.
  - When the tooth is carious, nonrestorable, and indicated for extraction, the tooth is recorded as M.
- F recordings:
  - Permanent and temporary fillings are recorded as F.
  - A tooth with a defective filling but without evidence of dental caries is recorded as F.

SCORING:

Tooth surfaces:

- Posterior teeth—each tooth has five surfaces examined and recorded: Facial, Lingual, Mesial, Distal, and Occlusal.
- Anterior teeth—each tooth has four surfaces for evaluation: Facial, Lingual, Mesial, and Distal.
- Missing posterior teeth—recorded as five surfaces. The number of surfaces that were carious before extraction usually cannot be determined.
- Total each component separately (D, M, F), then total D + M + F = DMF.

Table 19–29: Decayed, Missing, and Filled (For Primary and Mixed Dentitions)

INSTRUMENTS AND EQUIPMENT:

Adequate lighting, mouth mirror, explorer

PROCEDURE:

- Twelve teeth are observed by visual means and with the explorer (eight primary molars; four primary canines).

CRITERIA:

Identification of dental caries:

- The lesion is clinically visible and obvious.
- The explorer tip can penetrate into soft yielding material.
- Discoloration or loss of translucency typical of undermined or demineralized enamel is apparent.
- Explorer tip in a pit or fissure resists removal after moderate-to-firm pressure on insertion.

Recording: Each tooth is recorded once.

- d recordings:
  - When both dental caries and a restoration are present, the tooth is listed as d.
  - When a Crown is broken down as a result of dental caries, the tooth may be recorded as d.

Continues

Table 19–29: Continued

***Recording*: Each tooth is recorded once.**

- m recordings:
  - When the tooth has been extracted because of dental caries, the tooth is recorded as m.
  - When the tooth is carious, nonrestorable, and indicated for extraction, the tooth is recorded as m.
- f recordings:
  - Permanent and temporary fillings are recorded as f.
  - A tooth with a defective filling but without evidence of dental caries is recorded as f.

SCORING:
Total each component separately (d, m, f), then total d + m + f = dmf.

Table 19–30: Decayed Indicated for Extraction and Filled Teeth or Surfaces (for Primary and Mixed Dentitions)

INSTRUMENTS AND EQUIPMENT:
Adequate lighting, mouth mirror, explorer

PROCEDURE:

- Twenty teeth are evaluated.
- Tooth surfaces are observed by visual means and with the explorer.

CRITERIA:

***Identification of* Dental *caries*:**

- The lesion is clinically visible and obvious.
- The explorer tip can penetrate into soft yielding material.
- Discoloration or loss of translucency typical of undermined or demineralized enamel is apparent.
- Explorer tip in a pit or fissure resists removal after moderate-to-firm pressure on insertion.

***Recording*: Each tooth surface is recorded once**

- d recordings:
  - When both dental caries and a restoration are present, the tooth is listed as d.
  - When a Crown is broken down as a result of dental caries, the tooth may be recorded as d.
- e recordings:
  - When the tooth has been extracted because of dental caries, the tooth is recorded as e.
  - When it is carious, nonrestorable, and indicated for extraction, the tooth is recorded as e.
- f recordings:
  - Permanent and temporary fillings are recorded as f.
  - A tooth with a defective filling but without evidence of dental caries is recorded as f.

Continues

Table 19–30: Continued

SCORING:

Tooth surfaces:

- Posterior teeth—each tooth has five surfaces examined and recorded: Facial, Lingual, Mesial, Distal, and Occlusal.
- Anterior teeth—each tooth has four surfaces for evaluation: Facial, Lingual, Mesial, and Distal.
- Missing posterior teeth—recorded as five surfaces. The number of surfaces that were carious before extraction usually cannot be determined.
- Total each component separately (d, e, f), then total d + e + f = def.

Table 19–31: Dean's Classification for Dental Flurosis

INSTRUMENTS AND EQUIPMENT:

Adequate lighting

PROCEDURE:

- Examine teeth.

CRITERIA:

Normal (0) = The enamel presents the usual translucent semivitriform type of structure; surface is smooth and glossy, and usually of a pale, creamy white color

Questionable (.5) = The enamel discloses slight aberrations from the translucency of normal enamel, ranging from a few white flecks to occasional white spots; use when a definite diagnosis of the mildest form is not warranted and a classification of "normal" not justified

Very mild (1) = Small, opaque paper-white areas scattered irregularly over the tooth but not involving as much as 25% of the tooth surface; frequently included are teeth showing no more than about 1–2 mm of white opacity at the tip of the summit of the cusps of the premolars or second molars

Mild (2) = The white opaque areas of the enamel surfaces of the teeth are more extensive but do not involve as much as 50% of the tooth

Moderate (3) = All enamel surfaces of the teeth are affected, and the surfaces subjected to attrition show wear; brown stain is frequently a disfiguring feature

Severe (4) = All enamel surfaces are affected and hypoplasia is so marked that the general form of the tooth may be affected; major diagnostic sign is the discrete or confluent pitting; brown stains are widespread and teeth often present a corroded-like appearance

SCORING:

Negative	0 – 0.4
Borderline	0.4 – 0.6
Slight	0.6 – 1.0
Medium	1.0 – 2.0
Marked	2.0 – 3.0
Very marked	3.0 – 4.0

Thylstrup-Fejerskov Index of Fluorosis

This is a modification of Dean's somewhat arbitrary index. This modification has a stronger biological basis for assessment of fluorosis (Table 19–32).

Table 19–32: The Thylstrup-Fejerskov Index of Fluorosis

INSTRUMENTS AND EQUIPMENT:
Adequate light source, mirror, periodontal probe, cotton rolls, and air

PROCEDURE:
- The teeth are isolated and dried.
- Each tooth is individually scored using the following criteria.

CRITERIA:

0 = Normal translucency of enamel remains after prolonged air drying

1 = Narrow white lines located corresponding to the perikymata

2 = *Smooth surfaces*: more pronounced lines of opacity that follow the perikymata; occasionally confluence of adjacent lines; *Occlusal surfaces*: scattered areas of opacity < 2 mm in diameter and pronounced opacity of cuspal ridges

3 = *Smooth surfaces*: merging and irregular cloudy areas of opacity; accentuated drawing of perikymata often visible between opacities; *Occlusal surfaces*: confluent areas of marked opacity; worn areas appear almost normal but usually circumscribed by a rim of opaque enamel

4 = *Smooth surfaces*: entire surface shows marked opacity or appears chalky white; parts of surface exposed to attrition appear less affected; *Occlusal surfaces*: entire surface exhibits marked opacity; attrition is often pronounced shortly after eruption

5 = *Smooth and Occlusal surfaces*: entire surface shows marked opacity with focal loss of outermost enamel < 2 mm in diameter

6 = *Smooth surfaces*: Pits are regular and arranged in horizontal bands < 2 mm in vertical extension; *Occlusal surfaces*: confluent areas < 3 mm in diameter exhibit loss of enamel; marked attrition

7 = *Smooth surfaces*: loss of outermost enamel in irregular areas involving < half the tooth surface; *Occlusal surfaces*: change in the morphology

8 = *Smooth and Occlusal surfaces*: Loss of outermost enamel involving > half of the surface

5 = *Smooth and Occlusal surfaces*: Loss of main part of enamel with change in anatomic appearance of surface. Cervical rim of unaffected enamel is often noted.

SCORING:
Each tooth in mouth is individually scored.

Radiographic Approaches to Measuring Bone Loss

In general, the use of radiographs in the study of the epidemiology of periodontal disease would appear to overcome some of the criticisms of the more subjective clinical measurements. Radiographs present a permanent objective record of interdental bone levels; in longitudinal studies they may ensure less variability than poorly standardized evaluations by dental examiners, and they offer the only method available for making Crown and root measurements. Their disadvantages are that they are not useful in the Buccal or Lingual assessment of bone level. They do not provide adequate information on soft tissue attachment, and their value may be lost if improper angulation is used. Furthermore, obtaining radiographs of survey participants, without the intent of providing treatment if needed, is unethical.

Only a few indices have been specifically designed to evaluate the radiographic assessment of periodontal disease, but other, more precise techniques for making reasonably accurate measurements from radiographs have been developed. The Gingival-Bone Count Index records the gingival condition on a scale of 0 to 3 and the level of the crest of the alveolar bone. The strength of each of these radiographic indices is in epidemiologic surveys in which evaluation time is limited because of large study populations.

Periodontitis Severity Index (PSI)

The Periodontitis Severity Index assesses the presence or absence of periodontitis as the product of clinical inflammation (CIS) and interproximal bone loss (BLS) determined radiographically using a modified Schei ruler. Because of the need for periapical radiographs, the PSI is limited to longitudinal studies and lacks validation.

Other Indices Used in Dentistry

Miller Index of Tooth Mobility

The Miller Index of Tooth Mobility is important for assessing the extent of periodontal disease around a tooth. This index has been modified in many ways to be used for the assessment of the amount of movement due to periodontal destruction (Table 19–33).

Table 19–33: Miller Index of Tooth Mobility

INSTRUMENTS AND EQUIPMENT:
Adequate light source, two metal instrument handles

PROCEDURE:
- Two metal instruments' handles are placed on either side of the tooth to be tested.
- Move the tooth back and forth.

CRITERIA:
0 = No movement when force applied
1 = Barely distinguishable tooth movement
2 = 1 mm movement in any direction, or tooth can be depressed or rotated in the socket

SCORING:
Each tooth is given individual score.

Review Questions

Multiple Choice

Directions: Select the letter of the choice that *best* answers the question.

1. A mean PLI score of 2.8 for a population of children would indicate which of the following?
   a. An abundance of soft deposits
   b. A moderate accumulation of soft deposits
   c. A slight film of plaque on the tooth surface
   d. No plaque
2 The PHP index is designed to:
   a. evaluate plaque and calculus on specific tooth surfaces.
   b. score plaque on specific tooth surfaces.
   c. score plaque and gingivitis.
   d. score plaque, calculus, and gingivitis.
3. Which of the following is a disadvantage of the DMF index?
   a. It is time consuming.
   b. It is a sum of dissimilar items.
   c. It is difficult to determine true caries using these criteria.
   d. It measures cumulative experience and is not necessarily indicative of current caries activity.

4. The dental index that is most age specific is:
   a. OHI-S. b. PI.
   c. DMF. d. DEF.
5. The D in the DEF index represents:
   a. all decayed teeth indicated for filling.
   b. all decayed primary anterior teeth indicated for filling.
   c. all decayed primary teeth.
   d. all decayed primary canines and molars indicated for filling.
6. An index that consistently measures what it is intended to measure is said to be:
   a. reliable. b. valid.
   c. objective. d. acceptable.
7. The index that would be most useful to evaluate gingivitis is:
   a. PLI (Plaque Index).
   b. PHP (Patient Hygiene Performance).
   c. PI (Periodontal Index).
   d. GI (Gingival Index).
8. The OHI-S serves best as a (an):
   a. cumulative oral hygiene index.
   b. assessment of debris and calculus on individual teeth.
   c. treatment index.
   d. assessment index of gingivitis on individual teeth.
9. The Periodontal Disease Index (PDI) includes all of the following except:
   a. gingivitis index. b. calculus index.
   c. pocket depth. d. mobility index.
10. The Simplified Oral Hygiene Index (OHI-S) measures the amount of:
    a. plaque. b. plaque and stain.
    c. plaque and calculus. d. plaque and gingivitis.

Answers

1. **a,** 2. **b,** 3. **d,** 4. **d,** 5. **a,** 6. **a,** 7. **d,** 8. **b,** 9. **d,** 10. **c**

References

Adams, R. A., & Nystrom, G. P. (1986). A periodontitis severity index. *Journal of Periodontology*, 57(3), 176–179.

Ainarno, J., Barmes, D., Beagrie, G., Cutress, T., Martin, T., & Sardo-Infirri, J. (1982). Development of the World Health Organization (WHO) community periodontal index of treatment needs (CPITN). *International Dental Journal*, 32(3), 281–291.

Ainarno, J., & Bay, I. (1975). Problems and proposals for recording gingivitis and plaque. *International Dental Journal*, 25(4), 229–235.

American Academy of Periodontology and American Dental Association. (1972). *Periodontal Screening & Recording* . Sponsored by Procter & Gamble.

Bellini, H. T. (1974). A system to determine the periodontal therapeutic needs of a population. *Norske Tannlaegeforenings Tildend*, 84(7), 266–268.

Bellini, H. T., & Gjermo, P. (1973). Application of the periodontal treatment need system (PTINS) in a group of Norwegian industrial employees. *Community Dentistry of Oral Epidemiology*, 1(1), 22–29.

Burt, B. A., & Eklund, S. A. (1992). *Dentistry, dental practice and the community* (4th ed., pp. 52 and ff.). Philadelphia: W. B. Saunders Company.

Butler, B. L., Morejon, O., & Low, S. B. (1996). An accurate, time-efficient method to assess: Plaque accumulation. *Journal of the American Dental Association*, 127(12), 1763–1766.

Carlos, J. P., Wolfe, M. D., & Kingman, A. (1998). The extent and severity index: A simple method for use in epidemiologic studies of periodontal disease. *Journal of Clinical Periodontology*, 13(5), 500–505.

Carter, H. G., & Barnes, G. P. (1974). The gingival bleeding index. *Journal of Periodontology*, 45(11), 801–805.

Caton, J. G., & Polson, A. M. (1985). The interdental bleeding index: A simplified procedure for monitoring gingival health. *Compendium of Continuing Education in Dentistry*, 6(2), 88.

Ciando, S. G. (1986). Current status of indices of gingivitis. *Journal of Clinical Periodontology*, 13(5), 375–378.

Elliott, J. R., Bowers, G. M., Clemmen, B. A., & Rovelstad, G. H. (1972). Evaluation of an oral physiotherapy center in the reduction of bacterial plaque and periodontal disease. *Journal of Periodontology*, 43(4), 221–224.

Fischman, S. L. (1986). Current status of indices of plaque. *Journal of Clinical Periodontology*, 13(5), 371–374.

Fischman, S. L. (1988). Clinical index systems used to assess the efficacy of mouth rinses on plaque and gingivitis. *Journal of Clinical Periodontology*, 15(8), 506–510.

Fischman, S. L., Cancro, L. P., Pretara-Spanedda, P., & Jacobs, D. (1986). Distal mesial plaque index: A technique for assessing dental plaque about the gingiva. *Dental Hygiene*, 61(9), 404–409.

Gjermo, P. (1994). CPITN as a basic periodontal examination in dental practice. *International Dental Journal*, 44(5 suppl), 547–552.

Greene, J. C. (1963). Oral hygiene and periodontal disease. *American Journal of Public Health*, 53, 6 and ff.

Greene, J. C. (1973). The oral hygiene index: Development and uses. *Journal of Periodontology*, 38(6 suppl), 625–637.

Greene, J. C., & Vermillion, J. R. (1960). Oral hygiene index: A method for classifying oral hygiene status. *Journal of the American Dental Association*, 61(8), 172 and ff.

Greene, J. C., & Vermillion, J. R. (1964). The simplified oral hygiene index. *Journal of the American Dental Association*, 68(1), 7 and ff.

Horowitz, H. S., Driscoll, W. S., Meyers, R. J., Heifetz, S. B., & Kingman, A. (1984). A new method for assessing the prevalence of dental fluorosis—The tooth surface index of fluorosis. *Journal of the American Dental Association*, 109(1), 37–41.

Ismail, A. L., Burt, B. A., & Brunelle, I. A. (1987). Prevalence of dental caries and periodontal disease in Mexican American children aged 5 to 17 years: Results from southwestern HHANES, 1982–1983. *American Journal of Public Health*, 77(8), 967–970.

Kelly, J. E., & Harvey, C. R. (1979). *Basic dental examination findings of persons 1–74 years, United States 1971–1974*. PHS (Publication No. 79–1662, Series II, No. 214). Hyarsville, MD: U.S. Public Health Service. U.S. Department of Health, Education, and Welfare, National Center for Health Statistics.

Klein, H., Palmer, C. E., & Knutson, J. W. (1938). Studies on dental caries: I. Dental status and dental needs of elementary school children. *Public Health Reports*, 53(5), 751 and ff.

Lenox, J. A., & Kopezyk, R. A. (1973). A clinical system for scoring a patient's oral hygiene performance. *Journal of the American Dental Association*, 86(4), 849–852.

Lobene, R., Weatherford, T., Ross, W., Lamm, R. A., & Menaker, L. A. (1986). A modified gingival index for use in clinical trials. *Clinical Preventive Dentistry*, 8(1), 3–6.

Loe, H. (1967). The gingival index, the plaque index and the retention index systems. *Journal of Periodontology*, 38(6 suppl), 610–616.

Loe, H., & Silness, I. (1963). Periodontal disease in pregnancy. *Acta Odontologica Scandinavica*, 21(6), 533 and ff.

Mandel, I. D. (1974). Indices for measurement of soft accumulations in clinical studies of oral hygiene and periodontal disease. *Journal of Periodontal Research Supplement*, 14, 106–110.

Mandel, I. D. (1974). Indices for measurement of soft accumulations in clinical studies of oral hygiene and periodontal disease (continued). *Journal of Periodontal Research Supplement*, 14, 7–30.

Massler, M. (1967). The P-M-A index for the assessment of gingivitis. *Journal of Periodontology*, 38(6 suppl), 592–601.

Muhlemann, H. R. (1967). Psychological and chemical mediators of gingival health. *Journal of Preventive Dentistry*, 4, 6 and ff.

Muhlemann, H. R., & Mazor, Z. S. (1958). Gingivitis in Zurich school children. *Helvetica Odontologica Acta*, 2, 3 and ff.

Muhlemann, H. R., & Son, S. (1971). Gingival sulcus bleeding—A leading symptom in initial gingivitis. *Helvetica Odontologica Acta*, 15(2), 107–113.

Muhlemann, H. R., & Villa, P. (1967). The marginal line calculus index. *Helvetica Odontologica Acta*, 11(2), 175–179.

O'Leary, T. J. (1967). The periodontal screening examination. *Journal of Periodontology*, 38(6 suppl), 617–624.

O'Leary, T. J., Drake, R. B., & Naylor, J. E. (1972). The plaque control record. *Journal of Periodontology*, 43(1), 38 and ff.

Podshadley, A. G., & Haley, I. V. (1968). A method for evaluating patient hygiene performance by observation of selected tooth surfaces. *Public Health Reports*, 83(3), 259–264.

Quigley, G., & Hein, I. (1962). Comparative cleansing efficiency of manual and power brushing. *Journal of the American Dental Association*, 65(7), 26 and ff.

Ramfjord, S. P. (1959). Indices for prevalence and incidence of periodontal disease. *Journal of Periodontology*, 30(1), 51 and ff.

Ramfjord, S. P. (1967). The periodontal disease index (PDI). *Journal of Periodontology*, 38(6 suppl), 602–610.

Ramfjord, S. P. (1974). Design of studies or clinical trials to evaluate the effectiveness of agents or procedures for the prevention, or treatment of loss of the periodontium, *Journal of Periodontal Research*, 14, 78–93.

Russell, A. L. (1956). A system of classification and scoring for prevalence surveys of periodontal disease. *Journal of Dental Research*, 35(6), 350 and ff.

Russell, A. L. (1969). Epidemiology and the rational bases of dental public health and dental practice. In W. O. Young and D. F. Striffier (eds.), *The Dentist. His Practice, and His Community* (2nd ed.). Philadelphia: W. B. Saunders Company.

Schei, O., Waerhaug, J., Lovdal, A., & Arno, A. (1959). Alveolar bone loss as related to oral hygiene and age. *Journal of Periodontology*, 30, 7 and ff.

Schour, I., & Massler, M. (1948). Survey of gingival disease using the PMA Index. *Journal of Dental Research*, 27, 733 and ff.

Shapiro, S., Pollack, B. R., & Gallant, D. (1971). A special population available for periodontal research. Part B. A correlation and association analysis between oral hygiene and periodontal disease. *Journal of Periodontology*, 42(3), 161–165.

Sheiham, A., & Striffler, D. F. (1970). A comparison of four epidemiological methods of assessing periodontal disease. *Journal of Periodontal Research*, 5(2), 155–161.

Shick, R. A., & Ash, M. M. (1961). Evaluation of the vertical method of tooth-brushing. *Journal of Periodontology*, 32(10), 346 and ff.

Silness, P., & Loe, H. (1964). Periodontal disease in pregnancy. II. Correlation between oral hygiene and periodontal condition. *Acta Odontologica Scandinavica*, 22(1), 121 and ff.

Suomi, J. D., & Barbano, J. P. (1968). Patterns of gingivitis. *Journal of Periodontology*, 39(2), 71–84.

Suomi, J. D., Greene, J. C., & Vermillion, J. R. (1971). The effect of controlled oral hygiene procedures on the progression of periodontal disease in adults: Results after third and final year. *Journal of Periodontology*, 42(3), 152–160.

Ten-state nutrition survey 1968–1970. (1972). HSM (Publication No. 72–8131, Vol. 3.) Washington, DC: Health Services and Mental Health Administration, U.S. Department of Health, Education, and Welfare.

Thylstrup, A., & Fejerskov., O. (1978). Clinical appearance of dental fluorosis in permanent teeth in relation to histologic changes. *Community Dentistry of Oral Epidemiology*, 6(6), 315–328.

Turesky, S., Gilmore, N. D., & Glickman, I. (1970). Reduced plaque formation by the chloromethyl analogue of vitamin C. *Journal of Periodontology*, 41(1), 41–43.

Volpe, A. R. (1974). Indices for the measurement of hard deposits in clinical studies of oral hygiene and periodontal disease. *Journal of Periodontal Research*, 14, 31–60.

Volpe, A. R., Manhold, J. H., & Hazen, S. P. (1965). In vivo calculus assessment: A method and its reproducibility. *Journal of Periodontology*, 36, 292 and ff.

Wilkins, E. (1994). *Clinical practice of the dental hygienist* (7th ed.). Baltimore: Williams and Wilkins.

World Health Organization. (1978). *Oral health surveys: Basic methods*. (3rd ed.). Geneva: Author.

CHAPTER 20

Occlusion and Malocclusion

Key Terms

Angle's Classification of Malocclusion
Centric Occlusion
Class I Malocclusion
Class II Malocclusion or Distocclusion
Class II, Division 1 Malocclusion
Class II, Division 2 Malocclusion
Class III Malocclusion or Mesiocclusion
Convex
Crossbite
End-to-End Bite
Malocclusion
Midline Alignment
Occlusion
Openbite
Overbite
Overjet
Prognathic
Retrognathic
Terminus
Underjet

Introduction

Occlusion refers to the relationship of the mandibular and maxillary teeth when they come in contact. Occlusion is determined by the particular arrangement of opposing teeth (dental) but influenced by the position and relationship of the upper and lower jaws (skeletal). The maximum intercuspation of the maxillary and mandibular teeth, the habitual "bite" of an individual, is called **centric occlusion**. It is used as the basis for making preliminary assessments about the dentition. The concept of an "ideal" or "normal" occlusion is hypothetical but helpful for dental assessments, diagnosis, and treatment planning. Criteria for an "ideal" dental occlusion include a Class I molar and canine interdigitation, coincident dental midlines, 1 to 2 mm anterior and

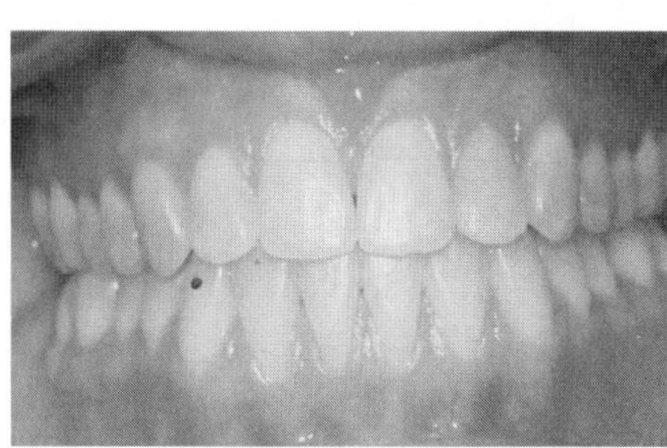

Universal System

#2 #3 #4 #5 #6 #7 #8 #9 #10 #11 #12 #13 #14
#31 #30 #29 #28 #27 #26 #25 #24 #23 #22 #21 #20 #19

Palmer System

7┘ 6┘ 5┘ 4┘ 3┘ 2┘ 1┘ └1 └2 └3 └4 └5 └6
7┐ 6┐ 5┐ 4┐ 3┐ 2┐ 1┐ ┌1 ┌2 ┌3 ┌4 ┌5 ┌6

ISO/FDI System

17 16 15 14 13 12 11 21 22 23 24 25 26
47 46 45 44 43 42 41 31 32 33 34 35 36

Figure 20–1 Photograph of an anterior view representing ideal occlusion, anterior midline alignment coincident, and a normal overbite

posterior **overjet**, and 1 to 2 mm anterior **overbite** (Plate 33 and Figure 20–1). These characteristics may be readily assessed during a dental examination in a general dental office. In dental specialty offices (orthodontics, prosthodontics, etc.), a more extensive assessment of occlusion is usually made prior to treatment to serve the specific clinical treatment planning needs of the specialty.

Malocclusion is an occlusion that deviates from the ideal. **Angle's Classification of Malocclusion** has been traditionally used to classify the anterior-posterior relationship of the maxillary and mandibular teeth in centric occlusion. The practitioner is cautioned to realize the simplistic nature of this classification, which describes the relationship in only one spatial plane, the anterior-posterior; the vertical and transverse spatial planes are not included in the Angle classification. The key teeth used in Angle's classification system are the first permanent molars. In an "ideal" occlusion, the Mesio-Buccal cusp of the maxillary first permanent molar is in the same vertical plane as the Mesio-Buccal (Buccal) groove of the mandibular first permanent molar. In this classification system, it is essential to compare the mandibular to the maxillary teeth because the mandible is the only movable bone in the head and face. The permanent canines are used to confirm the Angle classification when molar occlusion does not accurately depict occlusion status. In an ideal occlusion, the tip of the maxillary canine should occlude in the interproximal space position between the mandibular canine and mandibular first premolar (Figure 20–2).

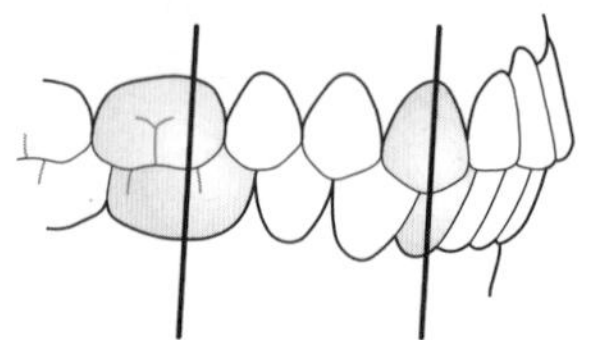

Figure 20–2 Normal "ideal" occlusion canine and molar relationship

Classifications of Malocclusion

Edward H. Angle identified three classifications of malocclusion: Class I, Class II, and Class III.

Class I Malocclusion

In a **Class I malocclusion** there is an " ideal," "normal," or "neutral" relationship of the opposing first permanent molars. Other alignment discrepancies may exist either within an arch (described in Chapter 18) or between the arches (Plate 34). "Perfect" occlusions, when observed, are customarily classified as Class I because of their "ideal" molar relationship.

Class II Malocclusion

In a Class II molar relationship, the Mesio-Buccal cusp of the maxillary first permanent molar is Mesial to the Mesio-Buccal (Buccal) groove of the mandibular first permanent molar by 2 mm or more. **Class II malocclusion** is also called a **distocclusion**, that is, the mandibular molar is Distal to its maxillary counterpart. Class II malocclusions may be further subcategorized into Division 1 and 2. In **Class II, Division 1** (Plate 35), the maxillary anterior teeth have excess overjet with a normal Labial-Lingual inclination. In **Class II, Division 2**, one or both of the maxillary central incisors are inclined lingually (Figure 20–3).

Class III Malocclusion

In a **Class III malocclusion**, the Mesio-Buccal cusp of the maxillary first permanent molar is Distal to the Mesio-Buccal (Buccal) groove of the mandibular

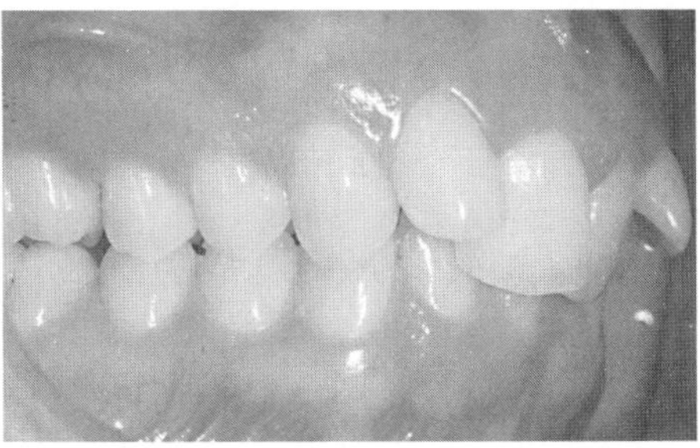

Figure 20–3 Class II, Division 2

Universal System
#3 #4 #5 #6 #7 #8 #9 #10
#30 #29 #28 #27 #26 #25 #24

Palmer System
6┘ 5┘ 4┘ 3┘ 2┘ 1┘ └1 └2
6┐ 5┐ 4┐ 3┐ 2┐ 1┐ ┌1 ┌2

ISO/FDI System
17 16 15 14 13 12 11 21 22
47 46 45 44 43 42 41 31 32

first permanent molar by 2 mm or more. Class III malocclusion is often called a **mesiocclusion**, that is, the mandibular molar is Mesial to its maxillary counterpart (Plate 37). When maxillary teeth are Lingual to the mandibular teeth, the condition is commonly referred to as an underjet (Plate 38).

Occlusion and Facial Profile

The observation of the facial profile of an individual may add more clarity to the classification of a malocclusion. Profile analysis provides additional information on the relationship of the arches and jaws to the upper face. In an "ideal" or Class I relationship of the jaws, the facial profile is slightly **convex**. An individual with a Class II malocclusion may have a **retrognathic** mandibular profile in which the lower jaw appears retruded in relation to the upper face, or a prognathic maxilla in which the upper jaw appears protruded relative to the upper face. In a Class III or "Mesial" malocclusion, the lower jaw may appear **prognathic** or protruded in profile or the upper jaw may be retrognathic or retruded relative to the upper face (Figure 20–4).

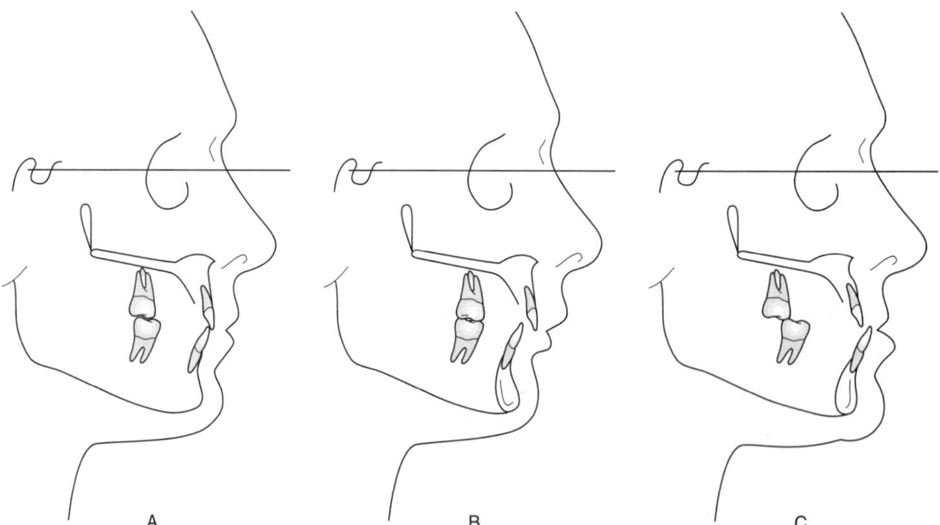

Figure 20–4 Facial profiles: (A) Convex (B) Retrognathic mandible (C) Prognathic mandible

Variations in Classification

In the clinical setting, there are several situations that may make Angle's classification difficult to use such as the presence of Crowns, bridges, and removable prosthetic appliances, or Missing teeth. If first permanent molars are Missing, then the canines are generally used to classify the occlusion. If premolars are Missing and there has been Mesial tilt or drift of the permanent molars, then the permanent canines should be used. If the molars are crowned or replaced with a bridge, then assessment of canine occlusion may supplement the anterior-posterior classification. If the individual is edentulous in one or both arches, the classification of occlusion is commonly determined by facial profile assessment. Frequently, the alignment of the teeth differs on right and left sides of the dentition. Angle's scheme accounts for unilateral occlusion problems by adding "subdivisions" to the classifications. However, in situations like this it is more practical to record the classification for both right and left sides.

Classification of Occlusion in Primary Dentitions

In a primary dentition (ages 2 to 6), the relationship of the Distal surfaces of the primary second molars are observed in centric occlusion. These surfaces are called the **terminus** or terminal plane. The terminus of the second primary molars in centric occlusion have predictive value in the development of the occlusion of the permanent or secondary teeth because the overall Occlusal pattern presented by an individual at an early age will often be maintained into adulthood (Figure 20–5).

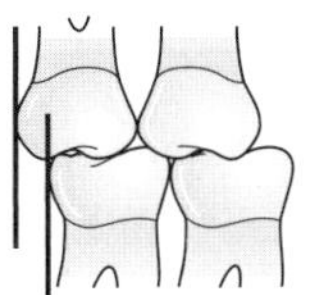

Figure 20–5 Primary second molar terminus

By age 3, the occlusion of the twenty primary teeth is frequently established. The relationship of the Distal terminal planes of opposing second primary molar teeth may be represented by one of three scenarios (Figure 20–6A, B, and C). A flush terminal plane means that the anterior-posterior position of the Distal surfaces of opposing primary second molars are in the same vertical plane. Distal-step terminal plane is a description given when the mandibular

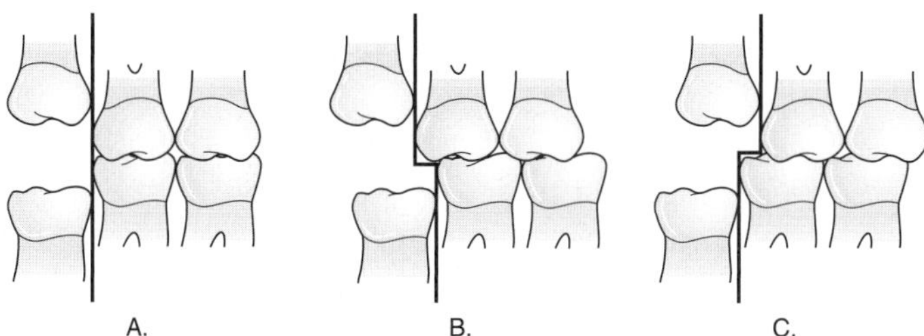

Figure 20–6 Illustrations representing primary molar terminus (terminal plane) of second primary molars in centric occlusion: (A) Flush (B) Mesial-step (C) Distal-step

second primary molar terminus is Distal to the maxillary primary terminus. Mesial-step terminus occurs when the terminal plane of the mandibular second primary molar is Mesial to the maxillary primary terminus.

Classifications of Occlusion During the Mixed Dentition

During childhood, the transitional phase of occlusion development is called the mixed dentition. An illustration of the development of first permanent molar relationships from primary dentition occlusion to initial interarch first molar occlusion contact at approximately age 7 to final occlusion at age 12 is shown in Figure 20–7. Research on occlusion has verified that the Distal-step terminus always leads to a Class II initial contact and final permanent first molar occlusion. Development of the occlusion from flush terminus, end-on,

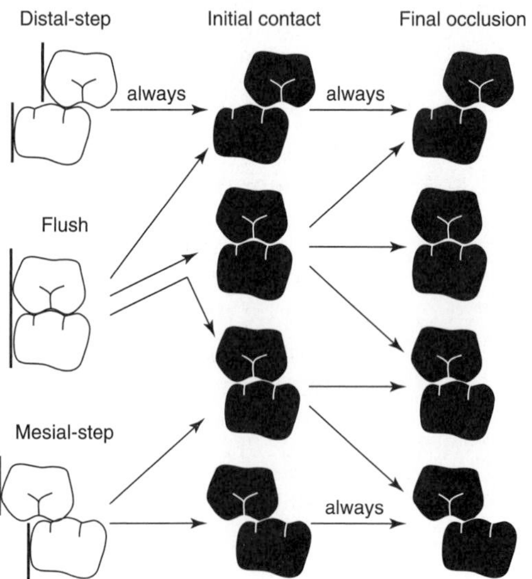

Figure 20–7 Illustration representing the development of occlusion from initial contact; outlined crown images represent three terminal plane relationships of primary second molars (about age 5 years); darkened crown images represent various permanent first molar relationships at initial occluding contact (about age 6.5 years); at full occlusion contact (about age 12 years) (Data from Arya 1973, Carlsen 1960, and Moyers 1973)

and Class I initial contact is highly variable. Long-term disposition of a Mesial-step terminus depends on the degree of the step. A mild Mesial-step primary occlusion often leads to a Class I permanent molar relationship at initial contact, although not predictably so. If the primary occlusion demonstrates an exaggerated Mesial-step, then initial contact and final permanent occlusion will always be a Class III.

Midline Alignment

Another characteristic of an "ideal" centric occlusion that may be assessed in the determination of occlusion/malocclusion is **midline alignment**. In an "ideal" dentition, the dental midlines between the maxillary and mandibular central incisors should be coincident (see Figure 20–1). When malalignment occurs between the midlines of the teeth, then the number of millimeters the mandibular arch is off to the right or left is recorded (Figure 20–8).

Overjet

The "ideal" overjet or horizontal overlap in centric occlusion is determined by measuring the number of millimeters between the Facial surface of the mandibular and the Incisal edge of the maxillary incisors in centric occlusion. In an ideal dentition, there are 1 to 2 mm of overjet. The millimeter markings on a periodontal probe are ideal for taking this measurement (Figure 20–9). Although the amount of overjet varies within the dentition, it is customary to record (only) the tooth and the largest amount of overjet.

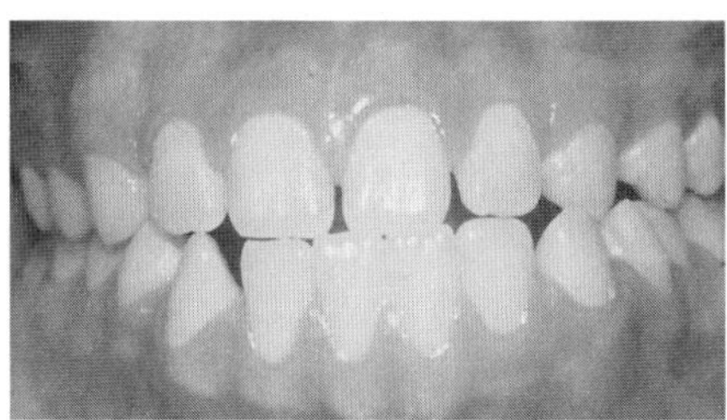

Figure 20–8 Photograph of anterior view shown with midline alignment that is not coincident

Universal System

#3 #4 #5 #6 #7 #8 #9 #10 #11 #12 #13

#31 #30 #29 #28 #27 #26 #25 #24 #23 #22 #21 #20 #19

Palmer System

6| 5| 4| 3| 2| 1| |1 |2 |3 |4 |5

7| 6| 5| 4| 3| 2| 1| |1 |2 |3 |4 |5 |6

ISO/FDI System

16 15 14 13 12 11 21 22 23 24 25

47 46 45 44 43 42 41 31 32 33 34 35 36

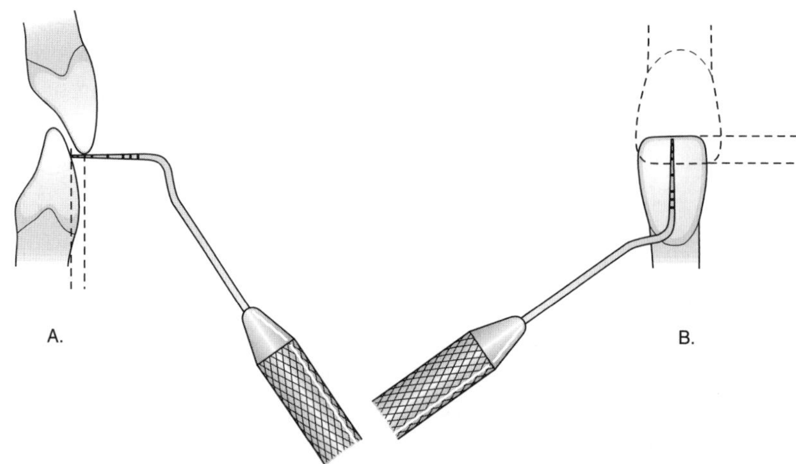

Figure 20–9
(A) Measuring overjet
(B) Measuring overbite

Overbite

The amount of overbite or vertical overlap in centric occlusion is determined by measuring the number of millimeters the maxillary anterior teeth vertically overlap the mandibular anterior teeth. Sometimes, word descriptors are used instead of millimeters. In an "ideal" dentition, there are 1 to 2 mm of overbite; the maxillary Incisal edges vertically overlap the Incisal third of the mandibular incisors in centric occlusion (see Plate 33 and Figure 20–1). "Moderate" overbite is 3 to 6 mm or the maxillary Incisal edges overlap the middle third of the mandibular incisors. "Excessive" or "deep" overbite is greater than 6 mm or when the overlap extends into the cervical third of the mandibular incisors or even beyond (Figure 20–10A and B).

End-to-End Bite

If the anterior teeth meet end to end or edge to edge, then there is no vertical overlap of the anterior teeth and it is referred to as **end-to-end bite** (Figure 20–11 and Plate 39).

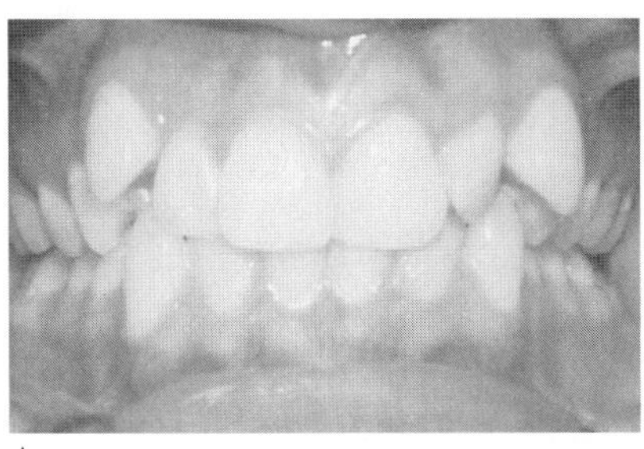

A.

Universal System

#3 #4 #5 #6 #7 #8 #9 #10 #11 #12 #13 #14
#30 #29 #28 #27 #26 #25 #24 #23 #22 #21 #20 #19

Palmer System

6| 5| 4| 3| 2| 1| |1 |2 |3 |4 |5 |6
6| 5| 4| 3| 2| 1| |1 |2 |3 |4 |5 |6

ISO/FDI System

16 15 14 13 12 11 21 22 23 24 25 26
46 45 44 43 42 41 31 32 33 34 35 36

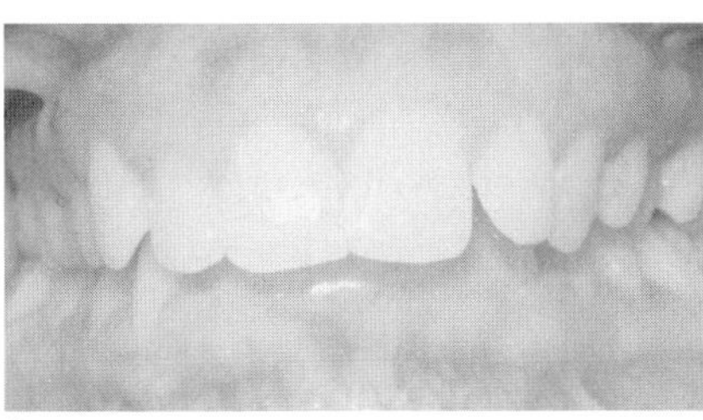

B.

Universal System

#3 #4 #5 #6 #7 #8 #9 #10 #11 #12 #13 #14
#30 #29 #28 #27 #26 #25 #24 #23 #22 #21 #20 #19

Palmer System

6| 5| 4| 3| 2| 1| |1 |2 |3 |4 |5 |6
6| 5| 4| 3| 2| 1| |1 |2 |3 |4 |5 |6

ISO/FDI System

16 15 14 13 12 11 21 22 23 24 25 26
46 45 44 43 42 41 31 32 33 34 35 36

Figure 20–10 Photographs of anterior views shown with overbites: (A) Moderate overbite (B) Excessive overbite

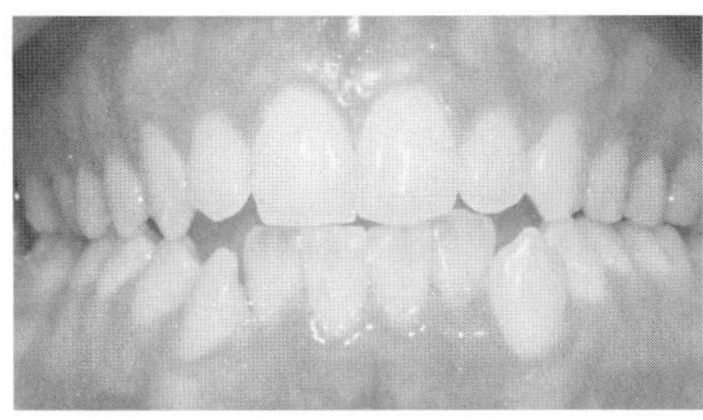

Universal System

#3 #4 #5 #6 #7 #8 #9 #10 #11 #12 #13 #14
#30 #29 #28 #27 #26 #25 #24 #23 #22 #21 #20 #19

Palmer System

6| 5| 4| 3| 2| 1| |1 |2 |3 |4 |5 |6
6| 5| 4| 3| 2| 1| |1 |2 |3 |4 |5 |6

ISO/FDI System

16 15 14 13 12 11 21 22 23 24 25 26
46 45 44 43 42 41 31 32 33 34 35 36

Figure 20–11 End-to-end-bite

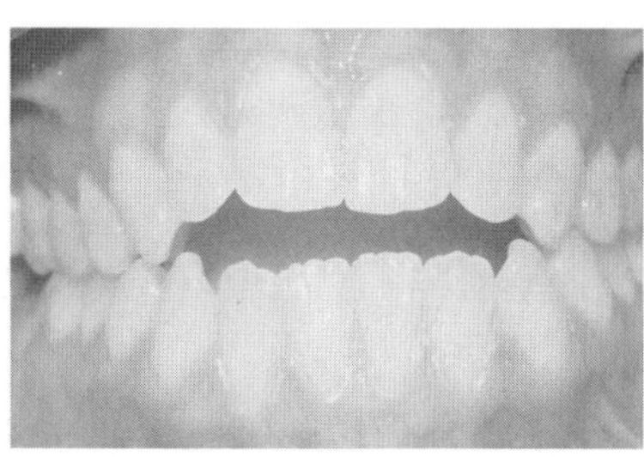

Figure 20–12 Openbite

Universal System
#3 #4 #5 #6 #7 #8 #9 #10 #11 #12 #13
#30 #29 #28 #27 #26 #25 #24 #23 #22 #21 #20

Palmer System
6| 5| 4| 3| 2| 1| |1 |2 |3 |4 |5
6| 5| 4| 3| 2| 1| |1 |2 |3 |4 |5

ISO/FDI System
16 15 14 13 12 11 21 22 23 24 25
46 45 44 43 42 41 31 32 33 34 35

Openbite

An **openbite** is present when there is a vertical overlap deficiency in centric occlusion (Figure 20–12 and Plate 40).

Crossbite

A **crossbite** occurs when the maxillary teeth do not have an "ideal" overjet or do not horizontally overlap the mandibular teeth. Crossbites can involve single teeth, a segment of teeth, quadrants, or involve the whole arch. Crossbites frequently occur because of malpositioning of a tooth (teeth) in the opposing arch. In the anterior dentition, a crossbite occurs when a mandibular tooth (teeth) is Facial rather than Lingual to the maxillary anterior teeth (Figure 20–13), a condition called **underjet**.

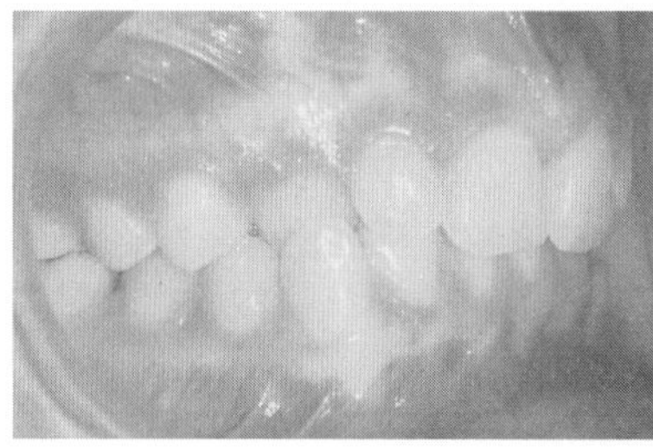

Universal System
#3 #4 #5 #6 #7 #8 #9 #10
#30 #29 #28 #27 #26 #25 #24

Palmer System
6| 5| 4| 3| 2| 1| |1 |2
6| 5| 4| 3| 2| 1| |1

ISO/FDI System
17 16 15 14 13 12 11 21 22
47 46 45 44 43 42 41 31

Figure 20–13 Anterior crossbite involving teeth #6 and #27

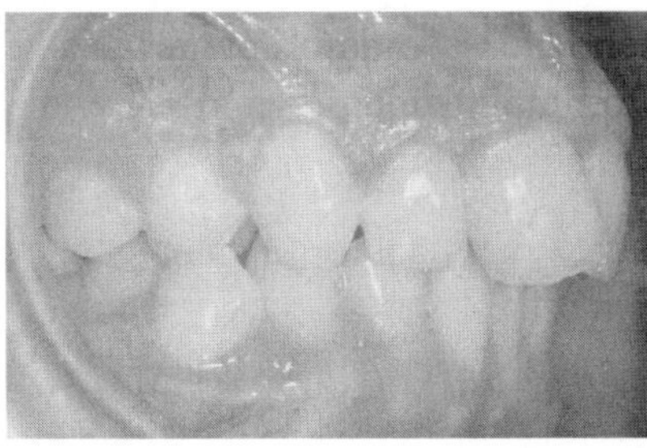

Universal System
#4 #5 #6 #7 #8 #9
#29 #28 #27 #26 #25 #24 #23

Palmer System
5| 4| 3| 2| 1| |1
5| 4| 3| 2| 1| |1 |2

ISO/FDI System
15 14 13 12 11 21
45 44 43 42 41 31 32

Figure 20–14 Posterior crossbite: single-tooth crossbite involving teeth #5 and #28

Crossbites in the posterior segments have more variations because of the possibilities with the intercuspation of multicusped posterior teeth. Normally, there is an intercuspation of the posterior teeth where the mandibular Lingual cusps contact the maxillary Occlusal surfaces in centric occlusion. In posterior crossbites, a number of possibilities can occur that alter the expected intercusping relationship (Figure 20–14).

In the clinical setting, openbites, end-to-end bites, and crossbites should be documented by indicating which teeth are involved and a description of the discrepancy.

Review Questions

Multiple Choice

Directions: Select the letter of the choice that *best* answers the question.

1. Which of the following is *not* a characteristic of an "ideal" centric occlusion?
   a. Coincident midlines
   b. Class I molar and canine relationships
   c. 1 to 2 millimeters of overjet
   d. 4 to 6 millimeters of overbite

2. The key teeth used to describe centric occlusion in a permanent dentition using Angle's Classification of Malocclusion are:
   a. permanent canines.
   b. permanent first molars.
   c. permanent second molars.
   d. permanent first molars and canines.
3. The key anatomical feature of the mandibular molar used in Angle's Classification of Malocclusion is the:
   a. Mesio-Buccal cusp.
   b. Mesio-Lingual cusp.
   c. Mesio-Buccal (Buccal) groove.
   d. Mesio-Lingual groove.
4. Which of the following statements best describes a Class II malocclusion?
   a. Distocclusion
   b. Mesiocclusion
   c. Neutrocclusion
   d. All of the above
5. What classification of malocclusion would be most likely to occur if the cusp tips of the permanent maxillary canines aligned with the cusp tip of the mandibular first premolar?
   a. Class I
   b. Class II, Division 1
   c. Class II, Division 2
   d. Class III
6. Which of the following is used to assess the occlusion of a child 4 years of age?
   a. The relationship of the Distal surfaces of the primary canines
   b. The cusp and groove relationships of the primary first molars
   c. The cusp and groove relationships of the primary second molars
   d. The terminus of the primary second molars
7. Class III permanent molar occlusion will likely have resulted from which of the following initial contacts of the permanent first molars?
   a. Flush primary terminus
   b. Distal-step primary terminus
   c. Mesial-step primary terminus
   d. An exaggerated Mesial-step primary terminus
8. The profile of the chin of a typical Class II, Division I malocclusion is:
   a. retrognathic.
   b. protruded.
   c. prognathic.

9. The vertical overlap of the maxillary to the mandibular anterior teeth is known as:
   a. overbite.
   b. overjet.
   c. underjet.
   d. crossbite.
10. Overjet is measured from the:
    a. Incisal edge of the most extreme maxillary central incisor to the Incisal edge of the mandibular central incisors in centric occlusion.
    b. Facial surface of the mandibular incisor to the Incisal edge of the most extreme maxillary central incisor in centric occlusion.
    c. Incisal edge of the maxillary incisors in relationship to the crown length of the mandibular incisors in centric occlusion.

Answers

1. **d,** 2. **b,** 3. **c,** 4. **a,** 5. **d,** 6. **d,** 7. **d,** 8. **a,** 9. **a,** 10. **b**

References

Angle, E. H. (1907). *Treatment of malocclusion of the teeth* (7th ed.). Philadelphia: SS White Dental Mfg. Co.

Bath-Balogh, M., & Fehrenbach, M. J. (1997). *Illustrated dental embryology, histology, and anatomy*. Philadelphia: W. B. Saunders Company.

Brand, R. W., & Isselhard, D. E. (1994). *Anatomy of orofacial structures*. St. Louis: The C. V. Mosby Company.

Darby, M. L., & Walsh, M. M. (1994). *Dental hygiene theory and practice*. Philadelphia: W. B. Saunders Company.

Du, S. Q., Rinchuse, D. J., Zullo, T. G., & Rinchuse, D. J. (1998). Reliability of three methods of occlusion classification. *American Journal of Orthodontics and Dentofacial Orthopedics*, 113, 463–470.

Karst, N. S., & Smith, S. K. (1998). *Dental anatomy, a self-instructional program*. San Mateo, CA: Appleton & Lange.

Lewis, S. J., & Lehman, I. A. (1929). Observations on growth changes in the teeth and dental arches. *Dental Cosmos*, 70, 480–499.

Moorrees, C. F. A. (1959). *The dentition of the growing child*. Cambridge: Harvard University Press.

Ngan, P., & Fields, H. W. (1997). Open bite: A review of etiology and management. *Pediatric Dentistry*, 19, 91–98.

Rinchuse, D. J., & Rinchuse, D.J. (1989). Ambiguities of angle's classification. *The Angle Orthodontist*, 59 (4), 295–298.

Tang, E. L., & Wei, S. H. (1993). Recording and measuring malocclusion: A review of the literature. *American Journal of Orthodontics and Dentofacial Orthopedics*, 103, 344–351.

Wilkins, E. (1994). *Clinical Practice of the Dental Hygienist*. Balitmore: Williams & Wilkins.

Woelfel, J. B., & Scheid, R. C. (1997). *Dental anatomy, Its relevance to dentistry*. Baltimore: Williams & Wilkins.

Woodall, I. (Ed.) (1993). *Comprehensive Dental Hygiene Care*. St. Louis: The C.V. Mosby Company.

CHAPTER 21

Dental Anomalies and Developmental Malformations

Key Terms

Amelogenesis Imperfecta
Anodontia
Concrescence
Dens In Dente
Dentinogenesis Imperfecta
Dilaceration
Distomolar
Enamel Hypoplasia
Enamel Pearl
Fusion
Gemination
Mesiodens
Paramolar
Peg-shaped lateral incisors

PRIMARY CODE	SECONDARY CODE
X = Missing	-A = Anomaly (in blue)
	SU (in diamond) = Supernumerary (blue outline)

Introduction

Dental abnormalities can occur from local, systemic, and hereditary factors during tooth development. These malformations may be present at birth and are referred to as congenital, or the defects become clinically apparent later in life.

Developmental Malformations During Tooth Germ Initiation

The developmental malformations that result during tooth germ initiation include the following:

- **Anodontia**. True anodontia is the absence of teeth that may affect either the Deciduous or permanent dentition.
- **Partial anodontia.** One or more Missing teeth that may affect either the Deciduous or permanent teeth.
- **Supernumerary teeth.** Extra teeth that occur in the maxilla or mandible and may resemble the shape of a normal tooth.
- **Accessory teeth.** Teeth in excess of the regular number and do not resemble the form of a normal tooth.
- **Mesiodens**. Small tooth located between the maxillary central incisor teeth that appears conical in shape (Figure 21–1A and B and Plate 41)
- **Distomolar**. Smaller than normal size tooth located Distal to the third molar (Figure 21–2).
- **Paramolar**. Small tooth located Buccal or Lingual to the molars.

Universal System
#3 A #5 C #7 #8 #9 #10 #11 #12 #13

Palmer System
6| E| 4| C| 2| 1|1 |2 |3 |4 |5

ISO/FDI System
16 55 14 53 12 11 21 22 23 24 25

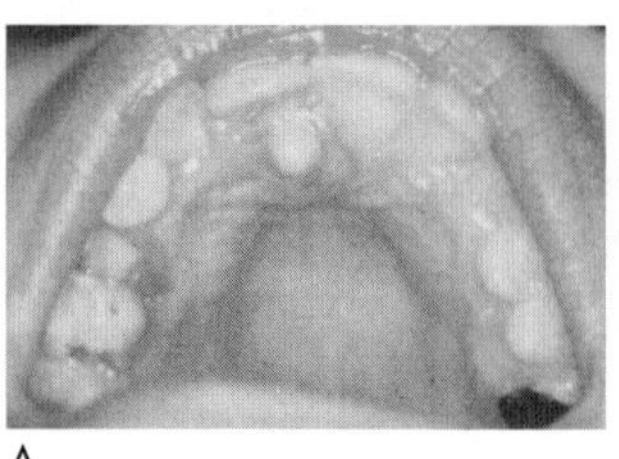

A.

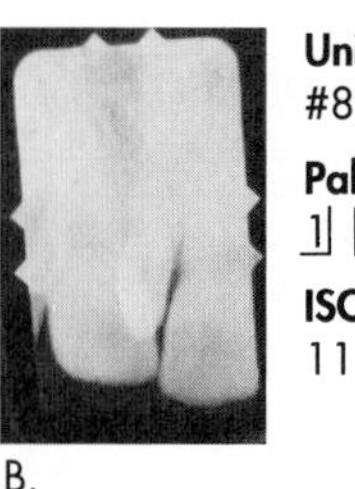

B.

Universal System
#8 #9

Palmer System
1| |1

ISO/FDI System
11 21

Figure 21–1 Mesiodens: (A) Photograph shown with an erupted accessory tooth between teeth #8 and #9 (B) Periapical radiograph shows the mesiodens appears as a radiopaque image (Courtesy Ronald E. Gier, DMD, MSD)

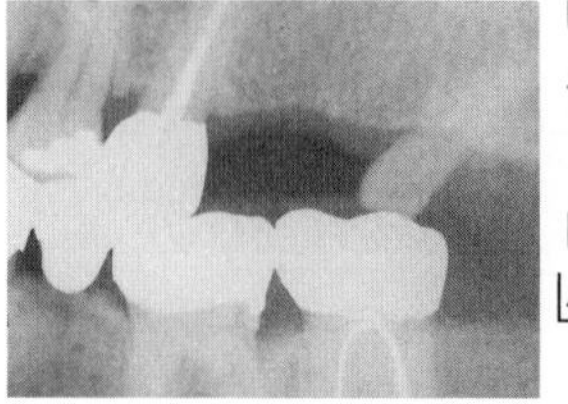

Figure 21–2 Bitewing radiograph shown of a distomolar on the posterior maxillary arch

Universal System
#12 #13 ↙
#19 #18

Palmer System
|4 |5 ↙
|6 |7

ISO/FDI System
24 25 ↙
36 37

Charting Supernumerary Teeth on Anatomic, Geometric, and Numeric Coding System Charts

To indicate the accessory tooth (mesiodens) located between teeth #8 and #9 shown in Figure 21–1 on the anatomic and geometric dental charts, locate the tooth designation numbers and use a blue pencil to draw a vertical diamond "◇" symbol between the tooth diagrams on the Lingual surface view. Print the uppercase letters "SU" inside ◇. To further indicate that the tooth is erupted, draw the point of the symbol so that it is positioned at the Incisal edge. To designate an Unerupted accessory tooth, draw the diamond symbol on the dental chart in the direction the tooth appears to be facing on the dental radiograph, located between the involved teeth adjacent to the root diagrams. Label the area "SU" (Figure 21–3A and B).

To indicate an accessory tooth on a numeric coding system chart, locate the tooth designation numbers and in the boxes located above or below the tooth number or on the vertical line between the tooth numbers draw and label the diamond symbol. To show that the tooth is either an erupted or

18	17	16	15	14	13	12	11	21	22	23	24	25	26	27	28
8	7	6	5	4	3	2	1	1	2	3	4	5	6	7	8
1	2	3	4	5	6	7	8	9	10	11	12	13	14	15	16
32	31	30	29	28	27	26	25	24	23	22	21	20	19	18	17
8	7	6	5	4	3	2	1	1	2	3	4	5	6	7	8
48	47	46	45	44	43	42	41	31	32	33	34	35	36	37	38

SU

A.

Figure 21–3 (A) Anatomic chart; accessory tooth (mesiodens) shown charted between tooth #8 and #9 and distomolar shown charted behind tooth #16

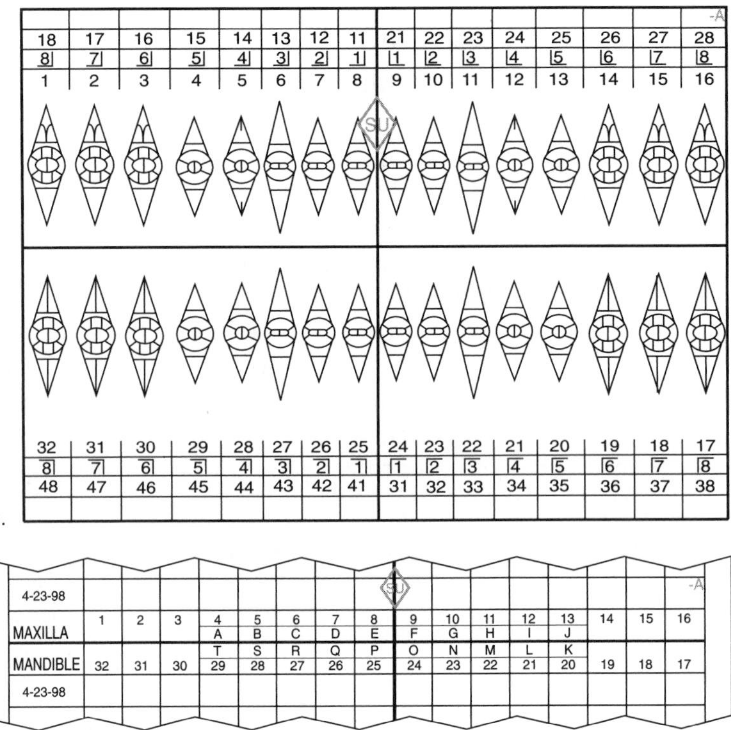

Figure 21–3 (B) Geometric chart (C) Numeric coding system chart; accessory tooth (mesiodens) shown charted between tooth #8 and #9 and distomolar shown charted behind tooth #16

Unerupted accessory tooth, follow the previously mentioned procedures (Figure 21–3C).

To indicate the distomolar shown in Figure 21–2 on all three charts, print the secondary code "-A" for Anomaly in the upper right corner of the box that designates the third molar (see Figure 21–3A, B, and C). In the progress notes, enter the tooth number of the involved tooth followed by the name of the developmental abnormality accompanied by a detailed description of the clinical features.

Developmental Malformations During Tooth Germ Morphodifferentiation

The developmental malformations that result during tooth germ morphodifferentiation include the following:

- **Peg-shaped lateral incisors**. Maxillary lateral incisor is narrow and conical in shape (Figure 21–4).
- **Dens in dente** (dens invaginatus). The enamel organ invaginates or infolds into the crown and produces a "tooth within a tooth" (Figure 21–5).
- **Gemination**. The inadequate division of a tooth germ that results in the incomplete formation of two teeth that appear as two crowns with a single root (Figure 21–6 and Plate 42).
- **Fusion**. Two adjoining tooth germs unite to form a tooth with a single crown that may or may not have two roots (Figure 21–7 and Plate 43).
- **Enamel pearl** or enameloma. Spherical-shaped mass of enamel located on the root surface at the furcation area that is formed as a result of displaced ameloblasts (Figure 21–8 and Plate 44).
- **Dilaceration**. Abnormal curvature of the roots that produces a very sharp bend (Figure 21–9).
- **Concrescence**. Two independently formed adjacent teeth form a single tooth by the fusion of the cementum.

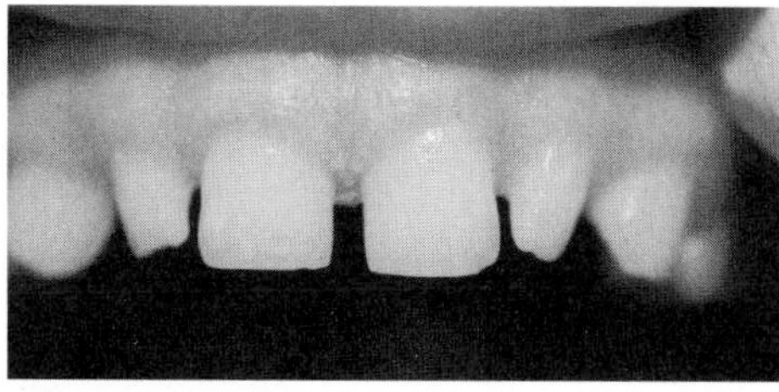

Universal System
#6 #7 #8 #9 #10 #11 #12

Palmer System
3| 2| 1| |1 |2 |3 |4

ISO/FDI System
13 12 11 21 22 23 24

Figure 21–4 Peg-shaped lateral incisors

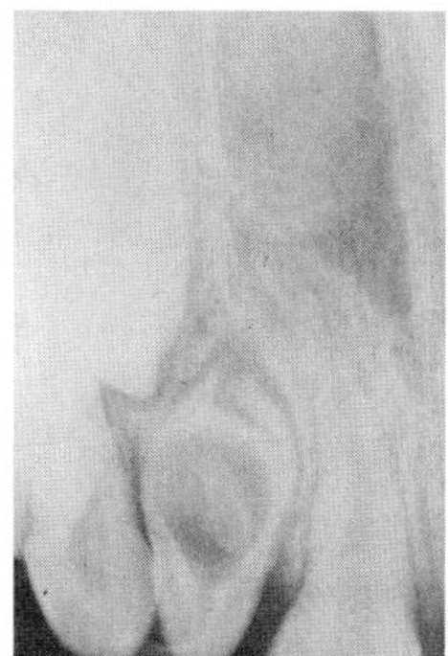

Universal System
#5
B #6 #7 #8

Palmer System
5|
D| 3| 2| 1|

ISO/FDI System
14
54 13 12 11

Figure 21–5 Dens in dente (Courtesy Ronald E. Gier, DMD, MSD)

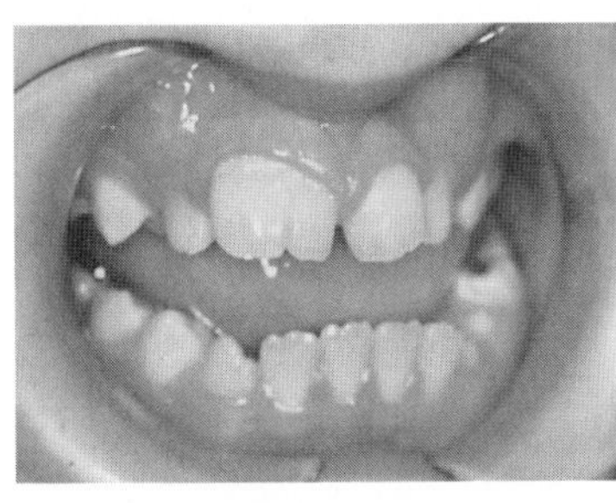

Figure 21–6 Gemination (Courtesy Ronald E. Gier, DMD, MSD)

Universal System

#5 #6 #7 #8 #9 #10 #11
#29 #28 #27 #26 #25 #24 #23 #22 #21 #20 #19

Palmer System

4| 3| 2| 1| |1 |2 |3
5| 4| 3| 2| 1| |1 |2 |3 |4 |5 |6

ISO/FDI System

14 13 12 11 21 22 23
45 44 43 42 41 31 32 33 34 35 36

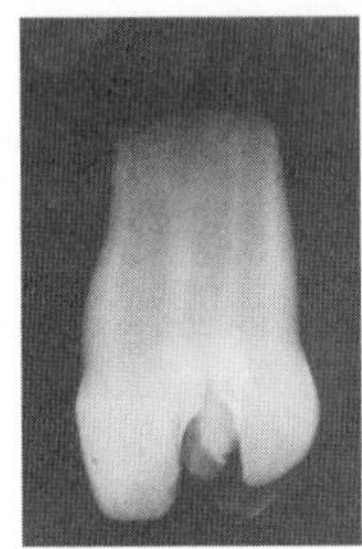

Universal System

(#6 #7)

Palmer System

(3| 2|)

ISO/FDI System

(13 12)

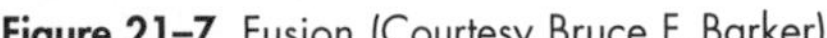

Figure 21–7 Fusion (Courtesy Bruce F. Barker)

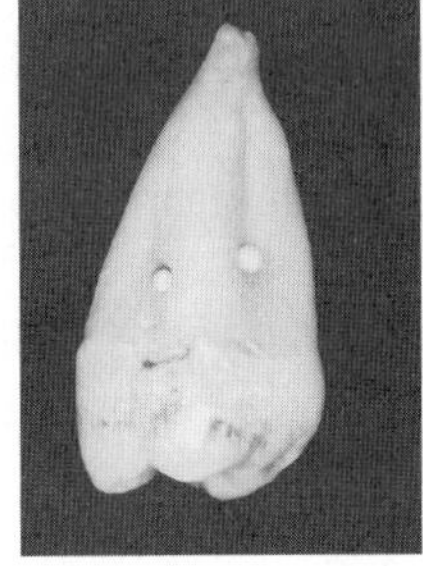

Universal System

#16

Palmer System

|8

ISO/FDI System

28

Figure 21–8 Enamel pearls

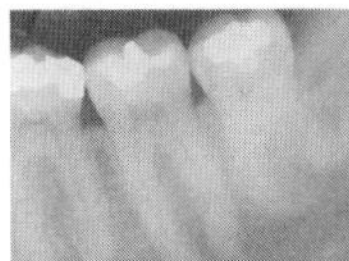

Universal System

#19 #18 #17

Palmer System

|6 |7 |8

ISO/FDI System

36 37 38

Figure 21–9 Dilaceration of the Mesial and Distal roots of the mandibular third molar (Courtesy Olsen Dental)

Developmental Malformations During Apposition of the Enamel and Dentin Matrices

The developmental malformations that result during the apposition of the enamel and dentin matrices include the following:

- **Enamel hypoplasia**. Incomplete development of ameloblasts that causes a reduction in the quantity and thickness of the enamel.
- Hereditary enamel hypoplasia. The condition is inherited as a dominant trait.
  - **Amelogenesis imperfecta**. Decreased calcification of enamel produces an extremely thin and fragile exterior tooth surface that fractures off easily (Plate 45).
- Hereditary dentin hypoplasia. Acquired through genetic transmission.
  - **Dentinogenesis imperfecta**. Progressive replacement of the pulp chambers and canals by atypical dentin until the areas are completely filled. The teeth are gray or brown and appear opalescent (Plate 46).
- Systemic enamel hypoplasia. Acquired through nutritional deficiencies or congenital syphilis.
  - Hutchinson's incisors. Abnormally shaped incisor teeth that broaden at the cervical and middle thirds then become narrower and notched at the Incisal edges.
  - Mulberry molars. Narrow and irregularly shaped crowns with numerous tiny rounded masses of enamel located on the Occlusal surfaces of permanent first molars.
- Local enamel hypoplasia. Hypocalcification that results from a bacterial infection or trauma.
  - Turner's tooth. Local trauma or infection on a Deciduous maxillary anterior tooth disrupts the ameloblast cells of the developing permanent tooth and produces a defect in the enamel as shown on tooth #8 in Figure 21–4.

Charting Developmental Malformations on Anatomic, Geometric, and Numeric Coding System Charts

To indicate localized or generalized developmental tooth abnormalities on the anatomic, geometric, and numeric coding system charts, locate the sections referred to as "Clinical" and "X-ray Examination." Use a black pen to enter the name of the developmental abnormality and the tooth numbers of the involved teeth accompanied by a detailed description of the clinical features.

Review Questions

Multiple Choice

Directions: Select the letter of the choice that *best* answers the question.

1. The developmental abnormality that appears as two crowns with a single root is called:
   a. concrescence. b. gemination.
   c. fusion. d. distomolar.
2. Small rounded masses of enamel located on the root surface are called:
   a. mesiodens. b. Epstien's pearls.
   c. enamel pearls. d. cementomas.
3. The developmental disturbance that results from the splitting of a single tooth germ is called:
   a. concrescence. b. gemination.
   c. fusion. d. distomolar.
4. The anomaly that produces a sharp bend in the root is called:
   a. dilaceration. b. concrescence.
   c. ankylosis. d. none of the above.
5. The term referred to as "tooth within a tooth" is:
   a. dentinogenesis imperfecta. b. dens in dente.
   c. amelogenesis imperfecta. d. gemination.
6. The absence of enamel on the teeth is the clinical feature of:
   a. amelogenesis hypoplasia. b. dentinogenesis imperfecta.
   c. hereditary dentin hypoplasia. d. amelogenesis imperfecta.
7. The developmental disturbance that affects the lateral incisors is known as:
   a. lateral pegs. b. peg-shaped laterals.
   c. microlateral. d. all of the above.

8. A congenital condition that results in mulberry molars and Hutchinson's incisors is:
   a. chicken pox.
   b. syphilis.
   c. meningitis.
   d. herpetic gingivostomatitis.
9. The term that implies the lack of teeth is:
   a. partial anodontia.
   b. Supernumerary.
   c. anodontia.
   d. microdontia.
10. The teeth involved may appear opalescent in which of the following developmental disturbances?
    a. Dens in dente
    b. Amelogenesis imperfecta
    c. Enamel hypoplasia
    d. Dentinogenesis imperfecta

Answers

1. **b,** 2. **c,** 3. **c,** 4. **a,** 5. **b,** 6. **d,** 7. **b,** 8. **b,** 9. **c,** 10. **d**

References

Dorland's pocket medical dictionary (28th ed.). (1994). Philadelphia: W. B. Saunders Company.

Haring, J. I., & Ibsen, O. A. C. (1992). Developmental disorders. In O. A. C. Ibsen and J. A. Phelan, *Oral pathology for the dental hygienist* (267–271, 395–399). Philadelphia: W. B. Saunders Company.

Hintze, H., & Wenzel, A. (1990). Accuracy of clinical diagnosis for the detection of dentoalveolar anomalies with panoramic radiography as validating criterion. *Journal of Dentistry for Children*, 119–123.

Jenkins, S., Addy, M., & Newcombe, R. (1989). Comparison of two commercially available chlorhexidine mouthrinses: II. Effects on plaque reformation, gingivitis, and tooth staining. *Clinical Reviews Dentistry*, 11, 12.

Thomas, C. L. (1997). *Taber's cyclopedic medical dictionary*. Philadelphia: F. A. Davis Company.

Villa, Vigil M. A., Arenal, A. A., & Gonzalez, M. A. R. (1989). Notation of numerical abnormalities by an addition to the F.D.I. system. *Quintessence International*, 20.

CHAPTER 22

Restorative Problems

Key Terms

Deficient Margin
Direct Restorations
Fractured Restoration
Indirect Restorations
Interface
Margin
Marginal Defects
Open Margin
Overhanging Margin
Undercontoured

PRIMARY CODE	SECONDARY CODE
M = Mesial	-S = Silver Amalgam (solid blue)
I = Incisal (#6–#11 and #22–#27)	FX = Fracture (in red)
O = Occlusal (#1–#5, #12–#16, #17–#21, and #27–#32)	• = and also
D = Distal	"/\" = deficient margin (in red)
F = Facial (#6–#11 and #22–#27)	"△" = open margin (in red)
B = Buccal (#1–#5, #12–#16, #17–#21, and #27–#32)	"▲" = overhanging margin (in red)
L = Lingual	
X = Missing	

Introduction

Dental restorations are classified as **direct restorations** when the restorative materials are placed directly into the cavity preparation, and **indirect restorations** are the restorations fabricated outside the mouth then inserted into the cavity preparation and cemented or bonded into place. Direct restorations are more likely to have deficiencies at the margins where the restorative material meets the tooth structures and they are referred to as **marginal defects.**

Marginal Irregularities

The junction where the tooth structure meets the restorative material is referred to as the **interface** or **margin** of the restoration. A small gap at this interface is acceptable if it does not exceed 50 micrometers. Figure 22–1 is an illustration of a clinically acceptable margin.

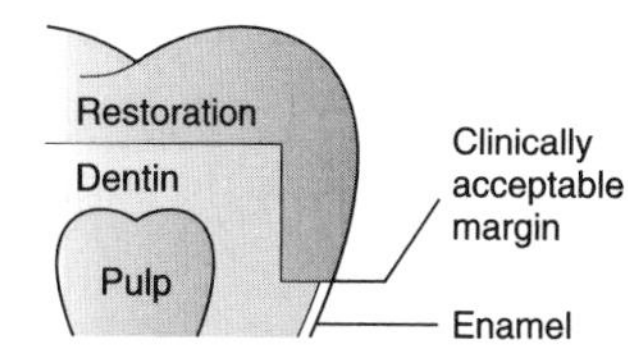

Figure 22–1 Acceptable margin

An **overhanging margin** of a restoration does not conform to the contour of the tooth and usually has an excessive amount of restorative material at the interface. A marginal overhang that involves the proximal tooth surface can be caused by improper placement of the matrix band and/or the wedge (Figure 22–2A). Figure 22–3 is a bitewing radiograph that shows a proximal overhang.

An **undercontoured** or **deficient margin** can be the result of a misdirected carving or misplaced matrix and/or wedge (Figure 22–2B). Figure 22–2C shows

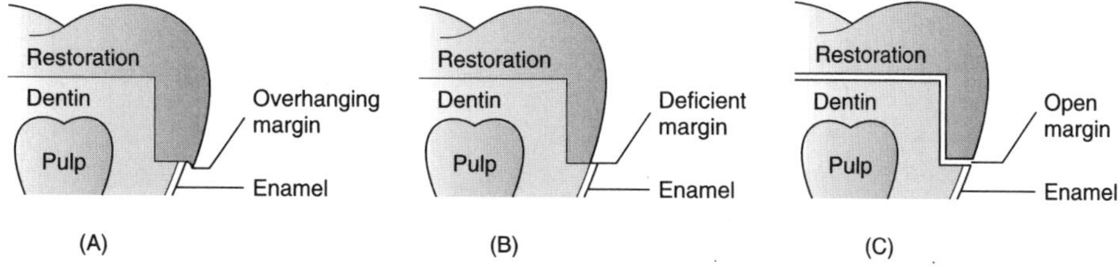

Figure 22–2 Defective margins: (A) Overhanging margin (B) Deficient margin (C) Open margin

an illustration of an **open margin**. This marginal defect has a distinct space between the wall of the cavity preparation and the restorative material.

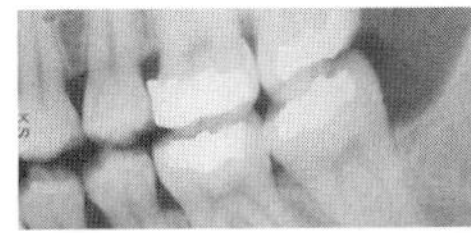

Figure 22–3 Bitewing radiograph shown with an overhanging margin on the Mesial surface of tooth #14

Universal System
#12 #13 #14 #15
#21 #20 #19 #18

Palmer System
|4 |5 |6 |7
|4 |5 |6 |7

ISO/FDI System
24 25 26 27
34 35 36 37

Fractured Restoration

Direct and indirect restorative materials are susceptible to becoming Fractured. A **Fractured restoration** can be the result of premature contacts and an increased biting force following the placement of a restoration, or from chewing or biting a very hard substance.

Fractured restorations are not always easily detected in the mouth or on dental radiographs. Figure 22–4 is a bitewing radiograph that does not show the Fractured restoration present on tooth #15. A photograph of the same area shows the Occlusal surface of tooth #15 with a Fractured Silver Amalgam restoration (Plate 47).

Figure 22–5 and Plate 16 are photograph of tooth #4 that is shown with an Occlusal surface Fracture and a section of the Silver Amalgam restoration missing.

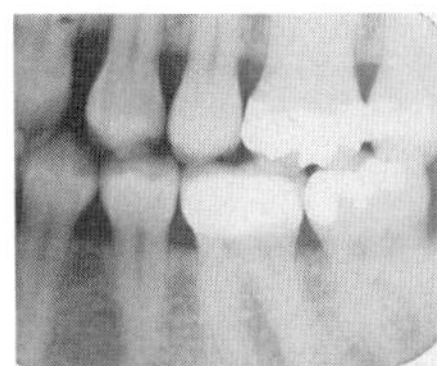

Figure 22–4 Bitewing radiograph that does not show the Fractured Silver Amalgam restoration on tooth #15

Universal System
#11 #12 #13 #14 #15
#21 #20 #19 #18

Palmer System
|3 |4 |5 |6 |7
|4 |5 |6 |7

ISO/FDI System
23 24 25 26 27
34 35 36 37

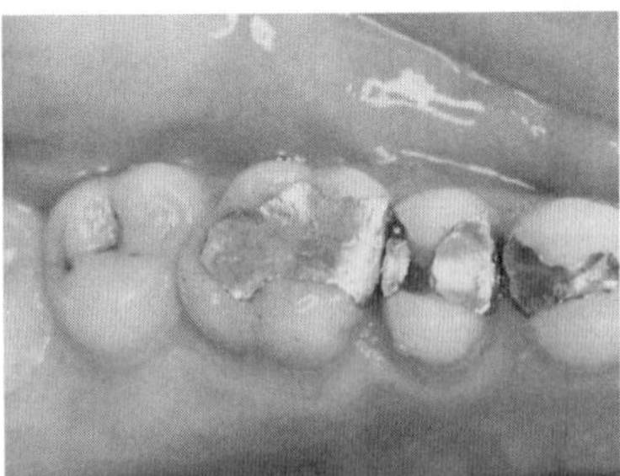

Figure 22–5 Photograph shown with a Fractured restoration on the Occlusal surface of tooth #4

Universal System
#2 #3 #4 #5

Palmer System
7| 6| 5| 4|

ISO/FDI System
17 16 15 14

Charting an Overhanging Margin, Deficient Margin, Open Margin, and Fractured Restoration on an Anatomic Chart

Figure 22–3 shows the Silver Amalgam restoration, MO-S, with proximal surface overhang that involves the Mesial surface of tooth #14. To chart an overhanging restoration on an anatomic chart, locate the tooth designation number and the diagram that depicts the Facial surface. With a red pencil adjacent to the involved tooth surface on the Facial view, draw a triangle and completely fill it in "▼." Tooth #14 is shown with a Mesial overhang in Figure 22–6.

To indicate an open margin, follow the same procedure used for the overhanging margin but do not fill in the triangle "▽." To indicate a deficient margin, also follow the previous procedures and do not connect the top and bottom of the triangle together "\/." Figure 22–6 shows tooth #15 with a MO-S restoration and a deficient margin on the Mesial tooth surface and tooth #16 with a MO-S restoration and an open margin on the Mesial tooth surface.

			FX												
18	17	16	15	14	13	12	11	21	22	23	24	25	26	27	28
8	7	6	5	4	3	2	1	1	2	3	4	5	6	7	8
1	2	3	4	5	6	7	8	9	10	11	12	13	14	15	16
32	31	30	29	28	27	26	25	24	23	22	21	20	19	18	17
8	7	6	5	4	3	2	1	1	2	3	4	5	6	7	8
48	47	46	45	44	43	42	41	31	32	33	34	35	36	37	38

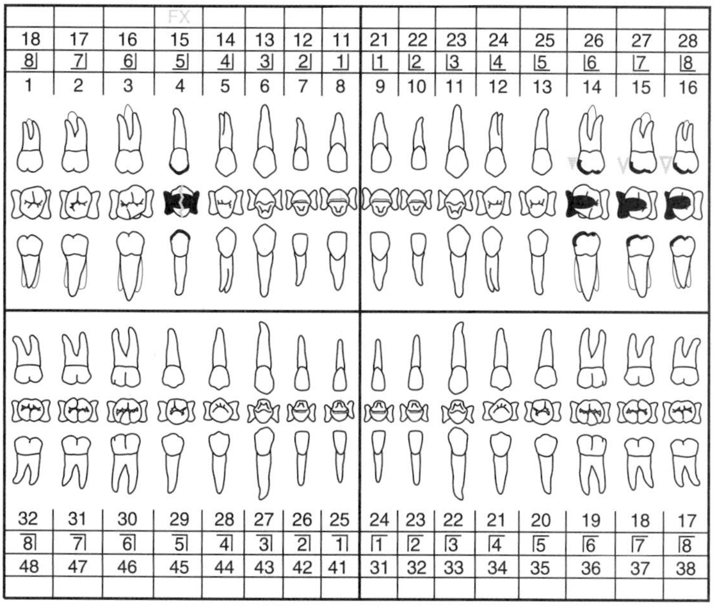

Figure 22–6 Anatomic chart shown with a Mesial overhanging margin on tooth #14, a Mesial deficient margin on tooth #15, a Mesial open margin on tooth #16, and a Fractured restoration on the Occlusal surface of tooth #4

To indicate a Fractured restoration on an anatomic chart, locate the tooth notation number and with a red pencil draw a zigzag line over the involved area and extend it out slightly from each side of the involved area; use only the Occlusal or Incisal surface view. In the box located above or below the tooth number, print the uppercase letters "FX" in red to indicate a Fracture. In Figure 22–5, the MOD-S restoration on tooth #4 is shown with an Occlusal Fracture and this is charted in Figure 22–6.

•

Charting an Overhanging Margin, Deficient Margin, Open Margin, and Fractured Restoration on a Geometric Chart

To chart an overhanging margin on tooth #14 using a geometric chart, locate the tooth notation number and adjacent to the involved tooth surface on the Buccal side use a red pencil to draw a triangle and fill it in completely (Figure 22–7). Follow the same procedure to indicate an open margin but do not fill in the triangle. Show a deficient margin by following the same procedure previously mentioned but do not connect the top and bottom of the triangle. Figure 22–7 is shown with a deficient margin on the Mesial of tooth #15 and an open margin located on the Mesial surface of tooth #16.

To indicate that tooth #4 has a MOD-S restoration with an Occlusal Fracture, use a red pencil to draw a zigzag line and extend it over and slightly past the involved area. In the box located above the tooth diagram, print the uppercase letters "FX" in red (see Figure 22–7).

Charting an Overhanging Margin, Deficient Margin, Open Margin, and Fractured Restoration on a Numeric Coding System Chart

To indicate an overhanging, deficient, and open margin on a numeric coding system chart, use black ink to enter the date above and below the last date entry. In the box above the existing restoration, use a red pencil to indicate

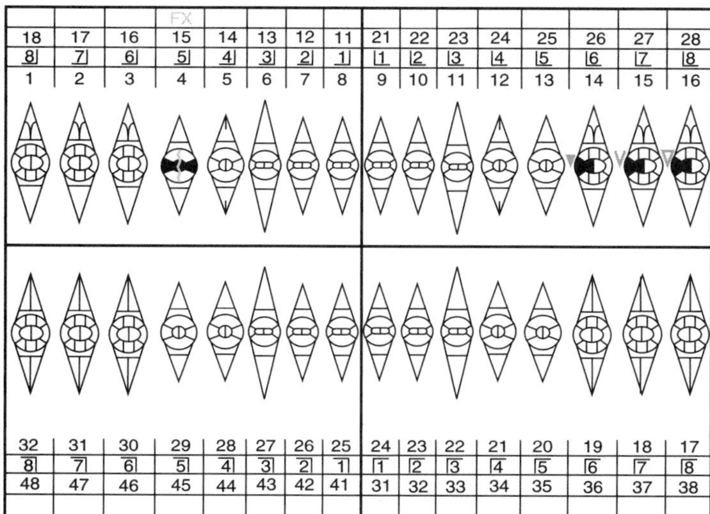

Figure 22–7 Geometric chart shown with a Mesial overhanging margin on tooth #14, a Mesial deficient margin on tooth #15, a Mesial open margin on tooth #16, and a Fractured restoration on the Occlusal surface of tooth #4

the involved tooth surface followed by a hyphen (-) then draw the appropriate symbol. Use the same triangle symbols as those that were formerly utilized to indicate overhang, deficient, and open margins.

When using a numeric coding system chart to indicate a Fractured restoration, locate the box above or below the previously entered restoration. Use a red pencil to print the letter(s) of the Fractured surface(s) separated by a hyphen (-) and followed by the uppercase letters "FX."

In Figure 22–8, the numeric coding chart is read as: on 4-23-95 tooth #4 had a Mesio-Occluso-Distal Silver Amalgam restoration (MOD-S) placed and teeth #14, #15, and #16 had Mesio-Occlusal Silver Amalgam restorations

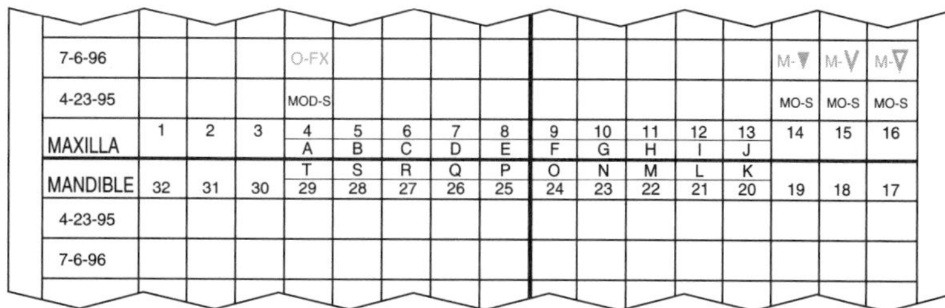

Figure 22–8 Numeric coding system chart shown with a Mesial overhanging margin on tooth #14, a Mesial deficient margin on tooth #15, a Mesial open margin on tooth #16, and a Fractured restoration on the Occlusal surface of tooth #4

(MO-S) placed. On 7-6-96 it indicates that tooth #14 has a Mesial overhanging margin, tooth #15 has a Mesial deficient margin, tooth #16 has an open margin involving the Mesial surface, and tooth #4 has an "O-FX"—a Fracture involving the Occlusal surface.

Review Questions

Matching

Directions: Place the uppercase letter(s) after the number to match each term with the statement that *best* defines it.

A Deficient margin
B Direct restorations
C Fractured restoration
D Indirect restorations
E Marginal defects
F Open margin
G Overhanging margin

1. ___ Marginal irregularities as a whole are referred to as
2. ___ Silver Amalgam and Resin
3. ___ A space located between the restoration and tooth structure
4. ___ Indicated by the excessive amount of restorative material
5. ___ Dental Crown and Gold Inlay
6. ___ Indicated by the decreased quantity of restorative material
7. ___ The letters "FX" are used
8. ___ A triangle filled in completely
9. ___ A broken triangle
10. ___ A zigzag line

Answers

1. **E,** 2. **B,** 3. **F,** 4. **G,** 5. **D,** 6. **A,** 7. **C,** 8. **G,** 9. **A,** 10. **C**

References

Brunsvold, M. A., & Lane, J. J. (1990). The prevalence of overhanging dental restorations and their relationship to periodontal disease. *Journal of Clinical Periodontology*, 17, 67–72.

Dorland's pocket medical dictionary (28th ed.). (1994). Philadelphia: W. B. Saunders Company.

Pack, A. R. C., Coxhead, L. J., & McDonald, B. W. (1990). The prevalence of overhanging margins in posterior amalgam restorations and periodontal consequences. *Journal of Clinical Periodontology*, 17, 145–152.

Rogo, E. J. (1995). Overhang removal: Improving periodontal health adjacent to class II amalgam restorations. *The Journal of Practical Hygiene*, 4(3), 15–23.

Thomas, C. L. (1997). *Taber's cyclopedic medical dictionary*. Philadelphia: F. A. Davis Company.

Glossary

1:1 (one-to-one) magnification-Term denoting a life-sized photograph, 1:1 or 100%. (Appendix A)

2:1 (two-to-one) magnification-Term denoting a twice life-sized photograph, 2:1 or 200%. (Appendix A)

ABFO #2-An "L" shaped scale developed by the American Board of Forensic Odontology for bite mark photography. (Appendix A)

abrasion-The mechanical wearing away and loss of tooth structure. (Chapter 17)

abutment-The teeth/tooth that support(s) a fixed or removable prosthesis. (Chapter 11)

acquired pellicle-Salivary glycoproteins that adhere to the teeth and structures in the oral cavity. (Chapter 15)

acrylic resin-Tooth-colored restorative material made from low molecular weight polymers. (Chapter 10)

acrylic ring-A ring made of the plastic methyl methacrylate that is used when excising a pattern injury from a cadaver. (Appendix A)

acute apical abcess-Rapid onset of inflammation caused by bacterial byproducts with necrosis at the infected pulp canal. (Chapter 16)

acute apical periodontitis-Rapid onset of inflammation of the apical region (alveolar process and tooth) producing pain and pressure. (Chapter 16)

air dry-Method for non-accelerated drying of wet or moist materials. This must be accomplished prior to packaging of the item. (Appendix A)

alloy-A mixture of two or more metals. (Chapters 5 and 6)

alternative light photography-Photographs made using a light source that is not normally considered part of the visible spectrum of light. This includes ultraviolet, both long- and shortwave, and infrared. Term can also be used when photography is accomplished using a commercially produced forensic light source called an Alternative Light Source (ALS) that has either a fixed wavelength or a tunable wavelength selection. (Appendix A)

aluminum shell crown-A temporary crown made from aluminum. (Chapter 8)

alveolar cortical plate defects-Absence of or defects in the alveolar cortical plate. (Chapter 15)

alveolar crest fibers-Part of the principal fiber apparatus; fibers that extend from the alveolar crest at an oblique angle to the cementum just apical to the CEJ. (Chapter 15)

alveolar mucosa-Loosely attached nonkeratinized epithelial tissue located inferior to the attached gingiva. (Chapter 15)

alveolar process-That part of the bone located in the maxilla and mandible that forms the tooth sockets and supports the teeth. (Chapter 1)

alveologingival fibers-Part of the gingival fiber apparatus; fibers that extend from the alveolar crest to the attached and free gingiva. Provides gingival support. (Chapter 15)

ameloblasts-Enamel-forming cells. (Chapter 1)

amelogenesis imperfecta-An inherited condition that produces enamel hypocalcification or hypoplasia. (Chapter 21)

American Dental Association Universal/National System-Tooth designation system in which the primary dentition utilizes continuous uppercase letters A through T and the permanent dentition utilizes continuous numbers 1 through 32. (Chapter 2)

anatomic chart-A charting form that shows the anatomy of the crown and root(s) of each tooth on three views: facial, incisal and occlusal, and lingual. (Chapter 3)

anatomic crown-The part of the tooth covered by enamel. (Chapter 1)

anatomic landmarks-Structures that appear on dental radiographs. (Chapter 4)

anatomic root-The part of the root covered by cementum. (Chapter 1)

Angle's Classification of Malocclusion-A system for classifying the anterior-posterior relationship of the maxillary and mandibular teeth in centric occlusion. (Chapter 20)

anodontia-Absence of teeth. (Chapter 21)

anterior-Anatomical term that refers to the front of. (Chapter 1)

anterior-In the front part of, in front of, or a frontal view. (Appendix A)

apical-Toward the root tip. (Chapter 1)

apical fibers-Part of the principal fiber apparatus; fibers extend from the cementum around the root apex to the adjacent alveolar bone tissue. Functions to resist forces from a vertical direction. (Chapter 15)

apical foramen-Opening in the end of the root tip through which the blood vessels and nerve pass. (Chapter 1)

apicoectomy-Surgical removal of the root apex of a tooth. (Chapter 16)

apposition-A layer of tissue upon another. (Chapter 1)

arch pattern-Curved pattern or pattern of individual tooth marks inflicted during the moment of a single bite. The curvature of the upper or lower jaw, which may be broad, narrow, round, or ovoid. (Appendix A)

arrested caries-A carious lesion that has stabilized. (Chapter 13)

artificial replacement-A prosthesis used to replace a missing body part. (Chapter 12)

assessment-The evaluation of individual dental care through the use of indices. (Chapter 19)

attached gingiva-Parakeratinized or keratinized epithelial tissue that extends from the free gingival groove to the mucogingival junction and is bound firmly to the cementum and alveolar bone tissue. (Chapter 15)

attrition-The loss of tooth structure that results from the forces of mastication. (Chapter 17)

attrition-Wearing away by friction. (Chapter 1)

bacterial plaque-Dense, nonmineralized, mass of colonized microorganisms that adhere firmly to the acquired pellicle. (Chapter 15)

bilateral bridge-A fixed partial denture with abutment teeth on each end. (Chapter 11)

bite mark-A patterned injury on the skin or a dental pattern in foodstuff or on inanimate objects. (Appendix A)

bitewing radiograph-Intraoral film that shows the alveolar bone and crowns of the teeth positioned together. (Chapter 4)

blade-Type of endosseous implant. (Chapter 11)

buccal-Toward the cheek. (Chapter 1)

buccoversion-Positioned toward the cheek (buccal). (Chapter 18)

cadaver-A dead body. (Appendix A)

calculus-Mineralized bacterial plaque that forms a solid mass and is covered by bacterial plaque. (Chapter 15)

canine-Positioned as the third tooth from the midline on the maxillary and mandibular arches and used for tearing and grasping; also referred to as cuspids. (Chapter 1)

cantilever bridge-A fixed partial denture with the pontic supported by single or double abutment on one end. (Chapter 11)

cavity-A hollow space. (Chapter 5)

cavity classification-A system of categorizing dental caries based on its location on the surface of the tooth. (Chapter 5)

cementoenamel junction (CEJ)-The union of the enamel of the crown of the tooth with the cementum of the root of the tooth. Located at the cervical region of the tooth. (Chapter 1)

cementum-A layer of bonelike tissue that covers the root of the tooth. (Chapter 1)

central incisor-The teeth located first from the midline on the maxilla and mandible. (Chapter 1)

centric occlusion-The maximum intercuspation of the maxillary and mandibular teeth, the habitual "bite" of the individual. (Chapter 20)

cervical line-The line formed by the union of the enamel and cementum in the neck region of the tooth. (Chapter 1)

charting-Recording the progress of a disease, condition of the teeth, or teeth that are missing. (Appendix A)

chrome clad-Type of finish placed on machinist's scale. The advantage of this finish is that it is practically impossible to photographically "washout" the detail during exposure. It also maintains a neutral gray tone when photographed. (Appendix A)

chronic apical abscess-Slow progression of the inflammatory response to bacterial infection. (Chapter 16)

chronic apical periodontitis-Slow progression of inflammation due to pressure of bacterial and other by-products. (Chapter 16)

chronic pulpitis-Slow progression of inflammation of the dental pulp; generally asymptomatic. (Chapter 16)

circular fibers-Part of the gingival fiber apparatus; fibers extend around the cervical region of the tooth to provide stability. (Chapter 15)

clasp-Metallic clips that surround abutment teeth on a removable partial denture. (Chapter 12)

Class I malocclusion-The "ideal" or normal relationship of the opposing first permanent molars. (Chapter 20)

Class II malocclusion or distocclusion-The mandibular first molar is distal to the maxillary first molar. (Chapter 20)

Class II, Division 1 malocclusion-The mandibular first molar is distal to the maxillary first molar and the maxillary anterior teeth have excess overjet with a normal labial-lingual inclination. (Chapter 20)

Class II, Division 2 malocclusion-The mandibular first molar is distal to the maxillary first molar and one or both maxillary central incisors are inclined lingually. (Chapter 20)

Class III malocclusion or mesiocclusion-The mandibular first molar is mesial to the maxillary first molar. (Chapter 20)

Classification of Cavities-Method for classifying dental caries developed by Dr. G. V. Black. (Chapter 13)

close focusing-Lens having the capability of producing image magnification greater than a normal lens, usually 1:8, to a range up to approximately half-life size (1:2). (Appendix A)

col-Nonkeratinized epithelial tissue located beneath the contact area between the facial and lingual papilla. (Chapter 15)

comparative analysis-Examination of one item to another, usually comparing characteristics to formulate a conclusion. (Appendix A)

comparison overlay technique-Method of applying a clear photographic overlay of suspect's teeth onto a color photograph of bite mark from victim or vice versa. (Appendix A)

complete denture-Removable prosthesis that replaces the maxillary and mandibular teeth. (Chapter 12)

composite resin-Tooth-colored restorative material made from organic polymers. (Chapter 10)

composite resin veneer-Tooth-colored restorative materials used primarily for anterior teeth that are made either by adding the substance in layers directly on the tooth surface or applying it indirectly on a model. (Chapter 10)

concrescence-Two independently formed adjacent teeth from a single tooth by fusion of the cementum (Chapter 21)

concussion-A traumatic injury that results from an impact and does not produce abnormal displacement or movement. (Chapter 14)

contrast control filters-Photographic filters used to attenuate specific wavelengths of light. When used with black and white film, these filters produce darker or lighter tones of gray on the film when reproducing visible colors; known as Wratten Series Filters. (Appendix A)

convex-The facial profile of an individual in an "ideal" or Class I relationship of the jaws appears curved. (Chapter 20)

copper-An element sometimes utilized for making dental amalgam. (Chapter 6)

cross bite-Malpositioned tooth (teeth) in relationship to the opposing arch. Anterior cross bite: mandibular anterior tooth (teeth) are facial rather than lingual to the maxillary anterior teeth (underjet). Posterior cross bite: mandibular posterior tooth (teeth) are facial to the maxillary posterior tooth (teeth) or the mandibular tooth (teeth) are lingual to the maxillary posterior tooth (teeth). (Chapter 20)

crown-That part of the tooth covered by enamel. (Chapter 8)

cusp-A rounded elevated structure located on the occlusal surface of posterior teeth. (Chapter 7)

cusp coverage-A restrictive material used to cover the cusps. (Chapter 7)

cyanoacrylate-Chemical name of substance used in glues similar to Superglue. (Appendix A)

deficient margin-A restoration with an undercontoured margin. (Chapter 22)

dehiscence-A defect in the alveolar process characterized by absence of the alveolar cortical plate and the formation of a cleft that is accompanied with soft tissue recession and an exposed root surface. (Chapter 15)

demineralization-The destruction of calcified structures of the teeth as a result of acid by-products released from bacterial plaque. (Chapter 17)

dens in dente-Invagination of the enamel organ into the dental papilla. (Chapter 21)

dental caries-A disease that affects the mineralized structures of the teeth. The disintegration of the calcified structures of the teeth (Chapter 5 and 13)

dental charts-Forms used to document dental patient's existing conditions, treatment, and progress. (Chapter 3)

dental implant-A device surgically inserted or grafted within or onto the bone of the maxilla or mandible to provide a support base for fixed or removable prosthesis or to replace missing teeth and includes: endosseous, subperiosteal, and transosteal implants. (Chapter 11)

dental kit-Term used in conjunction with a Polaroid CU-5 camera system. Kit has mirrors and positioning devices for extraoral and intraoral photographs of the mouth and teeth. (Appendix A)

dental prosthesis-A device used as an artificial replacement for missing teeth. (Chapter 11)

dental pulp-Vascular and nervous tissue located within the pulp cavity of the tooth. (Chapter 1)

dental stone-A nonporous form of calcined gypsum used for dental models. It is harder and denser than plaster of paris. (Appendix A)

dentin-Calcified tissue located beneath the enamel and the cementum of the tooth. (Chapter 1)

dentinocemental junction-The region where the dentin joins the cementum in the root. (Chapter 1)

dentinogenesis imperfecta-An inherited condition that affects the development of the dentin. (Chapter 21)

dentition-The type, arrangement, and number of teeth in the maxillary and mandibular arches. (Chapter 1 and Appendix A)

dentogingival fibers-Part of the gingival fiber apparatus; fibers extend from the cementum to the free gingiva. Provides support to the gingival tissues. (Chapter 15)

dentoperiosteal fibers-Part of the gingival fiber apparatus; fibers extend from the cementum transversely to the alveolar crest. (Chapter 15)

denture teeth-Artificial teeth that are used for the replacement of missing teeth. (Chapter 12)

depilatory cream-Over-the-counter product used to remove hair from skin. (Appendix A)

diastema-Natural space located between adjacent teeth. (Chapter 15)

dilaceration-Malformed root(s) with a sharp bend. (Chapter 21)

direct restorations-Restorative materials placed directly into a cavity preparation. (Chapter 22)

dislocation-A traumatic injury that causes the displacement of the tooth with a high degree of mobility. (Chapter 14)

distal-Away from the midline. (Chapter 1)

distilled water-Water that has been purified and refined through a distillation process. Not common tap water. (Appendix A)

distomolar-A supernumerary tooth that is smaller than normal located distal to the maxillary third molar. (Chapter 21)

DNA-Acronym for deoxyribonucleic acid. (Appendix A)

drift-A change in the position of the remaining teeth following the premature loss of a tooth or an extraction. (Chapter 18)

Duraclear-A transparent color photographic material that may be viewed as a transparency. (Appendix A)

Duratrans-A translucent color photographic material that may be viewed as a transparency or as a reflection print. (Appendix A)

early childhood caries-Rampant caries occurring in young children; also referred to as nursing caries. (Chapter 13)

enamel-Calcified tissue that covers the crown portion of the tooth and is considered the hardest substance in the body. (Chapter 1)

enamel hypocalcification-Deficient calcification of the enamel tooth structure. (Chapter 17)

enamel hypoplasia-Abnormal development of the enamel. (Chapter 21)

enamel pearl-Displaced masses of enamel located on the root surface of the tooth in the furcation region. (Chapter 21)

endodontics-A specialty in dentistry concerned with diseases of the dental pulp and periapical tissues. (Chapter 16)

endogenous-Originates from within the tooth from systemic disturbances. (Chapter 17)

endosseous implant-Device placed within the bone. (Chapter 11)

end-to-end bite-The anterior teeth meet edge to edge without any vertical overlap. (Chapter 20)

epithelium-Cells that form in a layer or layers and cover the surface of the body or line body cavities. (Chapter 15)

erosion-The loss of tooth structure due to a chemical process. (Chapter 17)

eruption-The movement of a tooth through the alveolar process and soft tissue into the oral cavity. (Chapter 1)

excision-To remove by cutting. A pattern injury may be recovered from a cadaver by excision. (Appendix A)

exemplars-Typical or representative example of the teeth and their condition. (Appendix A)

exfoliation-Loss of a primary tooth following root resorption. (Chapter 2)

exogenous-Originates outside the body from exposure to environmental agents. (Chapter 17)

external PC synch cord-An electronic cord that allows connection of the flash to the camera when the flash is not physically on the camera. Camera and flash stay in "synch" when camera takes photograph. Connection is via a post connector (PC) fitting located on the body of the camera or via a hot shoe adapter that has a PC fitting fabricated onto the adapter. (Appendix A)

extraction-Surgical removal of a tooth. (Chapter 14)

extraoral-Outside the mouth. (Appendix A)

extraoral radiograph-The film is positioned outside of the mouth. (Chapter 4)

extrinsic stain-Stain occurring on the external tooth surface that may be removed by toothbrushing, scaling, and polishing procedures. (Chapter 17)

extrusion-Migration of a tooth past the line of occlusion. (Chapter 18)

facial-The term that designates the outer surfaces of the maxillary and mandibular teeth collectively. (Chapter 1)

fenestration-A lack of bone tissue in the alveolar process characterized by a spherical-shaped defect in the alveolar cortical plate that is formed inferior to the remaining intact cortical plate, which exposes the root on either side of the facial or lingual surface. (Chapter 15)

first molar-In the primary dentition, on the maxillary and mandibular arches, the posterior tooth located in the fourth position from the midline. In the permanent dentition, on the maxillary and mandibular arches, the posterior tooth located in the sixth position from the midline. (Chapter 1)

fistula-A tract that forms from an abscess within the bone that leads to the outside of the surface of the gingiva into the oral cavity from which pus drains through. (Chapter 16)

fixed partial denture-Abutment teeth or implants that provide support for the replacement of missing teeth and is fixed into position. (Chapter 11)

fluorosis-During tooth development and formation, excessive fluoride intake results in deficient calcification of the enamel. (Chapter 17)

food impaction-Food particles forced into the gingival sulcus. (Chapter 15)

forensic odontologist-A dentist qualified in the use of dental science in forensic procedures. (Appendix A)

fracture-A break in a tooth or bone. (Chapter 14)

fractured restoration-A break in a restoration. (Chapter 22)

free gingival groove-A shallow depression that separates the marginal gingiva from the attached gingiva. (Chapter 15)

frenum-A fold of mucous membrane tissue that connects an immobile part to a semi- or less mobile part and controls movement of the part. (Chapter 15)

frontal-"Anterior"; in the front part or in front of. (Appendix A)

full cast crown-A restoration made from cast gold, or non-precious metal, and porcelain that replaces the natural crown of the tooth completely. (Chapter 8)

furcation-The anatomic region of multirooted teeth where the roots separate. (Chapter 15)

fusion-A single tooth is formed from two adjoining tooth germs. (Chapter 21)

gasket-A piece or ring of rubber. (Chapter 11)

gemination-The splitting of a tooth germ, which forms two partially or completely separated crowns. (Chapter 21)

geometric chart-A charting form that represents the teeth with stylized anatomy. (Chapter 3)

gingiva-Soft (gum) tissue composed of keratinized stratified squamous epithelium that covers the alveolar process and surrounds the teeth. (Chapter 1 and 15)

gingival fiber apparatus-Includes the alveologingival, dentogingival, dentoperiosteal, circular, and transeptal fibers. (Chapter 15)

gingival pocket-An increase in the sulcus depth due to inflammation and/or apical migration of the epithelial attachment. (Chapter 15)

gingival recession-Exposure of the root surface due to apical migration of the epithelial attachment (junctional epithelium). (Chapter 15)

gingivitis-Inflammation of the gingiva characterized by edema and redness due to bacterial plaque. (Chapter 15)

glass ionomer-Restorative material utilized for cement-based or tooth-colored restorations. (Chapter 10)

gold alloy-A mixture of copper, platinum, silver, and other trace metals added for hardness or strength. (Chapter 6)

gold crown-A full cast crown made from gold alloy. (Chapter 8)

gold foil-Restorative material derived from gold leaf. (Chapter 6)

gold inlay-A restoration cast from gold alloy that is contained within a tapered cavity preparation. (Chapter 6)

gold onlay-A restoration cast from gold alloy that covers the cusps and occlusal surfaces of posterior teeth. (Chapter 7)

guide number-Numerical system for rating relative light output of an electronic flash. The higher the number, the more power the flash has. The guide number is based on exposure achieved at a set distance measured either in feet or meters. (Appendix A)

gutta-percha-The restorative material used to fill and seal the root canal(s) of an endodontically treated tooth. (Chapter 16)

hemisection-Surgical removal of one half of the crown and root structures of a tooth. (Chapter 16)

Hexcelite-An orthopedic tape that is used for backing and reinforcing impression material. (Appendix A)

histodifferentiation-A process in which primitive cell types develop and mature into specific types of tissues. (Chapter 1)

histologic-Refers to the microscopic study of the structure of tissues. (Appendix A)

horizontal bone loss-Reduction in the height of bone tissue in an apical direction perpendicular to the long axis of the tooth. (Chapter 15)

horizontal fibers-Part of the principal fiber apparatus; fibers extend from the cementum on the middle third of the root transversely to the adjacent alveolar bone tissue. Provides stability for the tooth. (Chapter 15)

hot shoe-Device for holding and triggering an electronic flash. Usually located on top of the camera's viewfinder housing for 35 mm-styled cameras. (Appendix A)

hydroxyapatite-Calcium carbonate and calcium phosphate crystals found in bones and teeth. (Chapter 1)

hyperdontia-The state of having supernumerary teeth. (Chapter 21)

hypocalcification-The deficient calcification of the enamel tooth structure. (Chapter 17)

incipient carious lesion-A carious lesion occurring for the first time. (Chapter 13)

incisal-A surface on anterior teeth that forms a ridge and is used for cutting. (Chapter 1)

indices-The measurement of a given substance or condition compared to a fixed standard. (Chapter 19)

indirect restorations-Restorations that are fabricated outside the mouth. (Chapter 22)

infrabony pocket-The base of the pocket is apical to the alveolar crest. (Chapter 15)

interdental papilla-Projection of epithelial tissue (gingiva) between adjacent teeth. (Chapter 15)

International Standards Organization/Fédération Dentaire Internationale (ISO/FDI) System-Two-digit system for designating teeth. Permanent teeth are numbered by quadrants beginning with the upper right quadrant = Q-1 (11 through 18); upper left quadrant = Q-2 (21 through 28); lower left quadrant = Q-3 (31 through 38); and the lower right quadrant = Q-4 (41 through 48). Primary teeth are numbered by quadrants beginning with the upper right quadrant = Q-5 (51through 55); upper left quadrant = Q-6 (61 through 65); lower left quadrant = Q-7 (71 through 75); and the lower right = Q-8 (81 through 85). Numbers are pronounced as two-digits; that is, 21 read as two-one. (Chapter 2)

interproximal carious lesion-A carious lesion occurring just below the contact area. (Chapter 13)

interradicular fibers-Part of the principal fiber apparatus; fibers extend from the cementum throughout the furcation regions to the adjacent alveolar bone tissue. (Chapter 15)

intraoral-Within the mouth. (Appendix A)

intraoral radiograph-The film is positioned inside of the mouth. (Chapter 4)

intrinsic stain-Stain incorporated within the tooth structure. (Chapter 17)

intrusion-Apical migration of a tooth. (Chapter 18)

IR-Acronym for infrared. For photographic purposes, wavelengths used usually range from 700 nm to 890 nm, although the IR spectrum extends to 1000+ nm. (Appendix A)

irreversible-The measurement of a given substance or condition that cannot change. (Chapter 19)

ISO-Abbreviation for International Standards Organization (used to be ASA). When used in conjunction with film, it denotes a standard for the film's "speed" or sensitivity to light and exposure. The higher the ISO number, the more sensitive the film is and the less exposure that is required to produce an acceptable photograph. (Appendix A)

junctional epithelium-Located at the base of the gingival sulcus, the sulcular epithelium joins the epithelial tissue, which forms a band of nonkeratinized epithelial tissue that encircles the tooth and forms an attachment on the cementum. (Chapter 15)

Kennedy Classification System-A system for classifying types of edentulous situations. (Chapter 12)

Kodalith-A black and white photographic graphic arts film. Used to make overlays in the comparison overlay method. (Appendix A)

labial-A surface on an anterior tooth located toward the lips. (Chapter 1)

labioversion-Positioned toward the lip (labial). (Chapter 18)

lamina propria-All of the connective tissue structures located beneath the gingiva. (Chapter 15)

lateral-Pertaining to the side. (Appendix A)

lateral incisor-The anterior tooth located in the second position from the midline on the maxilla and mandible. (Chapter 1)

letter codes-Abbreviations to designate existing restorations or conditions; either primary or secondary. (Chapters 3 and 4)

lingual-Toward the tongue. (Chapter 1)

linguoversion-Positioned toward the tongue. (Chapter 18)

lining mucosa-Nonkeratinized epithelial tissue that covers the alveolar mucosa, lips, cheeks, soft palate, ventral surface of the tongue, and the floor of the mouth. (Chapter 15)

luxation-A traumatic injury to the supporting structures of the tooth that results in some mobility. (Chapter 14)

macro-An abbreviation for photomacrography, which denotes photographs made at magnifications larger than life size (1:1). (Appendix A)

malocclusion-Occlusion that deviates from the ideal. (Chapter 20)

malpositioned-Abnormal placement. (Chapter 18)

mandibular-Regarding the lower jaw (mandible). (Chapter 1 and Appendix A)

manual 35 mm SLR camera-This is a camera that requires setting the lens opening (aperture or f stop) and shutter speeds manually after obtaining a light meter reading. SLR is an acronym for single lens reflex. 35 mm designates the physical size of the film or film format. (Appendix A)

margin-The border or edge. (Chapter 22)

marginal defects-A fault located at the margin of the restoration where it meets the tooth structures. (Chapter 22)

marginal gingiva-Surrounds the cervical region of the tooth. It is not attached and forms the gingival sulcus. (Chapter 15)

Maryland bridge-A fixed partial denture with one pontic supported by metal retainers on both ends. (Chapter 11)

masticatory mucosa-Provides the covering for the hard palate and gingiva and consists of keratinized epithelium that is firmly attached to the underlying connective tissue. (Chapter 15)

maxillary-Regarding the upper arch. (Chapter 1)

medium view-Specific photograph of an area or items within an area that shows some detail about the area or items. Not close enough for individual details on items. (Appendix A)

mesial-Toward the midline. (Chapter 1)

mesiodens-An accessory tooth with an abnormal shape located between the maxillary central incisor teeth. (Chapter 21)

metric analysis-Examination of one item to another by measuring points of distance or unique properties of the items to formulate a conclusion. (Appendix A)

midline-An imaginary line parallel to the long axis of the body that divides the body into right and left halves. (Chapter 1)

missing-Regarding a tooth that is not visible clinically or not present on a radiograph. (Chapter 4)

mixed dentition-A combination of primary and permanent teeth that begins with the eruption of the first permanent tooth between the ages of 6 and 12. (Chapter 2)

mixing board-In video terms, an electronic device that allows multiple signals to be processed or "mixed" together to create images different from the single original source. (Appendix A)

mobility-Movement of a tooth in any direction. Normal physiologic mobility: small degree of movement is normal. Pathologic mobility: greater degree of movement is considered abnormal. (Chapter 15)

molar-Posterior tooth used for chewing. (Chapter 1)

morphogenesis-Developmental processes in which the forms of structures are established. (Chapter 1)

mucogingival junction-Scalloped line between the keratinized gingival epithelium and the alveolar mucosa. (Chapter 15)

multiple sutures-Using threadlike material, the process of joining an acrylic ring to the skin containing a pattern injury. Basically, it is looping the thread around the ring, through the skin until the entire circumference of the ring has been covered. (Appendix A)

necrotizing ulcerative gingivitis (NUG)-Severe gingival inflammation with bleeding, necrotic papilla that can have craterlike defects. (Chapter 15)

non-precious metal crown-A full cast crown made from non-precious metals. (Chapter 8)

non-restored-Regarding a tooth that does not have a restoration on it. A "virgin" tooth. (Chapter 4)

numeric coding system chart-A charting form depicted as a graph with individual boxes that represent the teeth. Charting codes and symbols are recorded in the boxes. (Chapter 3)

oblique fibers-Part of the principal fiber apparatus; fibers that extend from the cementum at the middle and apical thirds of the roots in an oblique direction that are coronally attached to the alveolar bone tissue. (Chapter 15)

occlusal-Biting surface of posterior teeth. (Chapter 1)

occlusal carious lesion-A carious lesion occurring on the occlusal tooth surface. (Chapter 13)

occlusion-The relationship of the mandibular and maxillary teeth when they come in contact. (Chapter 20)

odontoblasts-During tooth development, the dentin-producing cells that form the surface of the dental papilla. Following tooth eruption, dentin-forming cells line the pulp cavity and continue to produce dentin. (Chapter 1)

openbite-A vertical overlap deficiency in centric occlusion with the lack of incisal or occlusal contact. (Chapter 20)

open margin-A space located between the wall of the cavity preparation and the restoration. (Chapter 22)

osseointegration-The attachment between the dental implant and the bone. (Chapter 11)

overall view-Global-type photography that shows general locations without specific detail. (Appendix A)

overbite-The vertical length by which the maxillary anterior teeth overlap the mandibular anterior teeth. (Chapter 20)

overdenture-A removable complete denture supported by retained natural teeth or dental implants. (Chapter 12)

overhanging margin-A restoration that does not conform to the contour of the tooth. (Chapter 22)

overjet-The horizontal length between the linguo-incisal surfaces of the maxillary anterior teeth and the labioincisal surfaces of the mandibular anterior teeth. (Chapter 20)

panoramic radiograph-An extraoral radiograph of the maxilla and mandible that utilizes curved surface tomography. (Chapter 4)

paramolar-An accessory tooth located lingual or buccal to normal position. (Chapter 21)

partial cast crown-A restoration made from cast gold or non-precious metal and porcelain that replaces three or more surfaces of the crown of the tooth. (Chapter 8)

partially erupted-Regarding a tooth that has not completely erupted into the line of occlusion. (Chapter 4)

periapical radiograph-An intraoral radiograph that shows the entire tooth and surrounding bone. (Chapter 4)

periapical radiolucency-The radiolucent area observed on a dental radiograph located around the root apex of the tooth. (Chapter 16)

periodontal abscess-An acute clinical manifestation characterized by the accumulation of pus in the tissue due to a bacterial infection. (Chapter 15)

periodontal chart-A comprehensive recording form for the evaluation of probing depths, plaque, calculus, mobility, recession, attachment levels, occlusion, and gingival and periodontal conditions. (Chapter 3)

periodontal ligament-Collagen and fibrous connective tissues surrounded by an amorphous ground substance located in the periodontal space that encircle and attach the roots of the teeth to the alveolar bone tissue. (Chapter 15)

periodontal ligament (membrane)-Collagen and fibrous connective tissues located in the periodontal space that encircle and attach the roots of the teeth to the alveolar bone tissue. (Chapter 1)

periodontitis-Inflammation of the supporting structures and tissues of the teeth. (Chapter 15)

periodontium-Includes the gingiva, periodontal ligament, cementum, and bone. (Chapter 15)

permanent dentition-The thirty-two natural teeth, also referred to as secondary dentition. (Chapter 1)

photomacrography-Term used for photographs made at magnifications of 1:1 or greater (up to approximately 50:1) without the use of a microscope. (Appendix A)

pin-pontic-Utilizes two pins to secure the facing. (Chapter 8)

pit and fissure sealants-Resin material used to fill in the fissures and voids on the occlusal tooth surfaces of posterior teeth. (Chapter 10)

Polaroid-Photographic materials, color and black and white, that will give instant results. Company also manufactures numerous camera systems and accessories for photography. (Appendix A)

Polaroid CU-5 camera system-A modular camera made by the Polaroid Corporation that allows for selected fixed magnification photographs of items.

Has a "built-in" ring flash and may be purchased with an extraoral and intraoral dental kit consisting of mirrors and positioning devices. (Appendix A)

pontic-The artificial tooth that replaces a missing tooth on a fixed or removable partial denture. (Chapter 11)

porcelain-A ceramic material. (Chapter 4 and 11)

porcelain-fused-to-metal crown-A restoration that is made of gold or non-precious metal that covers the crown of the tooth and is completely or partially covered with a tooth-colored ceramic material. (Chapter 9)

porcelain inlay-An all-ceramic, tooth-colored restoration that fits into a tapered cavity preparation. (Chapter 10)

porcelain jacket crown-An all-ceramic, tooth-colored restoration that completely covers the crown of the tooth. (Chapter 10)

porcelain veneer-A custom made all-ceramic, tooth-colored restoration that is bonded to the facial surface of an anterior tooth. (Chapter 10)

posterior-Toward the rear or back. (Chapter 1)

premolars-Permanent teeth located in the fourth and fifth positions from the midline on the maxillary and mandibular arches and replace the primary first and second molars. (Chapter 1)

primary code-The first code utilized in charting procedures that includes an abbreviation for the anatomic surfaces of the teeth or existing conditions. (Chapter 4)

primary dentition-The first twenty teeth replaced by the permanent dentition. (Chapter 1)

principal fiber apparatus-Includes the alveolar crest, horizontal, oblique, apical, and interradicular fibers. (Chapter 15)

prognathic-The facial profile of an individual in a Class III malocclusion in which the lower jaw may appear protruded. (Chapter 20)

proximal-Near or adjacent to. (Chapter 1)

pulp canal-The channel in the root of the tooth that extends from the pulp chamber to the apex and contains the blood vessels and nerves (pulp). (Chapter 1)

pulp cavity-The cavity within the tooth that includes the pulp chamber and pulp canal. (Chapter 1)

pulp chamber-Cavity located in the center of the tooth that is connected to the pulp canal that contains the blood vessels and nerves (pulp). (Chapter 1)

pulpectomy-The complete removal of the pulp tissue. (Chapter 16)

pulp horns-Pointed extensions that arise from the corners of the pulp chamber and contain pulp tissue. (Chapter 1)

pulpitis-Inflammation of the pulp tissue. (Chapter 16)

pulpotomy-The partial removal of the dental pulp. (Chapter 16)

purple top EDTA tube-Tube used for collection of blood that contains the anticoagulant ethylenediaminetetra-acetic acid (EDTA). Distinguished from other blood tubes by the purple color top. (Appendix A)

quadrant-One of four corresponding regions, the maxillary and mandibular arches each consists of right and left quadrants. (Chapter 2)

radiation caries-Carious lesions that occur from the effects of radiation therapy. (Chapter 13)

radiograph-The effects of exposure to x-rays on a film following processing that produces a visual image. (Chapter 4)

radiolucent-The black regions on a radiograph. (Chapter 4)

radiopaque-The white regions on a radiograph. (Chapters 4 and 5)

Ramjford teeth-Six selected teeth (#3, #9, #12, #19, #25, and #28) that have been tested as reliable indicators for other regions of the oral cavity. (Chapter 19)

rampant caries-Carious lesions that are widespread and progress rapidly. (Chapter 13)

recurrent caries-Caries that are a continuation of the initial lesion or that occur adjacent to a dental restoration. (Chapter 13)

reflection print-Photograph that is "normally" viewed by reflected light as opposed to a "transparency" or "slide," which is viewed by transmitted light. (Appendix A)

reliability-The ability of a dental index or other measuring method to measure a condition or substance regarding the same subject repeatedly and can obtain the same results each time. (Chapter 19)

removable partial denture-An artificial replacement for associated structures and missing teeth in a partially edentulous jaw and is not fixed into position. (Chapter 12)

reparative dentin-Dentin formation in response to caries or trauma. (Chapter 1)

rest-A metallic device of a fixed or removable denture that contacts a remaining tooth or teeth and is used for stability. (Chapter 12)

restoration-The structural replacement for missing tooth structure(s). (Chapter 5)

retention core-A restorative material used to replace the significant loss of tooth structure that provides retention for a permanent restoration. (Chapter 16)

retention pin-A screw-type device inserted into the dentin to secure a silver amalgam restoration. (Chapter 5)

retention post-A dowel-like device placed into the tooth following the removal of the pulp to help anchor the permanent restoration. (Chapter 16)

retrofilling-Silver amalgam is placed into the apical region of the tooth to seal the end following an apicoectomy. (Chapter 16)

retrognathic-The facial profile of an individual in a Class II malocclusion in which the lower jaw appears retruded in relation to the upper face. (Chapter 20)

reversible-The measurement of a given substance or condition that can change. (Chapter 19)

reversible pulpitis-Following the placement and removal of an insulating agent, inflammation of the pulp tissue subsides. (Chapter 16)

root-That part of the tooth covered by cementum. (Chapter 1)

root amputation-Surgical removal of one or more roots of a multirooted tooth. (Chapter 16)

root form-Type of endosseous implant. (Chapter 11)

root surface caries-Carious lesion occurring on the surface of the root. (Chapter 13)

satin clad-Type of finish placed on machinist's scale. Advantage of this finish is that it is practically impossible to photographically "washout" the detail during exposure. It also maintains a neutral gray tone when photographed. (Appendix A)

scale-Measuring device. Used in forensic photographic terms, a measuring device that exhibits good accuracy and precision. (Appendix A)

scanner-An electronic device used to "copy" images into an electronic environment such as a computer or image processor. (Appendix A)

secondary code-The second code utilized in charting procedures that includes an abbreviation for existing conditions. (Chapter 4)

secondary dentin-Dentin formation in the pulp chamber and canal that occurs following eruption. (Chapter 1)

second molar-In the primary dentition, on the maxillary and mandibular arches, the posterior tooth located in the fifth position from the midline. In the permanent dentition, on the maxillary and mandibular arches, the posterior tooth located in the seventh position from the midline. (Chapter 1)

sextant-Any one of six regions. (Chapter 2)

silicate-Silicon dioxide used for dental materials. (Chapter 16)

silver-An element used for dental materials. (Chapter 6)

silver amalgam-A metal alloy and mercury combination that is used as a restorative material in a cavity preparation. (Chapter 5)

single-surface-One of the six anatomic surfaces of the teeth. (Chapter 5)

slow caries activity-Carious lesions that progress at a very slow rate. (Chapter 13)

specialized mucosa-Parakeratinized and keratinized epithelial tissue that covers the dorsal surface of the tongue. (Chapter 15)

splint-A device used to prevent movement. (Chapter 14)

stainless steel crown-A temporary crown. (Chapter 8)

Steele's-facing-Utilizes a single slot or groove to secure the facing. (Chapter 8)

sterile cotton swabs-Commercially produced cotton swab that is individually sealed in a sterile container and has not been previously opened or used. May have been subjected to ultraviolet light for sterilization. (Appendix A)

Stone model-A reproduction made by pouring dental stone or other material into a hollow imprint (impression) and letting it set. (Appendix A)

subperiosteal-The type of implant that is placed underneath the periosteum and on the alveolar bone tissue. (Chapter 11)

succedaneous-To succeed, the permanent teeth that replace the primary dentition. (Chapter 1)

sulcular epithelium-The medial surface of the marginal gingiva descends inferiorly toward the CEJ region. (Chapter 15)

suprabony pocket-The base of the pocket is coronal to the alveolar bone crest. (Chapter 15)

supraerupt-Regarding a tooth positioned above the line of occlusion. Extrusion. (Chapter 18)

surgical latex gloves-Tight-fitting latex gloves that provide a biohazard barrier. (Appendix A)

swabbing-Term used for acquiring a sample from a surface, especially when using a cotton swab. (Appendix A)

temporary crown-A prefabricated or custom made restoration used in the interim until a permanent restoration is warranted. (Chapter 10)

temporary restoration-A restoration used in the interim until a permanent restoration is warranted. (Chapter 16)

three-quarter crown-A restoration made from cast gold, or non-precious metal, and porcelain that replaces three fourths of the crown portion of the tooth except the facial surface. (Chapter 8)

tilt-The direction an impacted or unerupted tooth is leaning. (Chapter 18)

tooth avulsion-A traumatic injury that results in the removal of the tooth from the alveolar bone. (Chapter 14)

tooth notation systems-Numbers, letters, and symbols that designate the permanent and primary teeth. American Dental Association Universal/National System, Zsigmondy-Palmer Notation System, and Internationale Standards Oganization/Fédération Dentaire Internationale System. (Chapter 2)

torsiversion-Turned or rotated tooth. (Chapter 18)

transosseous implant-An implant placed through the alveolar bone tissue. (Chapter 11)

transseptal fibers-Part of the gingival fiber apparatus; fibers that extend from the cementum at the cervical region of one tooth across interproximally to an adjacent tooth. (Chapter 15)

traumatic injury-A wound resulting from trauma. (Chapter 14)

treatment partial-A temporary, removable prosthetic appliance that is a replacement for a missing tooth. (Chapter 12)

underjet-The maxillary teeth are lingual to the mandibular teeth (anterior cross bite). (Chapter 20)

unerupted-Regarding a tooth that has yet to erupt. Failure of a tooth to erupt due to space constraints. (Chapter 4)

UV-Acronym for ultraviolet. For photographic purposes, wavelengths used usually range from 360 nm to 400+ nm. Shorter wavelengths down to 305 nm can be used with special lenses. (Appendix A)

variability-A tendency to change. (Chapter 19)

veneer crown-A restoration that covers the natural crown portion of the tooth made from porcelain or composite resin. (Chapter 8)

vertical bone loss-Reduction in the height of crestal bone at an angle. (Chapter 15)

vinyl polysiloxane-A material used for taking accurate dental impressions. A puttylike material of base and catalyst that when mixed forms an elastic mold. (Appendix A)

virgin-Non-restored tooth. (Chapter 4)

wear facet-A worn and flattened area on a tooth surface that occurs as a result of attrition, bruxism, or malocclusion. (Chapter 17)

Zsigmondy-Palmer Notation System-Permanent teeth are numbered 1 through 8 in each of the four quadrants, beginning at the maxillary and mandibular central incisors of each quadrant. Each quadrant is designated by a symbol that encloses the tooth designation number: maxillary right = ┘, maxillary left = └, mandibular left = ┌, mandibular right = ┐. Primary teeth are identified with uppercase letters A through E in each of the four quadrants, beginning at the maxillary and mandibular central incisors of each quadrant. Each quadrant is designated by a symbol that encloses the tooth designation letter: maxillary right = ┘, maxillary left = └, mandibular left = ┌, mandibular right = ┐. (Chapter 2)

Index

I

J

K

L

M

N

U

V

W

Z